Diagnostic and Therapeutic Procedures in Gastroenterology

Clinical Gastroenterology

George Y. Wu, Series Editor

For other titles published in this series, go to
www.springer.com/series/7672

DIAGNOSTIC AND THERAPEUTIC PROCEDURES IN GASTROENTEROLOGY

An Illustrated Guide

Edited by

GEORGE Y. WU, MD

Professor, Department of Medicine
Director, Hepatology Section
Herman Lopata Chair in Hepatitis Research
University of Connecticut School of Medicine
Farmington, CT, USA

SUBBARAMIAH SRIDHAR

Professor, Department of Gastroenterology
Medical College of Georgia
Augusta, GA, USA

Humana Press

Editors
George Y. Wu, MD
Professor
Department of Medicine
Director, Hepatology Section
Herman Lopata Chair in Hepatitis Research
University of Connecticut School of Medicine
Farmington, CT
USA
wu@nso.uchc.edu

Subbaramiah Sridhar
Professor
Department of Gastroenterology
Medical College of Georgia
Augusta, GA
USA
ssridhar@mcg.edu

ISBN 978-1-58829-478-4 e-ISBN 978-1-59745-044-7
DOI 10.1007/978-1-59745-044-7
Springer New York Dordrecht Heidelberg London

Printed on acid-free paper

Humana Press is part of Springer Science+Business Media (www.springer.com)

Dedication

I would like to dedicate this book to my friend and mentor, James Freston, a great clinician and administrator, whose teaching and influence stimulated my career in medicine and gastroenterology (GYW).

To my parents who molded my life, to Professor Sir Ferguson Anderson (Glasgow, Scotland) and Professor Richard Hunt (McMaster University, Canada) who molded my career and to all gastroenterology fellows who are thinkers and not mere scope pushers for mind is a more powerful tool than endoscope (SS).

Foreword

The editors of a *Diagnostic and Therapeutic Procedures in Gastroenterology: An Illustrated Guide*, George Wu and Subbaramiah Sridhar, are to be congratulated on producing this important book, which addresses a previously unperceived, but very important, unmet educational need. With the explosion of endoscopic skills and the development of new approaches to diagnosis and treatment, much of our work in gastroenterology is now interventional in nature, either by the endoscopic route or with the assistance of ultrasound or CT. Moreover, while seriously ill or high-risk patients undergo their procedures within the hospital setting, many procedures are now conducted outside hospitals or on an ambulatory basis. Since the optimal management of patients with gastrointestinal disease often involves many disciplines, it is increasingly important that all those involved at various stages of care are aware of the details of the procedures and interventions that their patients may experience. This illustrated guide is providing just such information and it should be read and appreciated by referring physicians be they in primary care or general internists or surgeons. Moreover, this text should be especially useful to GI trainees and to nursing staff who can optimize ward care when well informed of the investigations and interventions that their patients with gastrointestinal problems undergo.

Drs. Wu and Sridhar have assembled an impressive array of distinguished contributors to address the management of a detailed range of GI conditions and procedures. The authors have drawn on their collective years of experience and assembled best evidence to present the current standards of care. This book should be read by those who perform these important and varied gastrointestinal procedures and by all those in their respective supporting roles. Patients with gastrointestinal disease will be the ultimate beneficiaries.

Richard Hunt
Farncombe Family Digestive Disease Research Institute
McMaster University Health Science Centre
Hamilton, Ontario
Canada

Preface

This volume was conceived with the intent to address common questions often raised by internists regarding details of gastrointestinal procedures. Because patients who undergo gastrointestinal procedures are frequently followed by their primary care providers and extenders, those providers should be familiar with pre- and post-procedural issues in order to select an optimal procedure, and provide appropriate post-procedure follow up. This volume follows in the mold of *An Internist's Illustrated Guide to Gastrointestinal Surgery* to provide a clear understanding of the concepts that underlie gastrointestinal procedures that is important for appropriate decision making for patients with diseases that require gastrointestinal procedures.

Over the past decade, there have been numerous advances in equipment and technical skills in performing gastrointestinal procedures. The field has generally become more invasive, in many cases supplanting surgical interventions. *Diagnostic and Therapeutic Procedures in Gastroenterology: An Illustrated Guide* is a comprehensive textbook describing procedures for the gastrointestinal tract in a simple way, with artistic illustrations to educate the physician about procedures, and to provide not only clear descriptions of the changes in the anatomy and physiology, but also to provide advice on medical management of the post-procedure patient. *Diagnostic and Therapeutic Procedures in Gastroenterology: An Illustrated Guide* describes in detail the indications, contraindications, anatomical alterations, and physiological alterations that result from various operations and procedures. Comparisons between alternative operations, complications, medical management issues, and costs are discussed. Clear, detailed, artist-rendered illustrations of the anatomy are included and, where appropriate, radiological images. This is a unique textbook, written primarily for primary care physicians, general internists, and students to educate them about those aspects of gastrointestinal procedures that are pertinent to an internist. It should also be a suitable textbook for medical students, residents, nurses and nurse practitioners, nutritionists, dietitians, and various subspecialists who take care of patients with gastrointestinal disorders.

George Y. Wu
University of Connecticut School of Medicine
Farmington CT
USA

Contents

Contributors

Kamran Ayub, M.D., MRCP (UK)
Visiting Clinical Associate Professor, University of Illinois at Chicago, Chicago IL, USA

Khalid Aziz, MBBS
Staff Physician Gastroenterology and Hepatology, Metrowest Medical Center, Framingham MA, USA

John Baillie, BSc(Hons), MB ChB, FRCP (Glasg.), FACG, FASGE
Section on Gastroenterology, Wake Forest University Health Sciences, Medical Center Boulevard, Winston-Salem NC, USA

Kenneth F. Binmoeller, M.D.
Medical Director, Interventional Endoscopy Service, California Pacific Medical Center, San Francisco CA, USA

John W. Birk, M.D.
Associate Professor of Medicine, Chief, Director, Division of Gastroenterology, Gastroenterology-Hepatology Fellowship Program, University of Connecticut Health Center, Farmington CT, USA

Sherman M. Chamberlain, M.D.
Assistant Professor of Medicine, Medical College of Georgia, Augusta GA, USA

Mark H. DeLegge, M.D., FACG, CNSP, AGAF, FASGE
Professor of Medicine, Division of Gastroenterology and Hepatology, Digestive Disease Center, Medical University of South Carolina, Charleston SC, USA

Peter V. Draganov, M.D.
Associate Professor of Medicine, Division of Gastroenterology, Hepatology and Nutrition, University of Florida, Gainesville FL, USA

Seth A. Gross, M.D.
Director of Advanced Endoscopy, Norwalk Hospital, Norwalk CT, USA

Joshua Hall, M.D.
Department of Gastroenterology, Medical College of Georgia, Augusta GA, USA

Muhammad K. Hasan, M.D.
Clinical Instructor and Attending in Gastroenterology, Medical University of South Carolina, Charleston SC, USA

Dennis M. Jensen, M.D.
VA Greater Los Angeles Healthcare System, UCLA Center for the Health Sciences, CURE Digestive Diseases Research Center, Los Angeles CA, USA

Joel R. Judah, M.D.
Department of Medicine, Division of Gastroenterology, University of Florida, Gainesville FL, USA

Antarpreet Kaur, MBBS
Internal Medicine Resident, University of Connecticut School of Connecticut, Farmington CT, USA

Richard A. Kozarek, M.D.
Executive Director, Director of GI Research, Digestive Disease Institute, Virginia Mason Medical Center, Clinical Professor of Medicine, University of Washington, Seattle WA, USA

Kristin Loening MacArthur, M.D.
Executive Board Member, South Marshall Women's Clinic, South Windsor CT, USA

Gustavo A. Machicado, M.D.
Clinical Professor, UCLA David Geffen School of Medicine, Los Angeles CA, USA

Shannon Marek, M.D.
Department of Gastroenterology, Medical College of Georgia, Augusta GA, USA

Koorosh MoezArdalan, M.D.
Gastroenterology Fellow, University of Connecticut, Farmington CT, USA

Nam Q. Nguyen, MBBS(Hons), FRACP, Ph.D.
Department of Gastroenterology and Hepatology, Royal Adelaide Hospital, Adelaide, Australia; Interventional Endoscopy Services, California Pacific Medical Center, San Francisco CA, USA

Akit Patel, M.D.
Baylor College of Medicine, Houston TX, USA

Sreeram V.J. Parupudi, M.D.
Visiting Associate Professor, Department of Internal Medicine (GI division), Texas Tech University Health Sciences Center, Lubbock TX, USA

Fadi Rahhal, M.D.
VA Medical Center, Augusta GA, USA

Joseph Romagnuolo, M.D., FRCPC, MSc(Epid), FASGE, FACG
Director of Clinical Research, Gastroenterology, Advanced ERCP and Endoscopic Ultrasound, Outcomes Research, Charleston SC, USA

Andrew S. Ross, M.D.
Medical Director, Gastrointestinal Research, Digestive Disease Institute, Virginia Mason Medical Center, Seattle WA, USA

Peter H. Rubin, M.D.
Clinical Associate Professor of Medicine, Mount Sinai Medical Center, New York NY, USA

Janak N. Shah, M.D.
Director of Pancreatic and Biliary Endoscopy, Division of Gastroenterology, VA Medical Center, San Francisco CA, USA

Prateek Sharma, M.D., FACP, FACG
Professor of Medicine, Program Director, Section Chief, Division of Gastroenterology and Hepatology, University of Kansas School of Medicine, VA Medical Center, Kansas City MO, USA

Nathan J. Shores, M.D.
Advanced Hepatology Fellow, Division of Hepatology, University of San Francisco (UCSF), San Francisco CA, USA

Mandeep Singh, M.D.
Fellow, Division of Gastroenterology and Hepatology, University of Kansas School of Medicine and Veterans Affairs Medical Center, Kansas City KS, USA

Prithvi Sreenivasan, M.D., MPH
Clinical Fellow in Gastroenterology, Norwalk Hospital, Norwalk CT, USA

Subbaramiah Sridhar, MBBS, MPH, FRCP(Edin), FRCP(Glasg), FRCP(Lond), FRSS(Lond), FRCPC, FACP, FACG, FASGE, AGAF, FAAG, MAAG
Professor, Department of Gastroenterology, Medical College of Georgia, Augusta GA, USA

Jessica Trevino, M.D.
Fellowship, Department of Gastroenterology, University of Alabama at Birmingham, Birmingham AL, USA

Frances Tse, M.D., MSc, FRCPC, LMCC
Faculty of Health Sciences, Health Research Methodology Program, McMaster University, Hamilton ON, Canada

Shyam Varadarajulu, M.D.
Assistant Professor, Attending Physician, University of Alabama School of Medicine, Children's Hospital, Birmingham AL, USA

Sachin Wani, M.D., FACP
Fellow, Division of Gastroenterology and Hepatology, University of Kansas School of Medicine and Veterans Affairs Medical Center, Kansas City KS, USA

Jerome D. Waye, M.D., FACP
Clinical Professor of Medicine, Chief, Gastrointestinal Endoscopy Unit, The Mount Sinai Hospital, New York NY, USA

George Y. Wu, M.D., Ph.D.
Professor, Director, Department of Medicine, Hepatology Section, Herman Lopata Chair in Hepatitis Research, University of Connecticut School of Medicine, Farmington CT, USA

1 Esophageal Strictures and Endoscopic Management

Nam Q. Nguyen and Janak N. Shah

Contents

Keywords: Esophageal, Strictures, Endoscopic, Management, Dilation

INTRODUCTION

Esophageal strictures are a relatively common problem in gastroenterology and are broadly divided into benign and malignant types. Recent data suggest that the overall incidence of new and recurrent esophageal strictures have decreased by about 10% and 30%, respectively, over the last decade (El-Serag 2006). This decline in the incidence of esophageal strictures is most likely due to the reduction in peptic-related strictures from the wide use of effective acid suppressive therapy with proton pump inhibitors (Guda and Vakil 2004). That noted, there does appear to be an increase in malignant strictures related to esophageal cancer, especially those located near the gastroesophageal junction (El-Serag 2006).

From: *Clinical Gastroenterology: Diagnostic and Therapeutic Procedures in Gastroenterology*,
Edited by: G. Y. Wu, S. Sridhar, DOI 10.1007/978-1-59745-044-7_1,

ETIOLOGY OF ESOPHAGEAL STRICTURES

Most benign esophageal strictures are caused by chronic inflammation leading to ulceration, formation of fibrous tissue, and collagen deposition (Spechler 1999). In the United States, gastroesophageal reflux disease (GERD) with resultant peptic injury is the most common cause of benign esophageal strictures (El-Serag 2006; Spechler 1999). Typically, these strictures are located near the gastroesophageal junction and are relatively short (1–2 cm) in length. Other common causes of benign esophageal strictures include anastomotic strictures, radiation injury, caustic ingestions, Schatzki rings, and esophageal webs (Pereira-Lima et al. 1999; Lew and Kochman 2002) (Table 1).

Approximately 20–30% of esophageal strictures are related to malignancy (Lew and Kochman 2002), with squamous cell carcinoma and adenocarcinoma of the esophagus comprising the two major histological types. Classically, squamous cell carcinoma arises from dysplastic squamous epithelium located in any part of the esophagus, and is related to heavy smoking. In contrast, the typical adenocarcinoma arises in a background of GERD and Barrett's esophagus, and is more commonly located towards the distal esophagus (Enzinger and Mayer 2003).

DIAGNOSTIC WORK-UP

Dysphagia to solids, liquids, or both is the main presenting complaint of patients with esophageal strictures. When approaching a patient with dysphagia, a detailed history can provide valuable insight as to the underlying cause of stricture in the majority of patients (Spechler 1999). Physical examination provides an assessment of patient nutritional status and potential tolerability from a medical standpoint for any invasive procedures that may be required for further diagnosis or treatment. However, clinical exam is usually not useful in identifying the cause of dysphagia. Specific laboratory tests are not necessary in the etiologic work-up of dysphagia, but a panel of routine serum tests (e.g. complete blood count, electrolytes, coagulation tests) may facilitate subsequent diagnostic and therapeutic procedural interventions.

Table 1
Common causes of esophageal strictures

Benign strictures	*Malignant strictures*
• Peptic stricture	• Squamous cell carcinoma
• Schatzki ring	• Adenocarcinoma
• Webs	• Extrinsic compression (e.g. malignant mediastinal lymph node, lung cancer, lymphoma)
• Postsurgical or anastomosis	
• Caustic injury	
• Radiation injury	
• Eosinophilic esophagitis	
• Extrinsic compression (e.g. benign inflammatory mediastinal lymph node, spine osteophyte, vascular compression)	

The two main tools that accurately identify the presence or absence of a stricture are barium contrast esophagram and upper GI endoscopy. For most patients, endoscopy is the preferred and only technique needed in evaluating dysphagia. Flexible endoscopy provides a platform to visually inspect the entire esophagus and upper GI tract, accurately identify the location and appearance of a stricture, perform tissue sampling if needed (e.g. biopsy of malignant-appearing strictures), and immediately treat a stricture using endoscopic dilation (Spechler 1999). Moreover, endoscopy without pre-procedure barium swallow appears to be cost-effective in patients with suspected esophageal obstruction in whom there is a high likelihood for endoscopic treatment (Esfandyari et al. 2002). However, pre-procedure contrast study may be useful in select circumstances, such as: (1) patients at high risk to undergo sedation for endoscopy due to medical comorbidities, (2) patients with higher likelihood for motility disorders (without a true obstruction), and (3) patients with suspected high-grade or anatomically complex strictures, in which a contrast study may provide useful information to the endoscopist for planning treatment. Given that the majority of patients do not require a preendoscopy contrast esophagram, the decision of whether to obtain this study is best left to the discretion of the endoscopist.

INDICATIONS FOR ENDOSCOPIC ESOPHAGEAL DILATION

Endoscopic esophageal dilation is the mainstay treatment for benign strictures and should be considered in all patients who are symptomatic with dysphagia and have luminal compromise on diagnostic endoscopy or contrast esophagram (Spechler 1999; Pereira-Lima et al. 1999). Most patients experience dysphagia when the esophageal luminal diameter is compromised to ≤13 mm. Thus, the goal of dilation therapy is to expand the lumen to at least 13–15 mm in diameter (Egan et al. 2006). Care is taken when dilating strictures that are related to eosinophilic esophagitis and caustic injury, as the risk of perforation may be higher with these types of strictures (Egan et al. 2006).

On the other hand, esophageal dilation has negligible benefit in treating malignant obstruction. Dilation rarely achieves durable relief of symptoms for patients with malignant strictures. However, endoscopic dilation is used to facilitate other types of diagnostic or therapeutic measures, such as endoscopic ultrasound for tumor staging or esophageal stent placement for palliation of unresectable tumor (Lew and Kochman 2002; Egan et al. 2006). These types of applications require only the minimum dilation diameter that would allow endoscope or instrument passage.

PATIENT PREPARATION FOR ESOPHAGEAL DILATION

Most patients are able to undergo endoscopy with esophageal dilation under conscious sedation. Pre-procedure cardiology clearance or anesthesia support during the procedure may be needed for patients with major medical comorbidities or those deemed high risk for endoscopy or conscious sedation. Anticoagulants are usually discontinued prior to the procedure to minimize bleeding risk during dilation. Antibiotic prophylaxis is not required for esophageal dilation. Although transient bacteremia may occur during endoscopy and endoscopic dilation, true infectious complications are rare, and thus antibiotic prophylaxis is no longer recommended even for patients at risk for infective endocarditis (Wilson et al. 2007).

Endoscopy and esophageal dilation is usually performed in an outpatient setting in either a hospital-based GI suite or ambulatory surgery center. Patients should fast for at least 6 h prior to procedure. After the procedure, patients usually spend ½ to 1 h in a recovery unit to monitor sedation effects prior to discharge home. There are no specific dietary restrictions after dilation for most patients. Adequate acid suppression with proton pump inhibitors after treating peptic strictures is an important measure to reduce stricture recurrence. No routine radiographic or laboratory tests are needed following dilation procedures.

ENDOSCOPIC DILATION TECHNIQUES

A number of techniques are available to dilate and treat esophageal strictures (Fig. 1). Two main types of dilators that are widely used today include (1) wire-guided, mechanical, push-type dilators, and (2) through-the-scope (TTS) balloon dilators (Taitelbaum et al. 2004). Specific models of dilators are available from several different manufacturers.

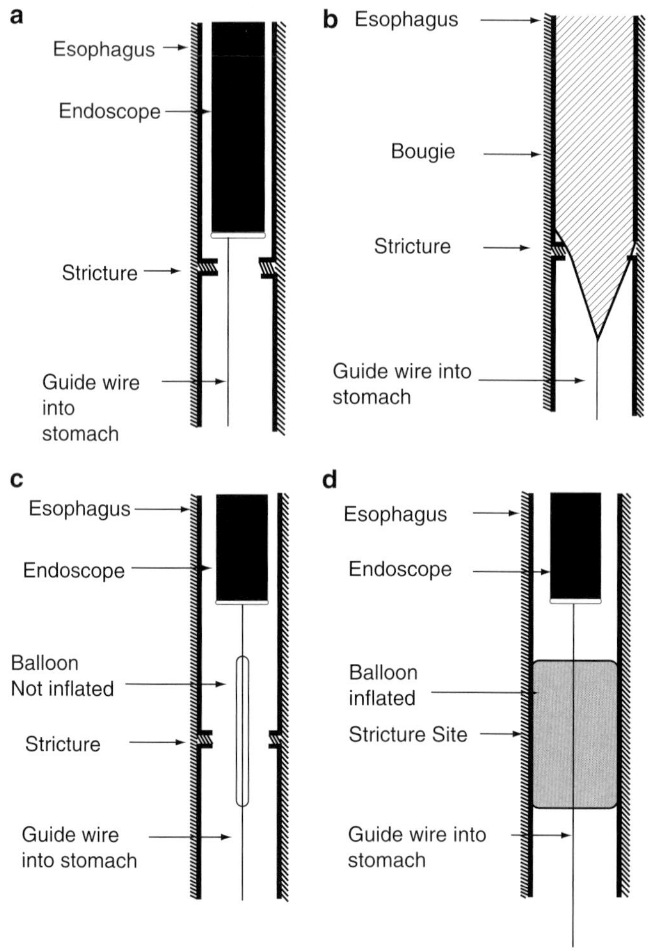

Fig. 1. Schematic of wire-guided, mechanical, push-type dilator (*top*) and balloon dilators (*bottom*). Mechanical dilator: (**a**) after endoscopic placement of a stiff wire across the stricture; (**b**) advancement of the tapered dilator disrupts the stricture. Balloon dilation: (**c**) deflated balloon dilator is placed across the stricture; (**d**) inflation of the balloon results in stricture dilation.

Tapered-tip, mechanical, push-type dilators (also commonly referred to as "bougie" dilators) come in wire-guided and nonwire-guided styles. The non-wire-guided type is rarely used nowadays due to risks of blind insertion. Wire-guided bougie-type dilators are composed of polyvinyl chloride, and have a central channel to allow passage over a guidewire. After endoscopic placement of a guidewire across the stricture, sequential bougie dilators are passed either blindly or under fluoroscopic guidance across the stricture. Dilation occurs as the increased diameter from the tapered section to the main body of the dilator crosses the stricture. Bougie style dilators will exert some downward longitudinal force along with radial force to disrupt the stenosis. Tactile feedback during passage may be appreciated by the endoscopist with this style of dilator. Several incremental dilator sizes are usually passed during one session (Fig. 2), but in general, most endoscopists follow the "rule of 3s" to minimize the risk of perforation (Egan et al. 2006; Lew et al. 2004).

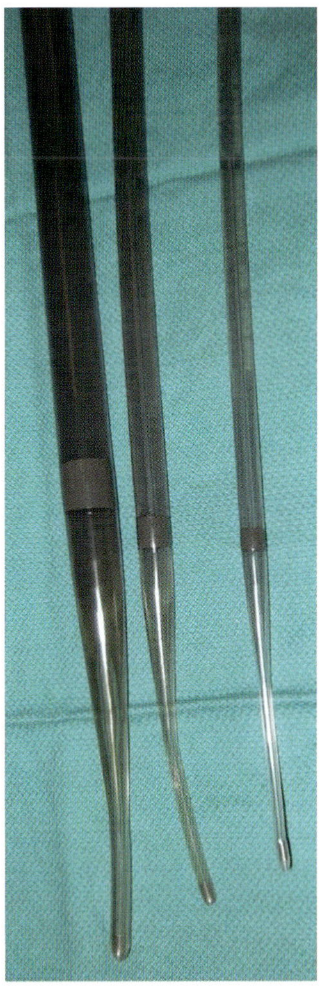

Fig. 2. Three distinct sizes of over-the-wire, mechanical, taper-tip dilators. Dilator size increases from right to left. A central channel for a guide wire is present to allow advancement of the dilator over a previously placed wire across the stricture. Dilation occurs as the increased diameter from the tapered section to the main body crosses the stricture. A radio-opaque black band facilitates dilation under fluoroscopy, if needed.

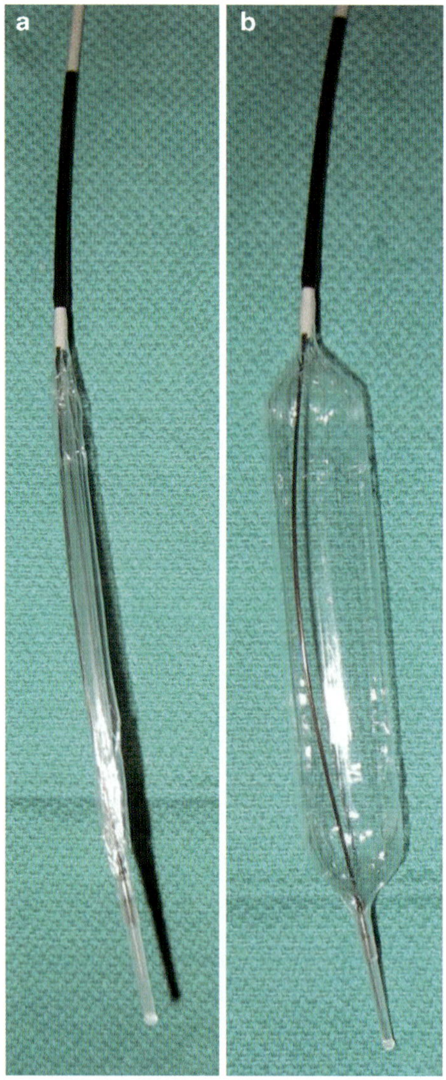

Fig. 3. (**a**) Deflated and (**b**) inflated balloon dilation catheter. After passage of a deflated balloon dilator across the stricture, inflation under pressure results in stricture dilation.

This generally accepted principle suggests that no more than three 1 mm incremental dilators should be passed after feeling moderate resistance.

Balloon dilation is performed by advancing a deflated balloon through the instrument channel of the endoscope (Fig. 3). The deflated catheter is placed across the stricture usually under direct endoscopic view. Fluoroscopy can be used to guide dilation, but is usually reserved for high-grade strictures that do not allow proper endoscopic visualization. Once the deflated balloon catheter is advanced traversing the stricture, the balloon is inflated with water (Fig. 4). This action results in the application of radial force, and disrupts the stricture. The inflation and stricture dilation can be visualized endoscopically. Balloons come in a variety of lengths and sizes, but most allow for multiple diameter, grade dilations using a single device (Taitelbaum et al. 2004).

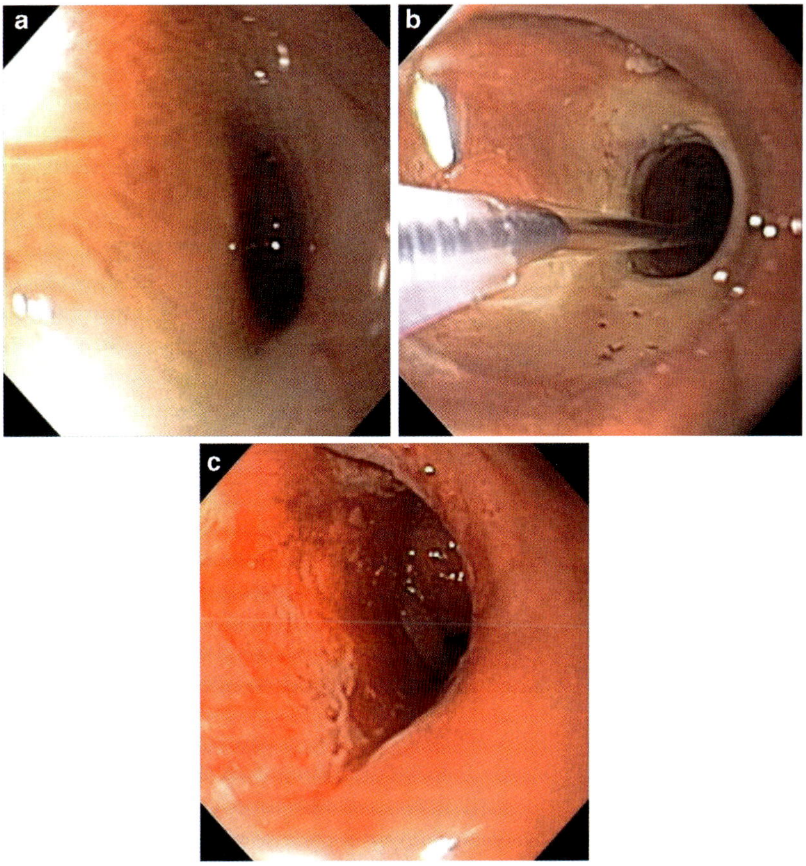

Fig. 4. Endoscopic images of esophageal stricture dilation with a balloon: (**a**) high-grade proximal esophageal stricture related following radiotherapy for squamous cell carcinoma. (**b**) dilation performed with balloon catheter. (**c**) a wider diameter is noted postdilation. Mild oozing post-dilation is of no clinical consequence.

Although bougie and balloon dilation differ in technical aspects, there are no demonstrated advantages or differences with respect to safety or efficacy between these techniques (Scolapio et al. 1999). One relative advantage of bougie is cost, as these dilators can be reused, whereas balloon dilators are for single use only.

The goal of dilation is to maintain a luminal diameter of at least 13–15 mm. Given the practice of graded increases in dilation diameters, interval dilation sessions may be required for narrow strictures. Most strictures will respond after 1–3 dilation sessions (Lew and Kochman 2002). The interval between dilation sessions usually varies between 1 and 3 weeks.

Some types of strictures are more difficult to treat with standard dilation. Published series have suggested that strictures that are anatomically complex (e.g. tortuous, narrow, long) or of non-peptic etiology are more likely to be refractory to standard dilation techniques (Lew and Kochman 2002; Shah 2006). Fortunately, other types of endoscopic treatments have emerged to circumvent these difficult strictures. Some of these techniques include steroid injection into strictures, electrosurgical incisions, and temporary esophageal stent placement.

COMPLICATIONS OF ESOPHAGEAL DILATION

The most dreaded complication of esophageal dilation is perforation. If there is concern for esophageal perforation, an esophagram or chest CT after ingestion of water-soluble contrast should be ordered. Fortunately, perforations are quite rare, occurring in 0.1–0.4% of procedures. If recognized early (during the procedure) and if the perforation is small, endoscopic techniques (e.g. clipping, temporary stent) and other conservative measures (e.g. antibiotics, nasogastric drainage) may allow healing without necessitating surgical repair. Large perforation often requires surgical treatment. Risk factors for perforation may include: anatomically complex strictures (e.g. high grade or long length), dilation of caustic or radiation-induced strictures, and endoscopist inexperience (Lew and Kochman 2002; Egan et al. 2006).

Self-limited oozing is almost universal after an esophageal dilatation as the procedure involves disruption of the mucosal and submucosal layers. Clinically significant bleeding, however, is rare and is limited to complex strictures related to either malignancy or radiation therapy. Aspiration is an infrequent complication of esophageal dilation, but may occur in patients with esophageal strictures who have food impactions or who develop total esophageal obstruction. Aggressive oral suctioning during the procedure may minimize this risk.

ALTERNATIVE MANAGEMENT

There are limited options for patients with strictures who do not respond to endoscopic treatment. Surgery may be considered on a case-by-case basis. Unfortunately, the underlying etiology of many of these difficult strictures (e.g. radiation or caustic injury) also makes surgical reconstruction a technically challenging endeavor. The other main option is to forgo establishment of luminal continuity and maintain hydration and nutrition through a gastrostomy tube. Fortunately, advances in dilation tools and other endoscopic techniques have minimized the need for these less-than-optimal alternative treatment strategies.

SUMMARY OF KEY POINTS

- The incidence of benign esophageal strictures is decreasing, most likely attributed to effective acid suppression medications. At the same time, esophageal cancer and malignant strictures seem to be increasing in incidence.
- Endoscopy is the main tool in evaluating patients with dysphagia, as it provides a platform for both diagnosis and treatment.
- Endoscopic dilation is an effective and safe tool to treat most benign esophageal strictures. Most strictures respond to endoscopic dilation techniques.

REFERENCES

El-Serag HB. Temporal trends in new and recurrent esophageal strictures in Department of Veterans Affairs. Am J Gastroenterol. 2006;101:1727–33.

Guda NM, Vakil N. Proton pump inhibitors and the time trends for esophageal dilation. Am J Gastroenterol. 2004;99:797–800.

Spechler SJ. AGA technical review on treatment of patients with dysphagia caused by benign disorders of the distal esophagus. Gastroenterology. 1999;117:233–54.

Pereira-Lima JC, Ramires RP, Zamin Jr I, Cassal AP, Marroni CA, Mattos AA. Endoscopic dilation of benign esophageal strictures: report on 1043 procedures. Am J Gastroenterol. 1999;94:1497–501.

Lew RJ, Kochman ML. A review of endoscopic methods of esophageal dilation. J Clin Gastroenterol. 2002;35:117–26.

Enzinger PC, Mayer RJ. Esophageal cancer. N Engl J Med. 2003;349:2241–52.

Esfandyari T, Potter JW, Vaezi MF. Dysphagia: a cost analysis of the diagnostic approach. Am J Gastroenterol. 2002;97:2733–7.

Egan JV, Baron TH, Adler DG, Davila R, Faigel DO, Gan SL, et al. Esophageal dilation. Gastrointest Endosc. 2006;63:755–60.

Wilson W, Taubert KA, Gewitz M, Lockhart PB, Baddour LM, Levison M, et al. Prevention of infective endocarditis: guidelines from the American Heart Association: a guideline from the American Heart Association Rheumatic Fever, Endocarditis and Kawasaki Disease Committee, Council on Cardiovascular Disease in the Young, and the Council on Clinical Cardiology, Council on Cardiovascular Surgery and Anesthesia, and the Quality of Care and Outcomes Research Interdisciplinary Working Group. J Am Dent Assoc. 2007;138(739–45):747–60.

Taitelbaum G, Petersen BT, Barkun AN, Chotiprasidhi B, Chuttani R, Liu J, et al. Tools for endoscopic stricture dilation. Gastrointest Endosc. 2004;59:753–60.

Lew RJ, Shah JN, Chalian A, Weber RS, Williams NN, Kochman ML. Technique of endoscopic retrograde puncture and dilatation of total esophageal stenosis in patients with radiation-induced strictures. Head Neck. 2004;26:179–83.

Scolapio JS, Pasha TM, Gostout CJ, Mahoney DW, Zinsmeister AR, Ott BJ, et al. A randomized prospective study comparing rigid to balloon dilators for benign esophageal strictures and rings. Gastrointest Endosc. 1999;50:13–7.

Shah JN. Benign refractory esophageal strictures: widening the endoscopist's role. Gastrointest Endosc. 2006;63:164–7.

2 Endoscopic Management of Barrett's Esophagus

Mandeep Singh, Sachin Wani, and Prateek Sharma

Contents

Keywords: Endoscopic, Management, Barrett's Esophagus, Surveillance

INTRODUCTION

Barrett's esophagus (BE) is a well-recognized premalignant condition for development of esophageal adenocarcinoma (EAC). It is defined as the displacement of the squamo-columnar junction proximal to the gastroesophageal junction, with the presence of intestinal metaplasia (IM) on biopsies (Wang and Sampliner 2008; Sharma et al. 2004). Chronic gastroesophageal reflux disease (GERD) is the most frequent identifiable risk factor for Barrett's esophagus (Wang and Sampliner 2008; Sharma et al. 2004). In Western populations, BE may be present in approximately 0.4–1.6% of adults, whereas in patients with chronic GERD, the prevalence is approximately 10–15% (Pondugula et al. 2007; Wani and Sharma 2007a). The frequency of EAC in the United States is gradually rising. It has been estimated that 14,550 new cases of esophageal cancer were diagnosed in 2006, with 13,770 deaths related to esophageal cancer, the majority diagnosed at an advanced stage (American Cancer Society 2006). Barrett's esophagus is considered to be one of the most important identifiable risk factors leading to development of EAC (Menke-Pluymers et al. 1993; Solaymani-Dodaran et al. 2004). Progression of BE to esophageal cancer involves a series

From: *Clinical Gastroenterology: Diagnostic and Therapeutic Procedures in Gastroenterology*,
Edited by: G. Y. Wu, S. Sridhar, DOI 10.1007/978-1-59745-044-7_2,

of pathological changes, from early nondysplastic columnar epithelium (ND BE) to low-grade dysplasia (LGD), high-grade dysplasia (HGD), and finally to cancer. The mortality associated with EAC is high, with a 5-year survival rate of only 15% (Pondugula et al. 2007; Cossentino and Wong 2003; Devesa et al. 1998).

At present, treatment aimed at BE may be the only way to control the rising incidence of EAC. Advances in endoscopic imaging are progressing at an increasingly rapid rate and may assist in the earlier detection of dysplasia and EAC within the Barrett's segment. Recently, results of endoscopic therapies (endoscopic resection and/or ablation) have been promising and have gained increased acceptance in the management of HGD and early EAC (Das et al. 2008).

In this chapter, an overview of the role of endoscopy in the diagnosis and management of BE, including the role of advanced imaging and endoscopic therapies, is provided.

ENDOSCOPY IN BARRETT'S ESOPHAGUS

The current standard to establish a reliable diagnosis of BE is by use of endoscopy with biopsy. There are no definitive risk factors to predict the occurrence of BE in the general population and, therefore, screening of the general population for BE is currently not recommended. Some of the proposed clinical and demographic predictors for BE development include age of more than 40 years, heartburn, long-standing GERD (more than 13 years), male gender, and obesity (mainly visceral) (Wang and Sampliner 2008; Pondugula et al. 2007). However, a critical review of Barrett's literature at the AGA Chicago workshop concluded that even in adults (whites or persons of other ethnicity), older than 50 years, who had had heartburn for 5–10 years, there was no evidence to support endoscopic screening for BE (Sharma et al. 2004). Similarly, recent American College of Gastroenterology practice guidelines for diagnosis and management of BE and the American Gastrointestinal Association position statement on the management of GERD could not offer any recommendation. There was insufficient evidence to justify endoscopic screening of BE and dysplasia in adults 50 years or older with >5–10 years of heartburn, to reduce mortality from EAC (Wang and Sampliner 2008; Kahrilas et al. 2008). Therefore, BE may be detected incidentally in patients without known risk factors (Gerson et al. 2002) and it may not be present in patients with potential risk factors for BE. The inability to predict BE prior to endoscopy even among high-risk groups poses a challenge to the formulation of appropriate guidelines for screening patients for BE (Wang and Sampliner 2008).

A precise localization of the gastro-esophageal and squamo-columnar junction (SCJ) (the Z-line) is important in the endoscopic diagnosis of BE. In the normal state, the SCJ is located distally at the gastro-esophageal junction (GEJ) and corresponds to the transition zone of stratified squamous epithelium (pale and glossy) to columnar epithelium (salmon-pink appearing). In patients with BE, the SCJ is displaced proximally in relation to GEJ (Fig. 1). A standard description for grading the BE segment includes its circumferential extent (the C value) and the maximum extent (the M value) based on the validated Prague C & M criteria (Sharma et al. 2006a). For a histological diagnosis, targeted biopsies of apparent lesions and a four-quadrant biopsy protocol every 1–2 cm should be followed (Sharma et al. 2006a). In patients with suspected BE, the presence of reflux esophagitis can mask its presence. These patients should be treated with high-dose proton pump inhibitor (PPI) therapy, and a repeat endoscopy should be performed within 3–6 months to

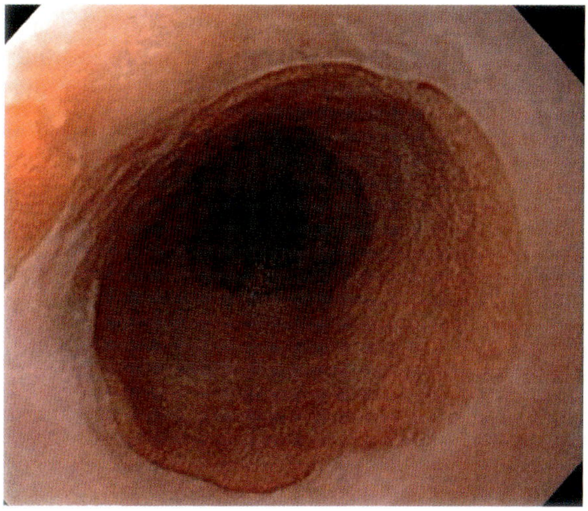

Fig. 1. Endoscopic view of Barrett's esophagus under white light endoscopy.

ensure healing of erosive esophagitis if BE is suspected. In a prospective study of 172 patients with reflux symptoms and erosive esophagitis, BE was detected in 14% of patients on repeat endoscopy after 3 months of PPI therapy (Hanna et al. 2006).

ENDOSCOPIC SURVEILLANCE

Identification of asymptomatic, early, and curable EAC in patients with BE forms the basis for regular surveillance endoscopy and biopsies. Despite lack of randomized clinical trials supporting its survival benefits, the vast majority of patients with BE are enrolled in surveillance programs. The ultimate goal of surveillance endoscopy is a reduction in cancer-related deaths by initiation of treatment at the pre-invasive stage of EAC (Falk et al. 2000; Corley et al. 2002). The surveillance interval is determined based on the grade of dysplasia, using a systematic four-quadrant 1–2 cm biopsy protocol, with advanced dysplasia requiring more frequent surveillance.

BE Without Dysplasia

In patients with BE without dysplasia (ND BE) on initial surveillance biopsies, the risk of progression to EAC is estimated to be approximately 0.5% annually (O'Connor et al. 1999; Sharma et al. 2006b). Barrett's patients with no dysplasia should undergo two surveillance endoscopies within 1 year, and if there is lack of dysplasia on subsequent biopsies, the surveillance interval may be widened to every 3 years. Absence of dysplasia on first two endoscopies does not rule out the possibility of BE progressing to HGD/EAC (Sharma et al. 2006b). The surveillance protocol should be modified if dysplasia is detected at any point during surveillance of BE without dysplasia.

BE with LGD

To make a definitive diagnosis of LGD, an expert opinion from a gastrointestinal pathologist is recommended, given the interobserver variability in making this diagnosis

(Montgomery et al. 2001a). Two different studies demonstrated that the likelihood of LGD progressing to HGD or cancer rose significantly when two or more gastrointestinal pathologists agreed on the diagnosis of LGD (Skacel et al. 2000; Montgomery et al. 2001b). Contrary to this statement, Lim et al. showed no difference in neoplastic progression of LGD regardless of consensus versus original diagnosis (Lim et al. 2007). Furthermore, the natural history of LGD is ill-defined with an annual incidence of cancer development ranging from 0.6% to 1.28% (Sharma et al. 2006b; Dulai et al. 2005). The unpredictable nature of LGD probably justifies the current use of surveillance in these patients. Once BE with LGD is confirmed, the first surveillance endoscopy is recommended at an interval of 6 months. If there is no evidence of high-grade dysplasia, yearly endoscopies are performed until two consecutive annual endoscopies are negative for dysplasia (Wang and Sampliner 2008). Use of more definitive diagnostic tools combined with innovative histopathological and novel endoscopic tools may impact the future practice of surveillance endoscopy in this group of BE patients.

BE with HGD

The presence of HGD carries with it a high risk of progression to EAC, with incidence of 6.5 per 100 patient-years and a 5-year risk exceeding 30% (Wang and Sampliner 2008; Rastogi et al. 2008; Buttar et al. 2001). Identification of HGD should also prompt a review by two expert gastrointestinal pathologists. The diagnosis of HGD on endoscopic biopsy does not completely rule out the possibility of occult EAC. A high possibility of co-existing EAC in these patients had been the rationale for performing prophylactic esophagectomy in HGD patients. However, in a recent systematic review, Konda et al. demonstrated an EAC prevalence of 12.7%, instead of the previously reported rate of 40%, in BE patients who underwent esophagectomy for HGD (Konda et al. 2008). Combined use of advanced imaging techniques, endoscopic ultrasonography, and endoscopic mucosal resection (EMR) can help in accurate staging of HGD and early EAC (Wang and Sampliner 2008). Most experts would recommend therapeutic intervention or intensive surveillance (every 3 months), once the diagnosis of HGD is established.

ADVANCED ENDOSCOPIC IMAGING OF BARRETT'S ESOPHAGUS

Use of standard white light endoscopy with random biopsies is currently the gold standard for diagnosing BE. Unfortunately, this is not target-sensitive, especially in the setting of short-segment BE. During standard endoscopy, biopsies obtained from short segments of columnar-appearing mucosa may identify intestinal metaplasia in only 40–60% of patients (Eloubeidi and Provenzale 1999). Similarly, the focal and patchy distribution of dysplastic and cancerous lesions within Barrett's segment lowers the sensitivity of standard biopsy techniques (Cameron and Carpenter 1997). Moreover, current endoscopic techniques are time-consuming, labor-intensive, involve high cost, and are limited by sampling errors.

To overcome these shortcomings, advanced endoscopic techniques have been developed to maximize the sensitivity and improve the overall accuracy in diagnosing various grades of Barrett's dysplasia and early cancer. The prognosis of esophageal neoplasia is dependent on the stage of disease at the time of diagnosis. The enhanced ability to identify EAC at preinvasive stage allows for early endoscopic therapeutic intervention in these patients that may reduce the morbidity and improve overall survival (Wani and Sharma 2007b). Use of advanced imaging techniques that highlight esophageal mucosal patterns facilitate in identification of metaplastic, dysplastic, and early cancerous lesions with better accuracy (Nelson et al. 2000).

In this section, we discuss the potential role of novel imaging techniques, including high-resolution/high-definition/magnification endoscopy, narrow band imaging (NBI), chromoendoscopy, autofluorescence imaging (AFI), and confocal endomicroscopy, in the management of Barrett's esophagus and/or early cancer.

High-Resolution/High-Definition/Magnification Endoscopy

High-resolution endoscopes are equipped with a high pixel density (600,000–1 million) charge-coupled device that enables a detailed visualization of the mucosal surface with its ability to discriminate lesions 10–71 μm in diameter. High-resolution endoscopy can be combined with magnification endoscopy that enlarges the video images up to 150×, using a movable lens at the tip of the endoscope. Typically, a cap is fitted onto the distal tip of the endoscope, allowing the mucosa in contact with the cap to be magnified without being affected by esophageal motility. Recently, the use of high-definition television (HDTV), which has a higher resolution than conventional endoscopes, has been explored. It can generate up to 1,080 scanning lines on a screen and increases image quality and allows projection onto a large screen while retaining image quality. Early mucosal lesions may be too small, focal, or patchy to be discriminated from normal surrounding tissues on standard endoscopy. However, use of high-resolution and magnification endoscopy allows for inspection of fine details of focal lesions that can represent early neoplastic lesions (Yao et al. 2006). Compared to standard endoscopy, high-resolution endoscopy appears to have higher sensitivity for detection of early neoplastic lesions in patients with BE (Kara et al. 2005a, b). Magnification endoscopy may be a useful adjunct to high-resolution endoscopy in characterization of mucosal and vascular pattern of Barrett's lesions.

Chromoendoscopy

This involves the application of different staining agents to enhance the characterization of esophageal mucosa and it is often combined with high-magnification and high-resolution endoscopy. The two types of chromoendoscopy stains used in the esophagus are vital stains and contrast stains. Vital stains (e.g. Lugol's solution, methylene blue, and toluidine blue) are absorbed by the surface epithelium, whereas contrast stains (e.g. indigo carmine) highlight the superficial mucosal pattern by accumulating in the pits and grooves of the tissue. Lugol's solution, methylene blue, and indigo carmine are the most commonly used stains in the esophagus. Lugol's solution is absorbed by the glycogen containing nonkeratinized squamous epithelium and accurately delineates the squamo-columnar junction by staining only the squamous part and leaving the columnar epithelium unstained. This demarcation allows better targeted biopsies of the Barrett's segment. This characteristic of Lugol's solution is also used to identify residual islands of Barrett's following ablation therapy (Overholt et al. 1999; Sharma et al. 2007a).

Methylene blue is actively absorbed by the intestinal metaplastic epithelium and can be useful in detecting intestinal metaplasia within the Barrett segment. Different studies conducted using methylene blue have shown varying results, with some demonstrating higher sensitivity (Canto et al. 2001; Sharma et al. 2001) and others showing low sensitivity in identifying intestinal metaplasia (Breyer et al. 2003). Canto et al. in a study of 45 BE patients who had over 500 methylene blue stained biopsies, demonstrated an overall sensitivity of 97% and specificity of 42% for detection of IM (Canto et al. 2001). A recent prospective randomized crossover trial of 48 patients compared the utility of methylene blue-directed biopsy with standard four-quadrant biopsy. Both the techniques were comparable for the diagnosis of IM and dysplasia; however, the mean number of biopsies required to diagnose these conditions was significantly lower with use of methylene blue (Horwhat et al. 2008). On the other hand, a randomized crossover study showed that random four-quadrant biopsies detected significantly more patients with dysplasia than methylene blue directed biopsies (Lim et al. 2006). Moreover, the methylene blue technique may not be suitable for routine surveillance of Barrett's epithelium because of time constraints and high interobserver variability of methylene blue-positive readings even among expert endoscopists (Meining et al. 2004). In addition, methylene blue has been implicated in causing DNA damage in Barrett's mucosa (Olliver et al. 2003).

Combining magnification with indigo carmine chromoendoscopy, studies have demonstrated different mucosal patterns such as ridged/villous, circular, and irregular/distorted patterns. Using this technique of magnification chromoendoscopy, the sensitivity, specificity, and positive predictive value of ridged/villous patterns for detecting intestinal metaplasia were 97%, 76%, and 92%, respectively, whereas the irregular/distorted pattern had a sensitivity of 100% for detecting high-grade dysplasia. However, indigo carmine magnification chromoendoscopy has been limited by its inability to clearly differentiate patterns of low-grade dysplasia from intestinal metaplasia (Sharma et al. 2003). A recent randomized crossover study showed that compared to high-resolution endoscopy, indigo carmine chromoendoscopy did not increase the sensitivity for detection of early neoplasia (Kara et al. 2005b). Application of acetic acid (1.5–3%) has been used to make the columnar mucosa look prominent by congestion of capillaries giving it a reddish appearance. In patients undergoing ablative therapy, acetic acid may be used to identify residual Barrett's epithelium (Guelrud and Herrera 1998). The use of chromoendoscopy cannot be recommended in routine clinical practice due to the difficulty in achieving complete and uniform application of dye on the mucosal surface, the need for dye-spraying equipment, lack of standardized mucosal patterns, inability to detect vascular patterns and abnormalities, and labor intensiveness and operator dependence. Finally, conflicting results of chromoendoscopy compared with significant improvements in the field of advanced imaging techniques has generally obviated the need for dye spraying for detection of metaplastic and dysplastic tissue.

Narrow Band Imaging

NBI is a novel technique that uses spectral narrow-band optical filters instead of the full spectrum white light (Gono et al. 2004). The penetration depth of light is dependent on its wavelength (i.e., the longer the wavelength, the deeper the penetration), visible blue light would penetrate only superficial areas of the tissue (Fig. 2a). Therefore, use of blue light with the help of a special narrow-band filter enables imaging of the superficial tissue structures with enhanced visualization of microvasculature and mucosal patterns. Combined use of NBI with magnification endoscopy has revealed distinct mucosal and vascular patterns

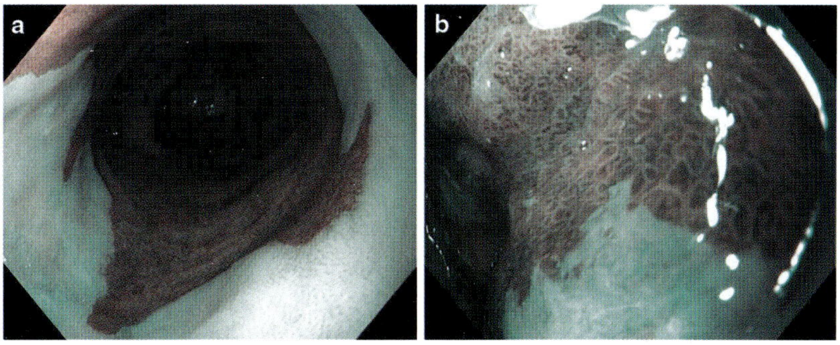

Fig. 2. (**a**) Endoscopic view of distal esophagus under narrow band imaging. (**b**) Endoscopic view of Barrett's esophagus under narrow band imaging showing irregular and distorted mucosal pattern.

that correspond to nondysplastic BE and BE with HGD (Kara et al. 2006a; Sharma et al. 2006c). In a prospective study, Sharma et al. assessed the potential of NBI images for predicting Barrett's histology in 51 patients. The authors graded NBI images into three distinct mucosal patterns, ridge/villous, circular, and irregular/distorted patterns (Fig. 2b), and vascular patterns into normal and abnormal patterns. The sensitivity, specificity, and positive predictive values of the ridge/villous pattern for diagnosis of intestinal metaplasia without high-grade dysplasia were 93.5%, 86.7%, and 94.7%, respectively. Similarly, the sensitivity, specificity, and positive predictive values of irregular/distorted pattern for high-grade dysplasia were 100%, 98.7%, and 95.3%, respectively. However, neither mucosal nor vascular patterns on NBI images were able to differentiate low-grade dysplasia from intestinal metaplasia (Sharma et al. 2006c). In another study, Kara et al. studied NBI images in 63 Barrett's patients and depicted three morphological patterns: irregular/disrupted mucosal patterns, irregular vascular patterns, and abnormal blood vessels. This study showed that areas of HGD had at least one of these abnormal patterns, and that the increase in frequency of abnormal patterns significantly correlated with increasing grades of dysplasia (Kara et al. 2006a). Whether NBI is better than chromoendoscopy in detecting HGD or early cancer in BE patients is not clear. In a randomized crossover trial of 28 patients, Kara et al. compared the efficacy of indigo carmine chromoendoscopy and NBI as adjuncts to high-resolution endoscopy in identifying Barrett's dysplasia or early cancer. There was no difference in the detection of high-grade dysplasia/early cancer between these two techniques (93% versus 86% sensitivity) and neither technique was superior to high-resolution endoscopy for neoplasia (Kara et al. 2005b). In a recent prospective, tandem endoscopy study involving 65 BE patients, NBI use increased the number of patients detected with HGD (18% versus 0%) compared to standard white light endoscopy. Furthermore, NBI-directed biopsies detected more dysplasia compared to biopsies obtained through standard endoscopy (Wolfsen et al. 2008).

Autofluorescence Imaging

This technique is based on the principle of light-tissue interaction where excitation of tissues with shorter wavelength light gives rise to emission of longer wavelength light (green to red spectrum), a phenomenon termed as "autofluorescence" (Fig. 3a).

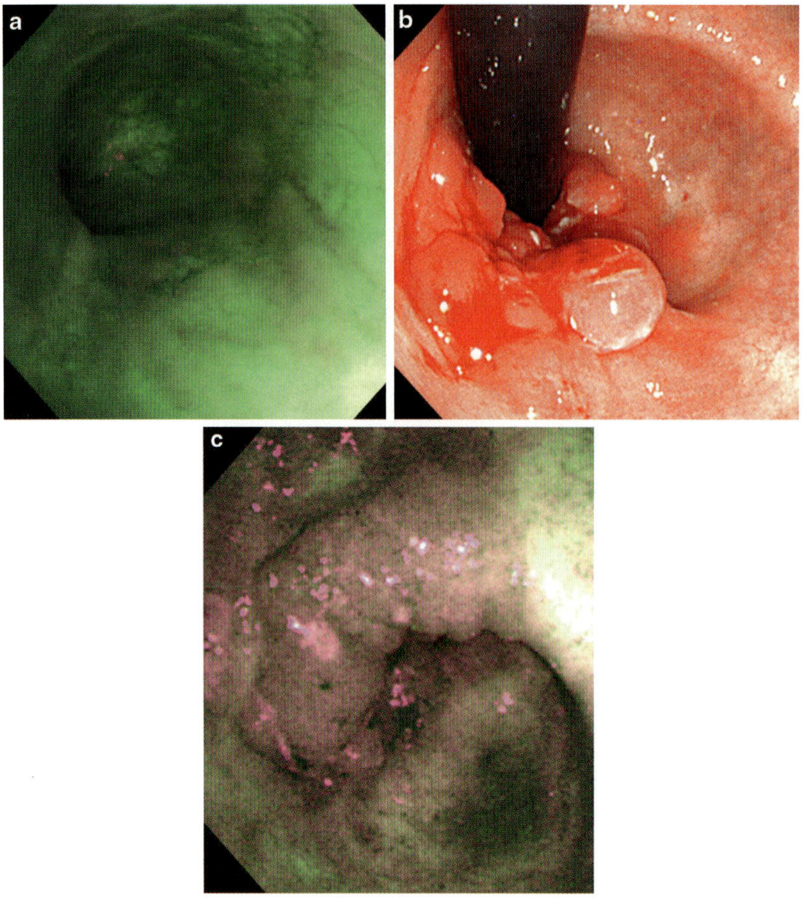

Fig. 3. (**a**) Endoscopic view of normal distal esophagus under autofluorescence imaging. (**b**) Endoscopic view of nodular esophageal cancer under white light endoscopy. (**c**) Endoscopic view of same lesion (Fig. 3b) under autofluorescence imaging (*AFI*).

The biological substances that emit fluorescent light are called fluorophores. In the gastrointestinal tract, submucosal collagen is the most important contributor to autofluorescence. The spectrum of autofluorescence differs in normal versus dysplastic and/or cancerous tissue because of molecular and architectural alterations. Malignant transformation of tissue is associated with emissions of relatively large wavelength of light (shift from green towards red spectrum) (Figs. 3b and c). This concept is used in identifying areas of dysplasia or cancer in Barrett's patients. In a feasibility study involving a prototype of HRE and AFI, it was demonstrated that AFI improved the detection rate of HGD, albeit with a positive predictive value of only 50% (Kara et al. 2005c). This led to a concept of multimodality imaging in BE, using AFI and NBI in a complementary fashion. In a proof-of-principle study, 20 BE patients with suspected or endoscopically treated HGD were initially examined by HRE and AFI, followed by NBI. AFI identified 47 suspicious lesions based on color blue/violet, only 28 of which had HGD, with a false-positive rate of 40%. Subsequent evaluation by NBI led to an overall reduction in the false-positive rate to 10%; 14 of the 19 false-positive areas had regular patterns on NBI (Kara et al. 2006b). In a multicenter trial of 84 patients with a similar trial design, AFI could identify all the HGD and early cancer lesions that were seen on high-resolution endoscopy. An additional 102 lesions were confirmed as HGD/EAC, giving AFI a false-positive rate of 81%. The false-positive rate was reduced to 26% after NBI examination. On a per-patient analysis, AFI detected all 16 patients with early neoplasia identified with high-resolution endoscopy and detected an additional 11 patients with early neoplasia who were not identified with high-resolution endoscopy. However, HGD/EAC was missed in three patients (10%) by advanced imaging modalities and was diagnosed only by random four-quadrant biopsies (Curvers et al. 2008b).

Confocal Laser Endomicroscopy

This novel technique allows subsurface microscopic mucosal analysis and in vivo histology during ongoing endoscopy. Confocal endomicroscopy involves stimulation of mucosal cells with laser light, which is reflected back through a pinhole and enables computer-aided generation of a cross-sectional microscopic image. A fluorescent contrast agent (mainly intravenous fluorescein) is used to attain high-contrast images during confocal endoscopy. Two approaches exist for in vivo microscopic imaging of the gastrointestinal tract with confocal laser endoscopy. One approach uses a Pentax Confocal Laser System that is integrated into the distal tip of a conventional videoendoscope enabling simultaneous confocal microscopy in addition to standard videoendoscopy. Magnification beyond 1,000× can be achieved, enabling visualization of cellular and subcellular elements, crypt architecture, mucosal cells and goblet cells in intestinal crypts, capillaries, and red blood cells with very high resolution and detail. During laser endoscopy, a single line laser delivers an excitation wavelength of 488 nm, and confocal images are generated at a scan rate of 0.8 frames/s to 1.6 frames/s. The field of view is 500×500 μm with an optical slice thickness of 7 μm and a lateral view of 0.7 μm (Kiesslich et al. 2006). Another approach for in vivo microscopic imaging involves a confocal laser microscope (CLM) miniprobe (Cellvizio, Mauna Kea technologies) that can be passed through the working channel of any standard endoscope. This miniprobe has a 2.5 mm outer diameter, mounted on which is a short (4 mm) transparent distant cap that helps in better targeting of the lesions. Like confocal endomicroscopy, the confocal miniprobe provides real-time microscopic surface and subsurface imaging of mucosa. Computer software using an image reconstruction algorithm allows dynamic single frame images into a single, larger, high-resolution static image, without compromising image quality.

In patients with suspected BE, the diagnosis can be confirmed by identifying and differentiating specialized columnar epithelium from gastric columnar epithelium because of the presence of goblet cells. It has also been shown to have high accuracy for the detection of HGD or cancer (Kiesslich et al. 2006). Based on vascular and cellular architectural characteristics of confocal microendoscopy images, Kiesslich et al. determined that images demonstrating regular-shaped capillaries visible only in deeper mucosa and regular columnar-lined epithelium with round glandular openings and a typical cobble stone appearance were suggestive of gastric-type epithelium, whereas regular capillaries present in the upper and deeper parts of the mucosal layer along with identification of dark mucin in goblet cells in the columnar-lined mucosa were diagnosed as intestinal metaplasia. Diagnosis of dysplasia or cancer was based on the identification of irregular capillaries in upper and deeper parts of mucosal layer with black cells that had irregular apical and distal borders and shapes on confocal images (Kiesslich et al. 2006). In another recent study by Pohl et al., the investigators conducted two phase clinical trials to evaluate an in vivo miniprobe CLM for the detection of invisible Barrett's neoplasia. These researchers established a CLM criteria for diagnosing Barrett's neoplasia, and demonstrated that fusion of glands was the most sensitive criterion for diagnosing advanced neoplasia, with a sensitivity of 80% and good interobserver agreement (kappa 0.6) (Pohl et al. 2008).

ENDOSCOPIC THERAPY IN BARRETT'S ESOPHAGUS

Patient Group to Be Treated

In spite of the striking increase in the incidence of EAC, the vast majority of patients with BE never develop EAC. The true incidence of EAC in BE is 0.5% per year with a lifetime cancer risk for a patient with ND BE in the range of 5–8% (Rastogi et al. 2008). Although endoscopic eradication of ND BE is attractive, there is no scientific evidence that this strategy decreases cancer risk. Wani et al., in a recent systematic review and meta-analysis, determined the cancer incidence in BE patients after ablative therapies and compared the rates to cohort studies of BE patients not undergoing ablation. The investigators showed that the greatest benefit was observed in BE patients with HGD (number needed to treat [NNT] 20), but the NNT in patients without dysplasia was prohibitively high (NNT 250). In addition, the need for surveillance is not eliminated and multiple sessions may be required (Wani et al. 2009). Until further information is available, we should follow the "primum nil nocere" principle. Endoscopic therapy for non-dysplastic Barrett's cannot be recommended at this time (Fig. 4).

PATIENTS WITH LGD

The rate of development of EAC in BE patients with LGD is unclear (range 0.6–1.6% per year) (Lim et al. 2007; Shaheen et al. 2000). This can be attributed to the highly variable natural history data of LGD frequently reported in a small number of patients, with short duration of follow-up (Wani et al. 2009). Other significant confounding variables include high interobserver variability among pathologists, difficulty in differentiating between prevalent and incident cases, and selection and referral bias (Montgomery et al. 2001a; Curvers et al. 2008a). The future lies in risk stratification and identification of those LGD patients most likely to progress to HGD/EAC. Until then, endoscopic therapies in LGD patients cannot be recommended as majority of them regress and have an overall lower incidence of cancer.

PATIENTS WITH HGD

Given the high rate of progression to EAC, patients with HGD is the group most likely to benefit from the various endoscopic therapies. The two main aggressive management approaches include surgical resection and complete endoscopic eradication of BE segment. Esophagectomy has traditionally been the standard treatment for patients with HGD. A number of proposed factors that favored this approach include high risk of HGD progressing to invasive cancer, resection of entire diseased esophageal segment with no

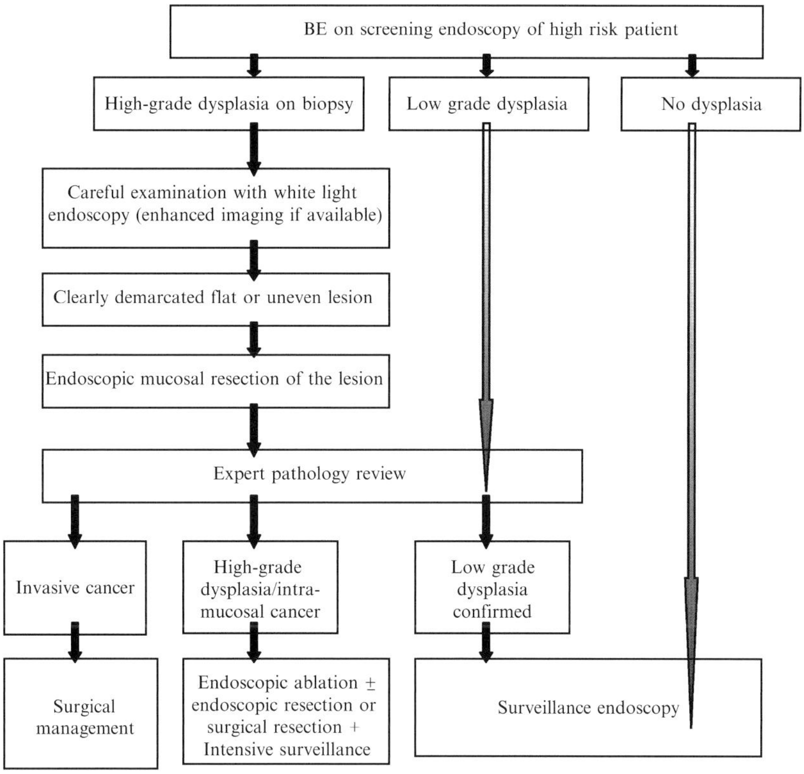

Fig. 4. Algorithm for BE management.

chances of development of BE and neoplasia in future, and results of studies demonstrating co-existing cancer in approximately 40% of esophagectomy specimens in patients with HGD (Heitmiller et al. 1996; Sharma et al. 2007b). However, recent studies provide better estimates of cancer incidence in this group of patients. A meta-analysis by Rastogi et al. showed the weighted incidence rate of EAC to be 6.6 per 100 patient years of follow-up in patients with HGD (Rastogi et al. 2008). Konda et al. demonstrated the true prevalence of occult adenocarcinoma to be 12.7%, which was much less than the earlier reported prevalence of 40% (Konda et al. 2008). Moreover, a finite risk of BE development exists after esophagectomy, and endoscopic surveillance may still be required post-surgery (Dresner et al. 2003). Finally, esophagectomy is associated with mortality rates of 3–5%, and morbidity rates of 20–50% even in high-volume and expert centers (59). Long-term survival in patients with HGD and early cancer treated with endoscopic therapy are comparable to those treated with esophagectomy. Prasad et al. in a retrospective cohort study showed that overall mortality in HGD patients treated with endoscopic therapy (PDT plus EMR) was 9% versus 8.5% in those patients who underwent esophagectomy during the same time period (Prasad et al. 2007). In another population-based study using the surveillance epidemiology and end results (SEER) databases, Das et al. demonstrated that long-term survival was not different in patients managed by endoscopic therapy compared to those treated with surgical resection (Das et al. 2008).

Pre-endoscopic Therapy Work-up

Different endoscopic techniques have been used for the eradication of BE. However, there are no definitive guidelines to specify these therapies for individual patients. Based on the extent of Barrett's HGD, presence and extent of EAC and availability of equipment, expertise of gastroenterologists, endoscopic therapy should be individualized. Histological confirmation of Barrett's by expert gastrointestinal pathologist, use of EUS, diagnostic EMR, and CT scan to stage EAC should be done.

Role of EUS

A critical factor in deciding between endoscopic therapy versus esophagectomy in patients with HGD and/or esophageal adenocarcinoma is accurate staging of the tumor (Lightdale 1999; Enzinger and Mayer 2003). Using TNM anatomical classification, EUS can provide the most accurate clinical staging of the depth of tumor invasion (T) and regional lymph-node metastasis (N) (Mallery and Van Dam 2000; Shumaker et al. 2002). However, results of EUS even with high-frequency ultrasound probes may be limited by its inability to sometimes differentiate HGD (T*is*), early adenocarcinoma confined to mucosa (T1m), and cancer invading the submucosa (T1sm) (Chak et al. 1997). In one study, 85% patients had correct EUS staging of cancer, one patient was understaged, and 6 others were overstaged on EUS (Larghi et al. 2005). For any suspicious mass lesion or lymph nodes, EUS fine-needle aspiration (FNA) should be performed.

Diagnostic EMR

For the success of endoscopic therapy, accurate staging is critical and such precision can only be achieved by EMR. The EMR specimens are significantly larger than biopsy samples, and they allow for more precise assessment of the depth of tumor invasion into the mucosa and submucosa (Fig. 5). Although EUS has been used to estimate cancer depth, its accuracy has varied in different studies. EMR may change the diagnosis of dysplasia grade. This was shown by Nijhawan and Wang where EMR diagnosed superficial EAC in

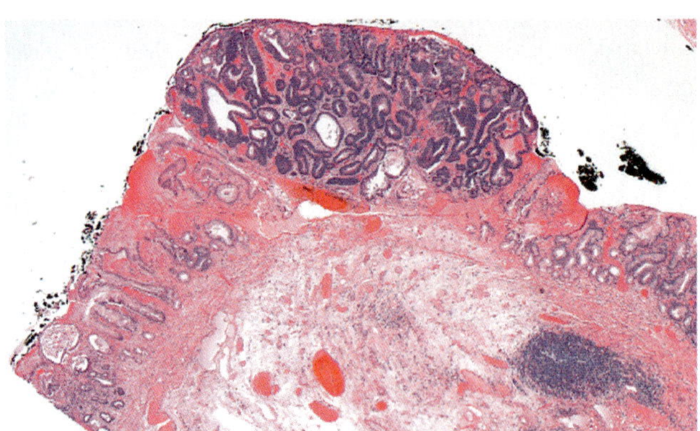

Fig. 5. Low-power microscopic view of tissue obtained by endoscopic mucosal resection showing mucosa and muscularis mucosae with dysplastic changes.

52% and HGD in 16% of the patients that resulted in change in diagnosis in 11 (44%) patients (Nijhawan and Wang 2000). In two additional studies, EMR downgraded previously diagnosed EAC in 9.5% patients and upgraded previous HGD to mucosal EAC in 18.5%, and to invasive EAC in 40% of study patients (Larghi et al. 2005; Nijhawan and Wang 2000). Thus, EMR provides a more accurate diagnosis than conventional biopsies and is useful in the staging of HGD and mucosal EAC.

Eradication Therapies for BE

Several eradication therapies (Table 1) have been developed in attempts to reverse BE and reduce cancer risk. These techniques are based on the hypothesis that injury of the metaplastic epithelium combined with vigorous acid suppression would lead to reversion of BE to squamous epithelium and reduce the risk of progression to cancer (Sampliner et al. 1996). Modalities include argon plasma coagulation (APC), multipolar electrocoagulation (MPEC), lasers (neodymium-yttrium aluminum garnet – Nd-YAG, potassium titanium phosphate – KTP), photodynamic therapy (PDT), and radiofrequency energy. Endoscopic mucosal resection (EMR) involves local snare extension of the lesion and has been used increasingly in recent years.

The long-term efficacy of different endoscopic techniques, in terms of eradicating BE and patient tolerability, is yet to be defined. These therapies can be used as single modalities or can be used in combination. All procedures are carried out in an outpatient setting under moderate sedation, and all of them require multiple sessions. The procedure time for

Table 1
Endoscopic ablatives techniques for management of Barrett's Esophagus

Thermal ablation
• Multipolar electrocoagulation (MPEC)
• Argon plasma coagulation (APC)
• Laser
• Neodymium-yttrium aluminum garnet (Nd:YAG)
• Argon
• Potassium titanyl phosphate (KTP)
• Heater probe
Nonthermal Ablation
• Photodynamic therapy (PDT)
• Porfimer sodium (used in USA)
• Hematoporphyrin derivative
• 5 Aminolevulinic acid (ALA)
• Cryotherapy
• Radiofrequency ablation
Mechanical
• Endoscopic mucosal resection (EMR)
• Jumbo biopsy forceps

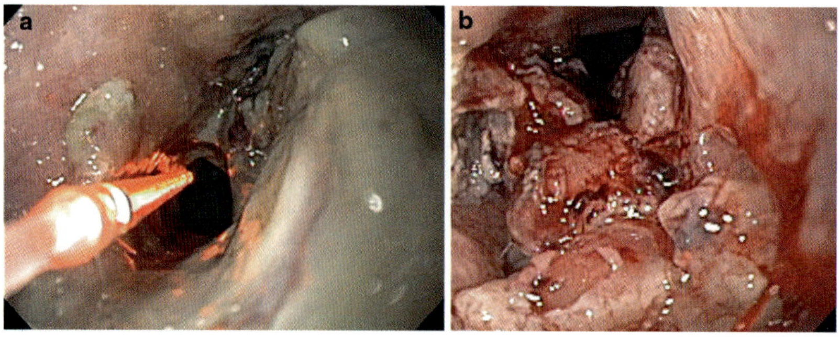

Fig. 6. (**a**) Endoscopic view showing photodynamic therapy probe in distal Barrett's esophagus. (**b**) Endoscopic view showing ablated Barrett's mucosa following PDT.

endoscopic therapies is variable, depending on the extent of BE, type of therapy used, and expertise of the gastroenterologist. Post-procedure, patients are instructed to take liquids/ soft diet only for the first 24 h and then advance their diet. Patients are advised not to take aspirin or other NSAIDs for approximately 7 days.

Photodynamic Therapy

This technique involves light-induced local injury of presensitized esophageal mucosa. The photosensitizer is administered by the oral or intravenous route and selectively sensitizes precancerous esophageal lesions. Ablation of these lesions is performed by endoscopically exposing Barrett's mucosa to light, resulting in mucosal damage from formation of highly reactive, unstable singlet oxygen species (Fig. 6a and b). Using different photosensitizers-porfimer sodium (used in the United States), hematoporphyrin derivative, and 5-aminolevulinic acid (5-ALA), PDT has been used most extensively and reported in randomized controlled trials. Several studies have shown its effectiveness in eliminating HGD. Overholt et al. in their long-term follow-up report (mean follow-up, 58.5 months) on 103 BE patients with neoplasia showed that HGD was eliminated in 94% of the patients (Overholt et al. 2003). Furthermore, in another randomized control trial, Overholt et al. assessed efficacy of PDT in HGD by comparing PDT plus omeprazole use in 138 patients to 70 patients on omeprazole only over a 2-year period. After a 5-year follow-up of these patients, the investigators showed that PDT was significantly more effective than omeprazole only in eliminating HGD (77% vs 39%, $p<0.0001$) and the likelihood of HGD progressing to cancer was also significantly lower after PDT compared to the omeprazole only group (15% vs 29%, $p=0.004$) (Overholt et al. 2007). Ablation therapy with PDT has also been used as an adjunct to EMR to eradicate the remaining BE segment, thus potentially reducing the risk of recurrent neoplastic lesions (Peters et al. 2006).

Radiofrequency Ablation

This is a relatively new technique for the ablation of BE, using either the circumferential HALO^{360} system or a focal HALO^{90} system (Figs. 7a through 7c). Interim results of a randomized, multicenter, sham-controlled trial of radiofrequency ablation for BE patients with dysplasia (LGD and HGD) showed that complete clearance of dysplasia and IM

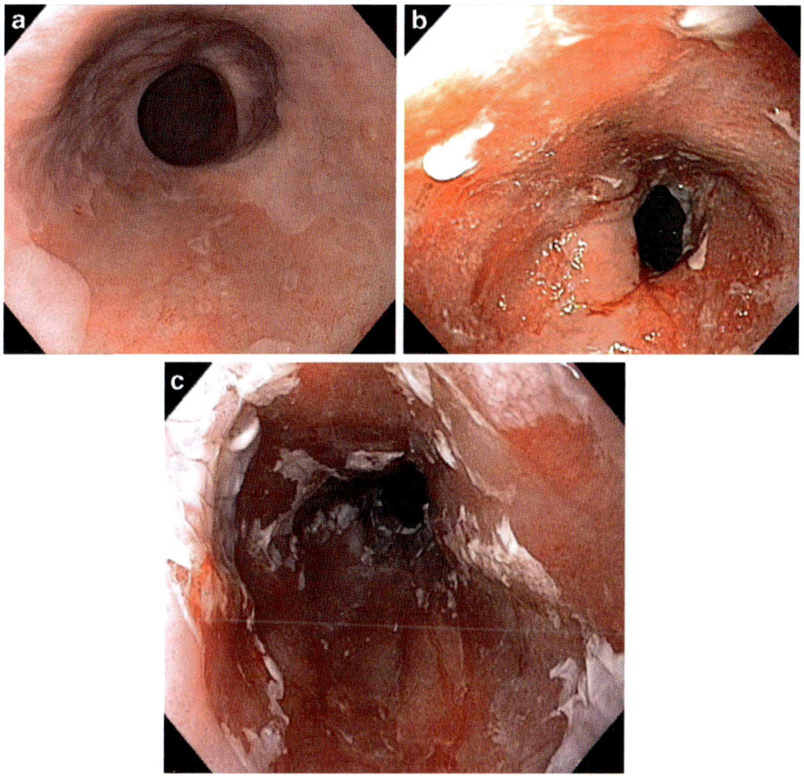

Fig. 7. (**a**) Endoscopic view showing Barrett's esophagus prior to radiofrequency ablation. (**b**) Endoscopic view of acutely ablated Barrett's mucosa following radiofrequency ablation. (**c**) Endoscopic view of ablated Barrett's mucosa after radiofrequency ablation.

occurred in 67% and 60% of HGD and 96% and 83% of the LGD patients, respectively, compared to 0% clearance in sham-controlled HGD and 33% clearance of dysplasia in sham-controlled LGD patients (Shaheen et al. 2008). In another study, Gondrie et al. assessed the safety and efficacy of stepwise circumferential and focal radiofrequency ablation (RFA) in 12 patients with flat HGD or residual dysplasia after EMR for HGD or intramucosal cancer. Complete remission of dysplasia and histological removal of BE was achieved in 100% patients. No recurrence of dysplasia was observed at median follow-up of 14 months (Gondrie et al. 2008). Pouw et al. used RFA in 44 patients, of whom 16 had early cancer and 12 had HGD. Circumferential and focal RFA was performed with prior endoscopic resection in 31 patients, and without that in 13 patients at 2-month intervals. Complete histological eradication of all dysplasia and IM was achieved in 43 (98%) patients. At 21-month follow-up, no recurrence of dysplasia was reported (Pouw et al. 2008). These results are encouraging and suggest that in expert hands, combination therapy of EMR with RFA is highly effective for HGD and early cancer in BE patients.

Cryotherapy

This technique utilizes compressed gas (nitrous oxide or carbon dioxide) to produce very cold temperature (–78 °C) to cause tissue injury. After development of a cryospray catheter, this technique has been used for endoluminal treatment of gastrointestinal lesions such as bleeding vascular malformations or superficial cancers (Pasricha et al. 1999; Kantsevoy et al. 2003). Animal model experimental studies have shown a dose-dependent effect of cryotherapy on esophageal mucosal ablation (Raju et al. 2005). Results of the first multicenter trial using cryotherapy ablation (low-pressure liquid nitrogen) for BE and early cancer in 77 patients suggests that cryotherapy is a safe and well-tolerated procedure (Greenwald et al. 2008).

Limitations of Ablative Therapies

Long-term studies suggest that complete eradication of BE may not be possible in all patients although post-ablation, the incidence of EAC declines in patients with HGD (Wani et al. 2009). The discrepancy in response to various ablative therapies is not clear, and may be attributed to the presence of residual IM, buried glands, patient factors, or lack of standardized patient selection with regard to ablative techniques. Post-ablation residual IM is not procedure-specific and has been reported using various ablative methods including MPEC, APC, PDT, and argon laser, Nd:YAG laser, and RFA therapy. Lugol's iodine chromoendoscopy may be used to enhance the targeting of columnar mucosa prior to thermal ablation, and at the end of ablation session to detect any residual islands/patches of untreated, previously unrecognized columnar tissue and at follow-up visits. All techniques except EMR are not diagnostic as they lack tissue for histopathological assessment of Barrett's.

Complications of Ablative Therapies

Most ablative techniques for Barrett's are associated with minor complications such as transient dysphagia, odynophagia, nausea, and vomiting and chest pain (Table 2). A few major complications may occur, with death reported very rarely. Complications from APC may also occur with increased frequency when there is unintended damage to deeper tissue of a targeted Barrett's segment, leading to pneumatosis, pneumoperitoneum, subcutaneous emphysema, pain, ulceration, stricture formation (Fig. 8), bleeding, perforation, and death. Application of porfimer sodium (long half-life) for PDT can cause prolonged skin photosensitivity (up to 6 weeks) to ultraviolet radiation, oral dehydration requiring intravenous fluid administration, and stricture formation. These complications were not seen when porfimer sodium was replaced with 5-ALA in clinical trials. Other complications of PDT include chest pain, pleural effusions, and atrial fibrillation. Major complications reported with Nd:YAG laser therapy include esophageal stricture formation and mild upper GI bleed, and minor complications such as nausea, vomiting, odynophagia, chest pain, fever, early dysphagia, and headache. Following RFA, complications such as transient fever, mild dysphagia, odynophagia, and perforation have been reported.

Most of the minor complications resolve spontaneously without the need for any intervention or observation in the hospital. Odynophagia can be treated with 1:1:1 mixture of diphenhydramine HCL:lidocaine:aluminum magnesium hydroxide. Chest pain can be treated with liquid acetaminophen 300 mg with 30 mg of codeine. For major complications like esophageal stricture, endoscopic dilation usually suffices and more aggressive treatment is needed only in patients with esophageal perforation and massive GI bleed. However, the endoscopist entering the arena of BE eradication therapies must be equipped and prepared to address all these complications.

Table 2
Complications reported after endoscopic ablative therapies for BE

Major
- Esophageal stricture formation
- Esophageal perforation
- Upper gastrointestinal bleeding
- Esophageal ulceration
- Cardiac arrhythmias (Atrial Fibrillation)
- Death

Minor
- Nausea/vomiting
- Sore throat
- Transient mild dysphagia
- Transient mild odynophagia
- Melena
- Fever
- Heartburn
- Chest pain
- Skin photosensitivity (specific to porfimer PDT)
- Headache
- Shortness of breath
- Small pleural effusions
- Subcutaneous emphysema
- Pneumomediastinum
- Pneumatosis
- Pneumoperitonium

Endoscopic Mucosal Resection or Mucosectomy

Therapeutic EMR

This eradication therapy is recommended in short segments of BE. Studies have shown that EMR is effective and safe in treating patients with early EAC (Fig. 9). Ell et al. in a non-blinded, non-randomized study involving 100 consecutive patients with low-risk EAC showed that complete remission was obtained in 99% at 1.9 months with no major complications, and at 36.7 month follow-up, 11% patients had recurrence of cancer (Ell et al. 2007). In an update involving a larger number of patients (total 349 patients) with HGD or mucosal EAC after therapeutic EMR, complete response was achieved in 96.6% patients with recurrence in 21.5% at follow-up. The risk factors that most frequently contributed to cancer recurrence were piecemeal resection, long-segment BE, no use of ablative therapy after complete remission of BE, and multifocal neoplasia (Pech et al. 2008). To overcome "piecemeal resection" as a risk factor for cancer recurrence, the role of circumferential

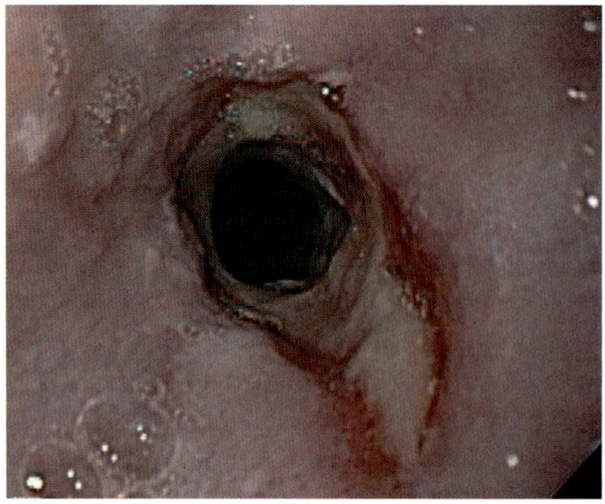

Fig. 8. Endoscopic view of distal esophageal stricture following endoscopic ablation therapy for Barrett's.

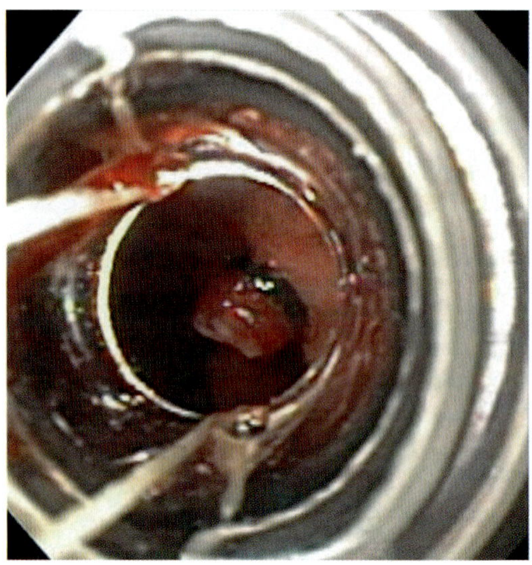

Fig. 9. Endoscopic view showing band technique for resection of nodular esophageal lesion.

EMR and combination therapy has been explored. This technique involves endoscopic resection of the entire BE segment, including the neoplastic lesion; this may provide more sustained treatment response during follow-up. Peters et al. evaluated the efficacy of this technique in 37 patients with early EAC. Early EAC was eradicated in all patients and complete removal of BE was achieved in 89% patients. During a follow-up of 11 months, no recurrence of neoplasia or BE was reported. However, circumferential EMR was associated with a 30–40% rate of esophageal stenosis that required endoscopic dilatations (Peters et al. 2006). Techniques for resection continue to evolve with introduction of endoscopic submucosal dissection, a method for en bloc resections of large neoplastic lesions.

Post-endoscopic Therapy BE Surveillance

Surveillance following eradication therapy is guided by the initial grade of dysplasia, and should include endoscopy with procurement of biopsies from the entire area of former Barrett's segment. Documentation of complete ablation with reasonable certainty on at least three consecutive surveillance endoscopies should be done. Periodic surveillance is still recommended to rule out recurrence of Barrett's at intervals not well defined due to paucity of data (Wang and Sampliner 2008). The results of different ablative techniques in achieving complete BE reversal are encouraging. Other than the presence of residual IM (Van Laethem et al. 2000), there are no other known predictors that may indicate sustained BE reversal or likely progression of BE to HGD and/or EAC (Pech et al. 2008). Although initial results of HGD ablation appear promising, the efficacy in reducing the incidence of cancer over long term is not clear (Ell et al. 2007).

SUMMARY OF KEY POINTS

- At present, endoscopy-guided diagnosis and eradication dysplastic BE appears to be the most feasible approach to curb the rapidly rising incidence of EAC.
- Advances in endoscopic imaging (high-resolution endoscopy, narrow-band imaging, autofluorescence, and confocal laser endomicroscopy) are progressing at an increasingly rapid rate, and may assist in the earlier detection of dysplasia and EAC within the Barrett segment.
- Recent results of endoscopic therapies (endoscopic resection and/or ablation) have been promising and have gained increased acceptance in the management of HGD and early EAC.
- Among different endoscopic techniques, diagnostic and therapeutic EMR, radiofrequency, and cryotherapy ablations are emerging as safe and effective therapies for eradication of dysplasia and/or mucosal EAC.
- Further research is required to better stratify screening of population at risk for BE development and also to predict BE progression to cancer.

REFERENCES

American Cancer Society. American cancer society: cancer facts and figures 2006. Atlanta: American Cancer Society; 2006.

Breyer HP, Silva De Barros SG, Maguilnik I, et al. Does methylene blue detect intestinal metaplasia in Barrett's esophagus? Gastrointest Endosc. 2003;57:505–9.

Buttar NS, Wang KK, Sebo TJ, et al. Extent of high-grade dysplasia in Barrett's esophagus correlates with risk of adenocarcinoma. Gastroenterology. 2001;120(7):1630–9.

Cameron AJ, Carpenter HA. Barrett's esophagus, high-grade dysplasia, and early adenocarcinoma: a pathological study. Am J Gastroenterol. 1997;92(4):586–91.

Canto MI, Setrakian S, Willis JE, et al. Methylene blue staining of dysplastic and nondysplastic Barrett's esophagus: an in vivo and ex vivo study. Endoscopy. 2001;33:391–400.

Chak A, Canto M, Stevens PD, et al. Clinical applications of a new through-the-scope ultrasound probe: prospective comparison with an ultrasound endoscope. Gastrointest Endosc. 1997;45(3):291–5.

Corley DA, Levin TR, Habel LA, Weiss NS, Buffler PA. Surveillance and survival in Barrett's adenocarcinomas: a population-based study. Gastroenterology. 2002;122(3):633–40.

Cossentino MJ, Wong RK. Barrett's esophagus and risk of esophageal adenocarcinoma. Semin Gastrointest Dis. 2003;14(3):128–35.

Curvers WL, Singh R, Wong Kee Song LM, et al. Endoscopic tri-modal imaging for detection of early neoplasia in Barrett's oesophagus; a multi-centre feasibility study using high-resolution endoscopy, autofluorescence imaging and narrow band imaging incorporated in one endoscopy system. Gut. 2008a;57:167–72.
Curvers W, Rosmolen W, Elzer B, et al. Low grade intraepithelial neoplasia in Barrett's esophagus: overdiagnosed but underestimated. Gastrointest Endosc. 2008b;67(5):M1324.
Das A, Singh V, Fleischer DE, Sharma VK. A comparison of endoscopic treatment and surgery in early esophageal cancer: an analysis of surveillance epidemiology and end results data. Am J Gastroenterol. 2008;103(6):1340–5.
Devesa SS, Blot WJ, Fraumeni Jr JF. Changing patterns in the incidence of esophageal and gastric carcinoma in the United States. Cancer. 1998;83(10):2049–53.
Dresner SM, Griffin SM, Wayman J, et al. Human model of duodenogastro-oesophageal reflux in the development of Barrett's metaplasia. Br J Surg. 2003;90(9):1120–8.
Dulai GS, Shekelle PG, Jensen DM, et al. Dysplasia and risk of further neoplastic progression in a regional Veterans Administration Barrett's cohort. Am J Gastroenterol. 2005;100(4):775–83.
Ell C, May A, Pech O, Gossner L, et al. Curative endoscopic resection of early esophageal adenocarcinomas (Barrett's cancer). Gastrointest Endosc. 2007;65(1):3–10.
Eloubeidi MA, Provenzale D. Does this patient have Barrett's esophagus? The utility of predicting Barrett's esophagus at the index endoscopy. Am J Gastroenterol. 1999;94(4):937–43.
Enzinger PC, Mayer RJ. Esophageal cancer. N Engl J Med. 2003;349(23):2241–52.
Falk GW, Ours TM, Richter JE. Practice patterns for surveillance of Barrett's esophagus in the United States. Gastrointest Endosc. 2000;52(2):197–203.
Gerson LB, Shetler K, Triadafilopoulos G. Prevalence of Barrett's esophagus in asymptomatic individuals. Gastroenterology. 2002;123(2):461–7.
Gondrie JJ, Pouw RE, Sondermeijer CM, et al. Effective treatment of early Barrett's neoplasia with stepwise circumferential and focal ablation using the HALO system. Endoscopy. 2008;40(5):370–9.
Gono K, Obi T, Yamaguchi M, et al. Appearance of enhanced tissue features in narrow-band endoscopic imaging. J Biomed Opt. 2004;9:568–77.
Greenwald BD, Horwhat JD, Abrams J, Lightdale CJ, Dumot J. Endoscopic cryotherapy ablation is safe and well-tolerated in Barrett's esophagus, esophageal dysplasia, and esophageal cancer. Gastrointest Endosc. 2008;67(5):AB76.
Guelrud M, Herrera I. Acetic acid improves identification of remnant islands of Barrett's epithelium after endoscopic therapy. Gastrointest Endosc. 1998;47:512–5.
Hanna S, Rastogi A, Weston AP, Totta F, Schmitz R, Mathur S, et al. Detection of Barrett's esophagus after endoscopic healing of erosive esophagitis. Am J Gastroenterol. 2006;101(7):1416–20.
Heitmiller RF, Redmond M, Hamilton SR. Barrett's esophagus with high-grade dysplasia. An indication for prophylactic esophagectomy. Ann Surg. 1996;224(1):66–71.
Horwhat JD, Maydonovitch CL, Ramos F, et al. A randomized comparison of methylene blue-directed biopsy versus conventional four-quadrant biopsy for the detection of intestinal metaplasia and dysplasia in patients with long-segment Barrett's esophagus. Am J Gastroenterol. 2008;103(3):546–54.
Kahrilas PJ, Shaheen NJ, Vaezi MF, et al. American Gastroenterological Association. American Gastroenterological Association Medical Position Statement on the management of gastroesophageal reflux disease. Gastroenterology. 2008;135(4):1383–91.
Kantsevoy SV, Cruz-Correa MR, Vaughn CA, Jagannath SB, Pasricha PJ, Kalloo AN. Endoscopic cryotherapy for the treatment of bleeding mucosal vascular lesions of the GI tract: a pilot study. Gastrointest Endosc. 2003;57(3):403–6.
Kara MA, Smits ME, Rosmolen WD, et al. A randomized cross-over study comparing light-induced fluorescence endoscopy with standard video endoscopy for the detection of early neoplasia in Barrett's esophagus. Gastrointest Endosc. 2005a;61:671–8.
Kara MA, Peters FP, Rosmolen WD, et al. High-resolution endoscopy plus chromoendoscopy or narrow-band imaging in Barrett's esophagus: a prospective randomized crossover study. Endoscopy. 2005b;37:929–36.
Kara MA, Peters FP, Ten Kate FJW, et al. Endoscopic video autofluorescence imaging may improve the detection of early neoplasia in patients with Barrett's esophagus. Gastrointest Endosc. 2005c;61:679–85.
Kara MA, Ennahachi M, Fockens P, et al. Detection and classification of the mucosal and vascular patterns (mucosal morphology) in Barrett's esophagus by using narrow band imaging. Gastrointest Endosc. 2006a;64:155–66.

Kara MA, Peters FP, Fockens P, et al. Endoscopic video-autofluorescence imaging followed by narrow band imaging for detecting early neoplasia in Barrett's esophagus. Gastrointest Endosc. 2006b;64:176–85.

Kiesslich R, Gossner L, Goetz M, et al. In vivo histology of Barrett's esophagus and associated neoplasia by confocal laser endomicroscopy. Clin Gastroenterol Hepatol. 2006;4:979–87.

Konda VJ, Ross AS, Ferguson MK, et al. Is the risk of concomitant invasive esophageal cancer in high-grade dysplasia in Barrett's esophagus overestimated? Clin Gastroenterol Hepatol. 2008;6(2):159–64.

Larghi A, Lightdale CJ, Memeo L, Bhagat G, Okpara N, Rotterdam H. EUS followed by EMR for staging of high-grade dysplasia and early cancer in Barrett's esophagus. Gastrointest Endosc. 2005;62(1):16–23.

Lightdale CJ. Esophageal cancer. American College of Gastroenterology. Am J Gastroenterol. 1999;94(1):20–9.

Lim CH, Rotimi O, Dexter SP, Axon AT. Randomized crossover study that used methylene blue or random 4-quadrant biopsy for the diagnosis of dysplasia in Barrett's esophagus. Gastrointest Endosc. 2006;64(2): 195–9.

Lim CH, Treanor D, Dixon MF, Axon AT. Low-grade dysplasia in Barrett's esophagus has a high risk of progression. Endoscopy. 2007;39(7):581–7.

Mallery S, Van Dam J. EUS in the evaluation of esophageal carcinoma. Gastrointest Endosc. 2000;52(6 Suppl):S6–11.

Meining A, Rösch T, Kiesslich R, Muders M, Sax F, Heldwein W. Inter- and intra-observer variability of magnification chromoendoscopy for detecting specialized intestinal metaplasia at the gastroesophageal junction. Endoscopy. 2004;36(2):160–4.

Menke-Pluymers MB, Hop WC, Dees J, van Blankenstein M, Tilanus HW. Risk factors for the development of an adenocarcinoma in columnar-lined (Barrett) esophagus. The Rotterdam Esophageal Tumor Study Group. Cancer. 1993;72(4):1155–8.

Montgomery E, Bronner MP, Goldblum JR, et al. Reproducibility of the diagnosis of dysplasia in Barrett esophagus: a reaffirmation. Hum Pathol. 2001a;32(4):368–78.

Montgomery E, Goldblum JR, Greenson JK, et al. Dysplasia as a predictive marker for invasive carcinoma in Barrett esophagus: a follow-up study based on 138 cases from a diagnostic variability study. Hum Pathol. 2001b;32(4):379–88.

Nelson DB, Block KP, Bosco JJ, et al. High resolution and high-magnification endoscopy: September 2000. Gastrointest Endosc. 2000;52(6 Pt 1):864–6.

Nijhawan PK, Wang KK. Endoscopic mucosal resection for lesions with endoscopic features suggestive of malignancy and high-grade dysplasia within Barrett's esophagus. Gastrointest Endosc. 2000;52(3):328–32.

O'Connor JB, Falk GW, Richter JE. The incidence of adenocarcinoma and dysplasia in Barrett's esophagus: report on the Cleveland Clinic Barrett's Esophagus Registry. Am J Gastroenterol. 1999;94(8):2037–42.

Olliver JR, Wild CP, Sahay P, Dexter S, Hardie LJ. Chromoendoscopy with methylene blue and associated DNA damage in Barrett's oesophagus. Lancet. 2003;362(9381):373–4.

Overholt BF, Panjehpour M, Haydek JM. Photodynamic therapy for Barrett's esophagus: follow-up in 100 patients. Gastrointest Endosc. 1999;49:1–7.

Overholt BF, Panjehpour M, Halberg DL. Photodynamic therapy for Barrett's esophagus with dysplasia and/or early stage carcinoma: long-term results. Gastrointest Endosc. 2003;58(2):183–8.

Overholt BF, Wang KK, Burdick JS, et al. International Photodynamic Group for High-Grade Dysplasia in Barrett's Esophagus. Five-year efficacy and safety of photodynamic therapy with Photofrin in Barrett's high-grade dysplasia. Gastrointest Endosc. 2007;66(3):460–8.

Pasricha PJ, Hill S, Wadwa KS, et al. Endoscopic cryotherapy: experimental results and first clinical use. Gastrointest Endosc. 1999;49(5):627–31.

Pech O, Behrens A, May A, et al. Long-term results and risk factor analysis for recurrence after curative endoscopic therapy in 349 patients with high-grade intraepithelial neoplasia and mucosal adenocarcinoma in Barrett's oesophagus. Gut. 2008;57(9):1200–6.

Peters FP, Kara MA, Rosmolen WD, et al. Stepwise radical endoscopic resection is effective for complete removal of Barrett's esophagus with early neoplasia: a prospective study. Am J Gastroenterol. 2006;101(7):1449–57.

Pohl H, Rosch T, Vieth M, et al. Miniprobe confocal laser microscopy for the detection of invisible neoplasia in patients with Barrett's esophagus. Gut. 2008 Oct;57(12):1648–53.

Pondugula K, Wani S, Sharma P. Barrett's esophagus and esophageal adenocarcinoma in adults: long-term GERD or something else? Curr Gastroenterol Rep. 2007;9(6):468–74.

Pouw RE, Gondrie JJ, Sondermeijer CM, et al. Eradication of Barrett Esophagus with early neoplasia by radiofrequency ablation, with or without endoscopic resection. J Gastrointest Surg. 2008;12(10):1627–36.
Prasad GA, Wang KK, Buttar NS, et al. Long-term survival following endoscopic and surgical treatment of high-grade dysplasia in Barrett's esophagus. Gastroenterology. 2007;132(4):1226–33.
Raju GS, Ahmed I, Xiao SY, Brining D, Bhutani MS, Pasricha PJ. Graded esophageal mucosal ablation with cryotherapy, and the protective effects of submucosal saline. Endoscopy. 2005;37(6):523–6.
Rastogi A, Puli S, El-Serag HB, Bansal A, Wani S, Sharma P. Incidence of esophageal adenocarcinoma in patients with Barrett's esophagus and high-grade dysplasia: a meta-analysis. Gastrointest Endosc. 2008;67(3):394–8.
Sampliner RE, Fennerty B, Garewal HS. Reversal of Barrett's esophagus with acid suppression and multipolar electrocoagulation: preliminary results. Gastrointest Endosc. 1996;44(5):532–5.
Shaheen NJ, Crosby MA, Bozymski EM, Sandler RS. Is there publication bias in the reporting of cancer risk in Barrett's esophagus? Gastroenterology. 2000;119(2):333–8. Review.
Shaheen N, Sharma P, Overholt BF, et al. A randomized, multicenter, sham-controlled trial of radiofrequency ablation (RFA) for subjects with Barrett's esophagus (BE) containing dysplasia: interim results of the Aim Dysplasia Trial. Gastroenterology. 2008;132:A-37.
Sharma P, Topalovski M, Mayo MS, et al. Methylene blue chromoendoscopy for detection of shortsegment Barrett's esophagus. Gastrointest Endosc. 2001;54:289–93.
Sharma P, Weston AP, Topalovski M, et al. Magnification chromoendoscopy for the detection of intestinal metaplasia and dysplasia in Barrett's oesophagus. Gut. 2003;52:24–7.
Sharma P, McQuaid K, Dent J, Fennerty MB, Sampliner R, et al. A critical review of the diagnosis and management of Barrett's esophagus: the AGA Chicago Workshop. Gastroenterology. 2004;127(1):310–30.
Sharma P, Dent J, Armstrong D, Bergman JJ, Gossner L, Hoshihara Y, et al. The development and validation of an endoscopic grading system for Barrett's esophagus: the Prague C & M criteria. Gastroenterology. 2006a;131(5):1392–9.
Sharma P, Falk GW, Weston AP, Reker D, Johnston M, Sampliner RE. Dysplasia and cancer in a large multicenter cohort of patients with Barrett's esophagus. Clin Gastroenterol Hepatol. 2006b;4(5):566–72.
Sharma P, Bansal A, Mathur S, et al. The utility of a novel narrow band imaging endoscopy system in patients with Barrett's esophagus. Gastrointest Endosc. 2006c;64:167–75.
Sharma VK, Wang KK, Overholt BF, et al. Balloon-based, circumferential, endoscopic radiofrequency ablation of Barrett's esophagus: 1-year follow-up of 100 patients. Gastrointest Endosc. 2007a;65:185–95.
Sharma P, Wani S, Rastogi A. Endoscopic therapy for high-grade dysplasia in Barrett's esophagus: ablate, resect, or both? Gastrointest Endosc. 2007b;66(3):469–74.
Shumaker DA, de Garmo P, Faigel DO. Potential impact of preoperative EUS on esophageal cancer management and cost. Gastrointest Endosc. 2002;56(3):391–6.
Skacel M, Petras RE, Gramlich TL, Sigel JE, Richter JE, Goldblum JR. The diagnosis of low-grade dysplasia in Barrett's esophagus and its implications for disease progression. Am J Gastroenterol. 2000;95(12):3383–7.
Solaymani-Dodaran M, Logan RF, West J, Card T, Coupland C. Risk of oesophageal cancer in Barrett's oesophagus and gastro-oesophageal reflux. Gut. 2004;53(8):1070–4.
Van Laethem JL, Peny MO, Salmon I, Cremer M, Devière J. Intramucosal adenocarcinoma arising under squamous re-epithelialisation of Barrett's oesophagus. Gut. 2000;46(4):574–7.
Wang KK, Sampliner RE. Practice Parameters Committee of the American College of Gastroenterology. Updated guidelines 2008 for the diagnosis, surveillance and therapy of Barrett's esophagus. Am J Gastroenterol. 2008;103(3):788–97.
Wani S, Sharma P. Management of dysplasia in Barrett's esophagus. Curr GERD Rep. 2007a;1(4):248–55.
Wani S, Sharma P. Endoscopic surface imaging of Barrett's Esophagus: an optimistic view. Gastroenterology. 2007b;133(1):11–3.
Wani S, Puli SR, Shaheen NJ, et al. Esophageal adenocarcinoma in Barrett's esophagus post endoscopic ablative therapy: a meta-analysis and systemic review. Am J Gastroenterol. 2009;104:502–13.
Wolfsen HC, Crook JE, Krishna M, et al. Prospective, controlled tandem endoscopy study of narrow band imaging for dysplasia detection in Barrett's Esophagus. Gastroenterology. 2008;135(1):24–31.
Yao K, Takaki Y, Ohara J, et al. Magnification endoscopy outlines the microvascular architecture and extent of Barrett's intramucosal carcinoma prior to endoscopic resection. Gastrointest Endosc. 2006;63:1064–10.

3 Gastrointestinal Tract Stenting

Andrew S. Ross and Richard A. Kozarek

Contents

Keywords: Gastrointestinal, Tract, Stenting, Esophageal, Enteral

INTRODUCTION

Enteral stent placement for disorders of the gastrointestinal tract has evolved significantly over the past decade. While the majority of enteral stent placement is still performed for malignant obstruction, advancements in endoscopic technique and device technology have opened the door for the use of enteral stenting for benign disease as well. This chapter focuses on the indications, techniques, and currently available technologies for stent placement in the esophagus, small intestine, and colon.

ESOPHAGEAL STENT PLACEMENT

Indications

The leading indications for esophageal stent placement are for palliation of complications related to esophageal malignancies. Up to one half of patients with esophageal cancer will present with stage IV (metastatic) disease. The majority of these patients will not survive beyond 12 months (Papachristou and Baron 2007; Dua 2007; Elton 2005; Enzinger and Mayer 2003). In this group of patients, the treatment goals are essentially directed toward improvement in quality of life: maintenance of esophageal luminal patency (and reduction in dysphagia), optimization of nutrition, and reduction in the risk of aspiration (and resultant pneumonia) (Dua 2007). In addition, this group of patients may be prone to the formation

From: *Clinical Gastroenterology: Diagnostic and Therapeutic Procedures in Gastroenterology*,
Edited by: G. Y. Wu, S. Sridhar, DOI 10.1007/978-1-59745-044-7_3,

of malignant tracheoesophageal fistulae (Cook and Dehn 1996; Kotsis et al. 1997; Kozarek et al. 1997; Raijman and Lynch 1997; Christie et al. 2001). These indications rarely exist in isolation in any given patient. However, esophageal stent placement is appropriate (and well suited) for each. Aside from dysphagia related to obstruction from intrinsic esophageal malignancies, extrinsic compression of the esophageal lumen can be observed in patients with various forms of lung cancer and mediastinal metastases. Self-expandable metal stent (SEMS) placement has been reported to be successful in relieving dysphagia resulting from extrinsic luminal compression (Bethge et al. 1998).

Self-expandable stent placement has also been utilized for the treatment of two benign diseases of the esophagus: perforation and anastomotic leaks in addition to refractory benign esophageal strictures (Papachristou and Baron 2007). Esophageal perforation, which may occur as a result of iatrogenic injury related to endoscopic therapy or spontaneous rupture (Boerhaave syndrome), is often associated with significant morbidity when repaired surgically (Papachristou and Baron 2007). In addition, abscess formation and mediastinitis can occur if these are left untreated (Zwischenberger et al. 2002). The placement of a completely covered SEMS or self-expandable plastic stent has emerged as an alternative therapeutic option in these cases (Siersema et al. 2003; Kiernan et al. 2006; Radecke et al. 2006; Freeman et al. 2007a). Esophageal leaks following esophagectomy and anastomotic breakdown following bariatric surgery have also been reported to be successfully managed using completely covered SEMS or self-expanding plastic esophageal stents without the need for operative intervention (Hunerbein et al. 2004; Yano et al. 2008; Tuebergen et al. 2008; Yano and Mittal 2007; Kauer et al. 2008; Profili et al. 2008; Schubert et al. 2005; Langer et al. 2005; Freeman et al. 2007b).

Contraindications

There are very few contraindications to esophageal stent placement. Severe cardiorespiratory compromise, which may limit the safe performance of upper gastrointestinal endoscopy, is an absolute contraindication to the placement of an esophageal stent. Uncontrolled coagulopathy and esophageal varices are additional contraindications.

Tumors located in the mid to upper esophagus raise important clinical issues with regard to compression of the tracheobronchial tree. The radial expansion force associated with SEMS placement across tumors in this location has the theoretical risk of causing airway obstruction (De Olabozal et al. 2001; Kawasaki et al. 2003; Farivar et al. 2004; Dasgupta et al. 1998). Although not a contraindication to esophageal stent placement, a chest CT scan should be obtained and reviewed with a thoracic surgeon prior to SEMS placement in patients with mid- to upper esophageal tumors. In some case, bronchoscopy with placement of a tracheal or bronchial stent may be indicated prior to, during, or immediately following esophageal stent placement (Fig. 1).

The risk of stent migration (see Complications) is typically lowest in patients with intrinsic strictures of the esophagus. Although not a contraindication, esophageal leaks or perforations where no intrinsic luminal narrowing is present should be stented with caution, proper informed consent, and with the use of clips (see Technique) to decrease the risk of stent migration.

An area of controversy, which remains a relative contraindication to esophageal stent placement, is in patients who are undergoing chemotherapy and/or radiotherapy, with or without intent for a subsequent operation (Kinsman et al. 1996; Siersema et al. 1998;

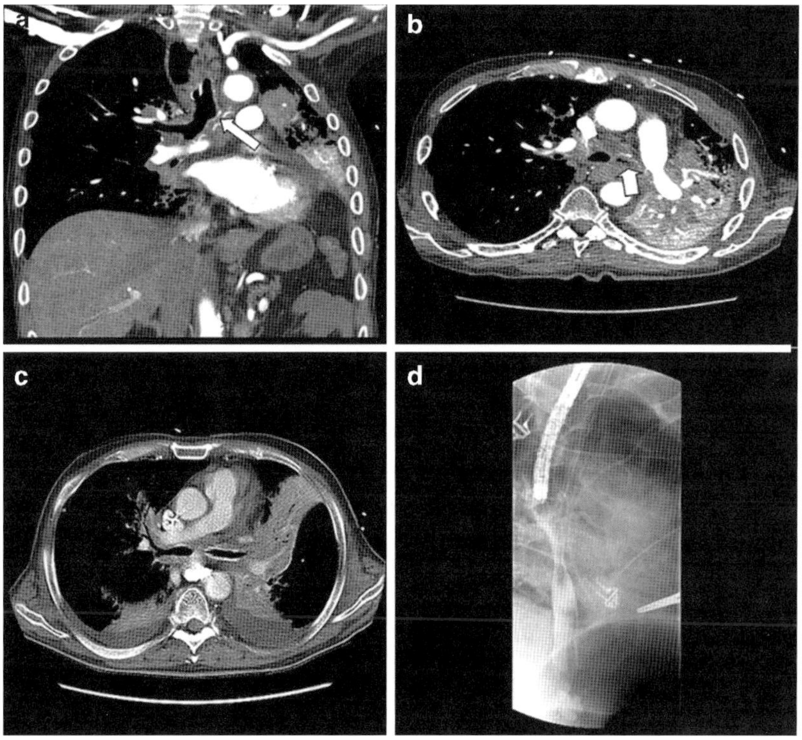

Fig. 1. Chest CT scan demonstrating left main stem bronchus (*arrows*) and proximal esophageal obstruction secondary to a squamous cell carcinoma of the lung (**a** and **b**). A bronchial stent was placed (**c**) following which an Ultraflex™ (Boston Scientific, Natick, MA) esophageal stent was successfully deployed (**d**) across the esophageal obstruction.

Bartelsman et al. 2000; Ginsberg 2007). Concern exists from a surgical perspective with regard to the possibility of removing a "permanent" SEMS at the time of surgery in addition to risking bleeding and esophageal perforation related to device insertion in a patient who is a good surgical candidate (Siddiqui et al. 2007a). In addition, as tumors respond to therapy, stent migration may occur. Finally, the safety of stent placement in the setting of concurrent radiation therapy has been questioned although not thoroughly investigated. The placement of SEMS following unsuccessful chemotherapy or radiation also remains controversial. Although a large observational study involving 200 patients failed to show an increase in major complications following SEMS in this group of patients (Homs et al. 2004a), a retrospective analysis suggested that a history of chemoradiotherapy was associated with major stent complications with an odds ratio of 5.6 (Papachristou and Baron 2007; Homs et al. 2004a). Given this controversy, use of SEMS prior to chemoradiotherapy is largely dictated by local practice bias.

Technique

The technique for endoscopic placement of esophageal stents, both plastic and metal, is relatively straightforward. Selection of appropriate candidates from the standpoint of medical stability and the ability to tolerate an endoscopic procedure is imperative. As for any endoscopic procedure, patients should be fasting for at least 6 h prior to the procedure. The choice of anesthetic is based on local practice bias. However, in our experience, the majority of procedures can be performed using conscious sedation with narcotic analgesics and a benzodiazepine. Patients being considered for esophageal stent placement due to a perforation or anastomotic breakdown following bariatric surgery should be approached with caution as these individuals are typically obese, and have poor oral airways. In these individuals or others with multiple medical comorbidities, consultation with an anesthesiologist is recommended.

For patients with malignant disease, an upper endoscopy to define the proximal and distal margins of the tumor is the first step in esophageal stent placement. The total length of the stricture will help to determine the length of the desired stent. In the event that the upper endoscope cannot be passed beyond the esophageal stricture, careful esophageal dilation should be performed to allow passage of the endoscope beyond the tumor in order to obtain proper measurements. Although esophageal dilation techniques are beyond the scope of this chapter, controlled radial expansion balloon dilators may be preferable to bougies for this purpose as the former allow direct visualization of the stricture and a more "controlled" dilation. Fluoroscopy, while mandatory for esophageal stent placement, may be helpful when dilating malignant esophageal strictures.

The proximal and distal margins of the stricture can be marked using a variety of methods. Endoscopic clips can be applied or contrast dye can be injected into the submucosa. A less desirable (but cheaper) approach consists of marking the level of the endoscope externally using a radio-opaque object (such as a paper clip or hemostat). For malignant disorders, the stent should be deployed 2 cm above the proximal tumor margin to decrease the risk of distal stent migration. Once the tumor has been measured and the proximal and distal margins marked, a wire guide should be placed across the stenosis into the stomach; the endoscope is then removed leaving the wire guide in place.

For malignant lesions, the type of stent (i.e., covered versus uncovered; anti-reflux, length and diameter) will depend on the lesion itself. In general, we prefer to place the stent with the largest diameter possible. A smaller stent diameter may be used for lesions within the cervical esophagus in order to decrease the possible "foreign body" sensation associated with stent placement in this location. For most lesions, a partially or fully covered SEMS is preferable to an uncovered stent in order to prevent the tumor in-growth and tissue hyperplasia. A covered stent should also be utilized for the treatment of malignant tracheoesophageal fistulas. The major drawback to partially or fully covered stents is the increased risk of stent migration. An uncovered stent may be selected for extrinsic compression or in patients with a history of stent migration. For lesions in the distal esophagus where the stent may cross the gastroesophageal junction, an antireflux stent may be selected. Stents placed in this location obliterate the natural reflux barrier and patients almost invariably develop reflux of gastric contents into the proximal esophagus or oropharynx; specifically designed "antireflux" stents may help to decrease symptoms. With regard to length, stents should be long enough to cover the desired lesion. Because endoscopic measurements may be slightly inaccurate, it is best to err on the side of a longer (rather than shorter) stent in order to decrease the risk of failing to palliate the obstructing lesion.

Once the appropriate stent has been selected, deployment is straightforward. The stent is advanced over the wire guide and the outer markings of the stent aligned with the proximal and distal margins of the stricture, recognizing that most SEMS foreshorten by 30–40%

with deployment. Release of the stent (which varies by device) can then proceed under fluoroscopic control. Post-deployment endoscopy can be performed to ensure proper stent positioning; in the case of fully covered metal stents, proximal repositioning, using grasping forceps, can be accomplished with ease in most cases. Partially covered stents can be repositioned with some difficulty, in most cases, immediately after deployment, especially when the deployed stent is a distal release device (Papachristou and Baron 2007). The same cannot be said for completely uncovered stents. An endoscope can be used to visualize post-deployment final position. However, the endoscope should not be passed through a tight "waist" in the stent in order to decrease the risk of stent dislodgement.

As is the case for malignant indications, esophageal stent placement for benign indications is technically straightforward. Typically, a contrast-enhanced radiograph or CT scan is indicated prior to esophageal stent placement for benign indications. This will allow the endoscopist to identify the exact location and extent of the stricture, leak, or perforation. Upper endoscopy is then performed to further define the proximal and distal margins of the stricture or defect, which can be marked using any of the three methods outlined above. A wire guide is then placed into the stomach following which the endoscope is removed leaving the wire guide in place. For benign indications, a self-expanding plastic stent or fully covered metal stent should be selected in order to allow removal at a later date. Deployment is performed under fluoroscopic control in most cases (see below).

The risk of migration is highest in patients with benign indications for esophageal stent placement (Papachristou and Baron 2007; Holm et al. 2008). Refractory benign esophageal strictures have different characteristics in comparison to their malignant counterparts. Although occasionally problematic (i.e., stent occlusion), in-growth of tumor into the stent helps to anchor it in position. In addition, malignant strictures tend to be longer than most benign strictures. Finally, for perforations and anastomotic leaks, there is no stricture to hold a stent in place (and, therefore, this indication has the highest risk of migration). Several measures can be taken to reduce the risk of stent migration. First, the stent with the largest possible diameter should be selected. The length of the stent should be long enough to bridge the stenosis, leak, or perforation. For the latter two indications, we tend to select the longest stent available as an additional (potential) safeguard against stent migration. Finally, endoscopic clips can be applied to the proximal end of the stent in an attempt to maintain stent position (Baron 2007).

Complications

Immediate or early procedure-related complications following esophageal stent placement occur in up to 10% of individuals (Papachristou and Baron 2007; Baron 2007). These include aspiration, airway compromise, malpositioning of the device, entrapment of the stent delivery system, dislodgement of the stent, hemorrhage, severe chest pain, nausea, and esophageal perforation. Careful intraprocedural airway management, including utilization of general anesthesia if necessary, can reduce the risk of aspiration. As discussed above, patients with stridor, wheezing, or mid- to upper esophageal tumors should undergo CT of the chest, prior to stent placement, to evaluate for airway compromise, which may be exacerbated by stent placement. As with all therapeutic endoscopic procedures, an INR of 1.5 or less is desired for elective esophageal stent placement to reduce the risk of bleeding.

Late (or delayed) complications include bleeding and fistula formation from stent erosion, severe gastroesophageal reflux, stent migration, and obstruction secondary to tissue in-growth or food bolus impaction (Papachristou and Baron 2007; Baron 2007; Siersema 2006). Some malpositioned or migrated stents can be repositioned or removed, using grasping forceps, inflated balloon catheter, or a polypectomy snare. On occasion, migrated stents may be left in the stomach and a new stent placed (Papachristou and Baron 2007; Rollhauser and Fleischer 1999). The decision to remove a migrated stent should ideally be made based on the patient performance status as this is not without risk. But, leaving a migrated stent within the stomach is associated with a small (but definite) risk of migration into the small intestine with resultant perforation or obstruction. Stents that become occluded secondary to tumor in-growth can be treated with argon plasma coagulation or placement of a second stent through the first (stent-within-stent design). Food bolus impaction can typically be treated endoscopically.

Postoperative Care

A liquid diet can be resumed immediately for patients with malignant indications for esophageal stent placement. Diet can then be advanced as tolerated to a goal of reaching puree status; advancement beyond this level places the patient at risk for stent occlusion by large food particles. For patients in whom stents are placed for malignant tracheoesophageal fistula, esophageal perforation, or anastomotic leak, our practice is to withhold an oral diet until an esophagram (using water soluble contrast) is obtained 24 h following stent deployment to ensure both proper positioning of the stent and closure of the leak.

Patients in whom stents are deployed across the EG junction require special attention. Because the natural barrier to reflux of gastric contents is rendered incompetent by the placement of the esophageal stent across the EG junction (unless using a prosthesis with an antireflux valve), aspiration remains a significant risk in these patients. For these individuals, twice daily proton pump inhibitors are prescribed indefinitely. We also suggest that these patients do not eat in close proximity to bedtime (2–3 h) and that the head of the bed is elevated to at least 30° at all times. This can be accomplished most easily by a specially designed wedge pillow available at most medical supply stores.

Outcomes

Although the concept of endoprosthesis placement for the palliation of malignant dysphagia has been around since the late nineteenth century, the use of stenting for palliation of malignant esophageal obstruction did not increase in popularity until over a century later, with the introduction into clinical practice of the self-expanding metal stent (SEMS) (Dua 2007; Domschke et al. 1990; Frimberger 1983; Fleischer and Bull-Henry 1992). The ideal modality for the treatment of any patient with metastatic cancer and limited survival should meet the following criteria: wide availability (i.e., ease of use), minimal side effects, minimal complications, rapid symptom improvement, and minimal need for re-intervention (Dua 2007). With respect to esophageal malignancies, SEMS meet the majority of these criteria.

For malignant disease, SEMS placement is technically possible in nearly all patients in whom it is attempted. SEMS placement may not be possible if the wire guide or stent introducer cannot be placed across the esophageal stenosis (Papachristou and Baron 2007; Dua 2007). Indeed, this is a rare event. A 2004 review of 415 patients with advanced esophageal cancer in Great Britain found that the technical success rate for SEMS placement ranged from 96% to 100% (Radiology., B.S.o.I. ROST: Registry if Iesophageal Stenting, first report 2004). In addition to high rates of technical success, SEMS are highly efficacious in their ability to palliate dysphagia and close malignant fistulae. Multiple case series and meta-analyses performed over the past 20 years suggest immediate improvement in clinical symptoms in 90–100% of patients (Cook and Dehn 1996; Christie et al. 2001; Bethge et al. 1998; Raijman et al. 1994, 1998; Song et al. 1994; Fiorini et al. 1995; De Palma et al. 1995, 1999; Moores and Ilves 1996; Lam et al. 1999; Toikkanen et al. 2000; Cordero and Moores 2000; Vakil et al. 2001; Razzaq et al. 2001; McGrath et al. 2001; Kostopoulos et al. 2003; Johnson et al. 2006; Costamagna et al. 2006; Sundelof et al. 2007; Xinopoulos et al. 2005). Despite these high technical and initial clinical success rates, the need for re-intervention remains significant with up to 1/3 of patients experiencing recurrent dysphagia from tumor in-growth or tissue hyperplasia at the proximal or distal stent margins.

A variety of different esophageal stents are currently available worldwide. Covered SEMS have been demonstrated to be superior to fixed-diameter plastic stents and uncovered SEMS for malignant indications (Vakil et al. 2001). This is due to the fact that covered SEMS prevent the in-growth of tumor, which has been reported in a significant percentage of patients with uncovered SEMS (De Palma et al. 1996). While there are a variety of currently available prostheses, no single manufacturer's covered SEMS has been proven superior to the others' for palliation of malignant esophageal disease (Papachristou and Baron 2007).

A covered self-expandable plastic stent (SEPS) (Polyflex, Boston Scientific, Natick, MA) has been introduced into the marketplace and, in Europe, is less costly than its metallic counterparts. A recent prospective randomized trial from Italy studied the use of covered SEPS versus covered SEMS for palliation of malignant esophageal dysphagia (Conio et al. 2007). Although there was no difference in palliation of dysphagia between the two groups, significantly more complications including stent migration were seen in the SEPS group. Other studies have yielded similar findings (Conigliaro et al. 2007; Eickhoff et al. 2005). Despite this, the idea of covered SEPS placement for malignant disease has appeal in patients who may require neoadjuvant therapy, but also have severe dysphagia. These stents could be subsequently removed once therapy is complete and prior to surgery (Ginsberg 2007).

Despite the superiority of covered SEMS over their uncovered counterparts for malignant esophageal disorders, they are not without their own limitations. Because of the decrease in tumor intercalation into the prosthesis, completely or partially covered SEMS are prone to migration. In one recent trial, stent migration was observed in 17% of patients who had covered SEMS placement for malignant disease (Homs et al. 2004b). In an attempt to decrease the risk of migration, some have advocated utilizing stents with a larger diameter. A recent prospective study in patients with dysphagia from obstructing gastroesophageal junction or esophageal malignancies found that larger caliber covered SEMS were associated with a decreased risk of stent migration, tissue overgrowth, or food bolus impaction (Verschuur et al. 2006).

Recurrent dysphagia requiring repeat intervention occurs in up to 30% of patients, following SEMS placement. Patients in whom stents are occluded by tumor in-growth can be treated with repeat stent placement or argon plasma coagulation (Papachristou and Baron 2007). Moreover, although SEMS provide rapid relief of dysphagia, the results of a single randomized trial comparing single-dose brachytherapy to SEMS for incurable esophageal cancer suggest that brachytherapy provides more durable (albeit slower) relief of symptoms (Homs et al. 2004b). In centers where brachytherapy is available, some authors have suggested that patients be referred for SEMS or brachytherapy depending on a prognostic model. SEMS are placed in patients with a poor prognosis (rapid onset of symptom relief) while those patients with an intermediate or good prognosis are referred for brachytherapy (slower onset of relief, longer sustainability) (Homs et al. 2004b). Besides brachytherapy, other alternative techniques to SEMS placement include local endoscopic techniques such as laser ablation, argon plasma coagulation, and photodynamic therapy (Eickhoff et al. 2005).

BENIGN DISEASE

The use of SEPS and, more recently, completely covered SEMS for benign indications is currently evolving. As opposed to their metallic counterparts, SEPS can be easily removed or repositioned, making them an ideal candidate for treating benign esophageal lesions such as strictures and iatrogenic perforations, and postoperative anastomotic leaks. A number of case series have now demonstrated the clinical efficacy of using SEPS for benign indications (Siersema et al. 2003; Kiernan et al. 2006; Radecke et al. 2006; Freeman et al. 2007a, b; Hunerbein et al. 2004; Yano et al. 2008; Tuebergen et al. 2008; Yano and Mittal 2007; Kauer et al. 2008; Profili et al. 2008; Schubert et al. 2005; Langer et al. 2005; Repici et al. 2004). Although most studies suggest promising results (albeit with limited sample sizes), a recent review from the Mayo Clinic suggests otherwise (Holm et al. 2008). Eighty three SEPS were successfully placed in 30 patients for benign indications. Stent migration occurred in almost 82% of patients who underwent SEPS for benign esophageal strictures, 75% of patients with anastomotic strictures, 59% of patients with anastomotic leaks, and in 29% of patients with radiation-induced strictures. Long-term symptomatic improvement following stent removal occurred in only 6% of all procedures. Given these findings, appropriate candidate selection, proper device placement, and close follow-up are indicated in patients considered for SEPS or completely covered SEMS placement for benign disease.

Available Devices

There are a large variety of esophageal stents currently available in the marketplace. Table 1 lists the characteristics of various covered SEMS which are currently available in the USA. As mentioned previously, there are no data to suggest clinical superiority of any one manufacturer's device over another for any indication.

Two additional stents are worth mentioning. The Polyflex (Boston Scientific, Natick, MA) stent is the only currently available SEPS in the USA. This device is composed of polyester mesh embedded in silicone; it is completely covered. The stent is available in a number of diameters and lengths, the largest diameter being a 25 mm flare at the proximal end. The device must be assembled prior to deployment and the delivery system is rather large, with a diameter of 12–14 mm. The Niti-S stent (Taewoong-Medical, Seoul, South

Table 1
Covered esophageal stents currently approved for use by the U.S. Food and Drug Administration

	Ultraflex™	*Z-Stent®*	*Alimaxx™*	*Evolution®*	*Wallflex™*
Stent material	Nitinol	Stainless Steel	Nitinol	Nitinol	Nitinol
Covering	Partial	Partial, full and anti-reflux	Full	Partial	Partial
Delivery system (F)	16	28	21	24	28
Length (cm)	10,12,15	6,8,10,12,14	7,12,15	8,10,12.5,25	12, 15
Proximal flare diameter (mm)	23,28	21,25	23,27	25	23,28
Distal flare diameter (mm)	N/A	N/A	21,25	N/A	N/A
Lumen diameter (mm)	18,23	18,22	18,22	20	18,28
Release	Proximal/ distal	Distal	Distal	Distal	Distal
Degree of shortening (%)	30–40	0–10	0	35	30–40
Manufacturer	Boston Scientific	Cook Medical	Alveolus	Cook Medical	Boston Scientific

Korea) is currently not available in the USA. This stent is a double-layered stent with an outer tube composed of nitinol and an inner layer fashioned from polyurethane. This combination prevents stent migration by allowing tumor in-growth and intercalation into the outer mesh while at the same time reducing recurrent dysphagia by having a completely covered inner core (Verschuur et al. 2006).

ENTERAL STENT PLACEMENT

Indications

Obstruction of the gastric outlet or duodenum is commonly seen with malignant neoplasms of the pancreatic head, bile duct, proximal small intestine and major papilla, gastric antrum as well as by malignant mesenteric lymphadenopathy and, rarely, metastatic disease or local extension of colonic neoplasms (Alam et al. 2003). Gastric outlet obstruction complicating pancreatic cancer occurs in up to 15% of all cases (Chopita et al. 2007). Recurrent tumor or stricture in the afferent limb following a Whipple resection and radiation therapy for pancreatic cancer can lead to the development of an "afferent limb syndrome" resulting in biliary obstruction and cholangitis. This represents an additional indication for enteral stent placement.

Besides malignant disease, enteral stents have occasionally been utilized in patients with benign etiologies of gastric outlet obstruction, namely, peptic strictures, inflammatory strictures from gastroduodenal Crohn's disease, and annular pancreas amongst others. The rapid improvements in endoscopic balloon dilation technologies and minimally invasive surgery, however, have significantly limited the use of enteral stents for benign indications (Chopita et al. 2007; Nagy et al. 1995; Rhodes et al. 1995).

Contraindications

There are few contraindications to enteral stent placement for malignant gastric or duodenal outlet obstruction. Patients who are medically unfit for endoscopic procedures should not undergo enteral stent placement. Enteral stent placement is also contraindicated in patients with uncontrolled coagulopathy and in individuals with life expectancy of less than 4–6 weeks. Localized intestinal perforation in the setting of malignancy represents a contraindication to enteral stent placement. Finally, enteral stents should not be placed in patients with multiple sites of distal intestinal obstruction (i.e., carcinomatosis) as relief of the proximal point of obstruction is unlikely to provide palliation in these individuals (Gupta and Freeman 2008).

Technique

Self-expanding metal stents for malignant gastric or duodenal outlet obstruction are usually placed endoscopically with fluoroscopic control. However, they can be placed by radiologists using fluoroscopy alone. Endoscopic delivery has the advantage of real-time investigation of the obstructing lesion and direct visualization of stent positioning and deployment. Most patients presenting with malignant gastroenteric obstruction will have had imaging with either a CT or contrast-enhanced radiograph (Fig. 2). Although such studies are useful for preprocedural planning, identification of the location and extent of the obstructing lesion, as well as determination of the presence of distal points of intestinal obstruction, it is not imperative that they be obtained prior to performing the procedure (Gupta and Freeman 2008).

Nasogastric decompression is imperative prior to the initiation of conscious sedation or the induction of general anesthesia. Patients with severe gastric outlet obstruction are also prone to gastroparesis (see below). As a result of both the intestinal obstruction and poor gastric contractility, several liters of fluid or semisolid gastric contents may be retained, making the risk of aspiration in a nondecompressed patient significant. We usually prefer at least 24 h of nasogastric decompression or endotracheal intubation prior to endoscopic stent placement.

Once conscious sedation is achieved or general anesthesia induced, insertion of the endoscope typically begins with the patient in the left lateral decubitus position. The choice of endoscope depends on the location of the lesion: proximal lesions can be handled utilizing a therapeutic (3.7 mm working channel) upper endoscope or duodenoscope (4.2 mm working channel), while those distal to the second portion of the duodenum typically require the use of an adult colonoscope. If the obstruction can be passed using the endoscope, this should be done with extreme caution as the majority of enteral stents can be placed without crossing the stenosis. Balloon dilation is rarely indicated, except when required to pass a duodenoscope for performance of ERCP during the same procedure (see below) (Gupta and Freeman 2008).

In the event that the stenosis is not crossed, a balloon catheter can be used to inject contrast beyond the obstruction so that the length of the stricture can be defined and an appropriate length stent selected (Fig. 2). A wire guide can then be placed through the stenosis into the distal bowel. The selected stent should be approximately 3–4 cm longer than the length of the stenosis to ensure adequate coverage on either side of the stricture (Gupta and Freeman 2008). Once the proper length stent is selected and advanced into position over the wire guide, deployment can proceed under endoscopic and fluoroscopic control. Most devices tend to deliver distally when released; therefore, gentle countertension is used to ensure proper deployment, and ultimately, positioning. In some cases, direct visualization of the proximal margin of the stricture is not possible during deployment. This is especially true for lesions at the apex of the duodenum where the acute angulation and "straightening" of the endoscope as the stent is passed through the working channel forces the endoscope tip into the stomach. In such cases, placement of an endoscopic clip

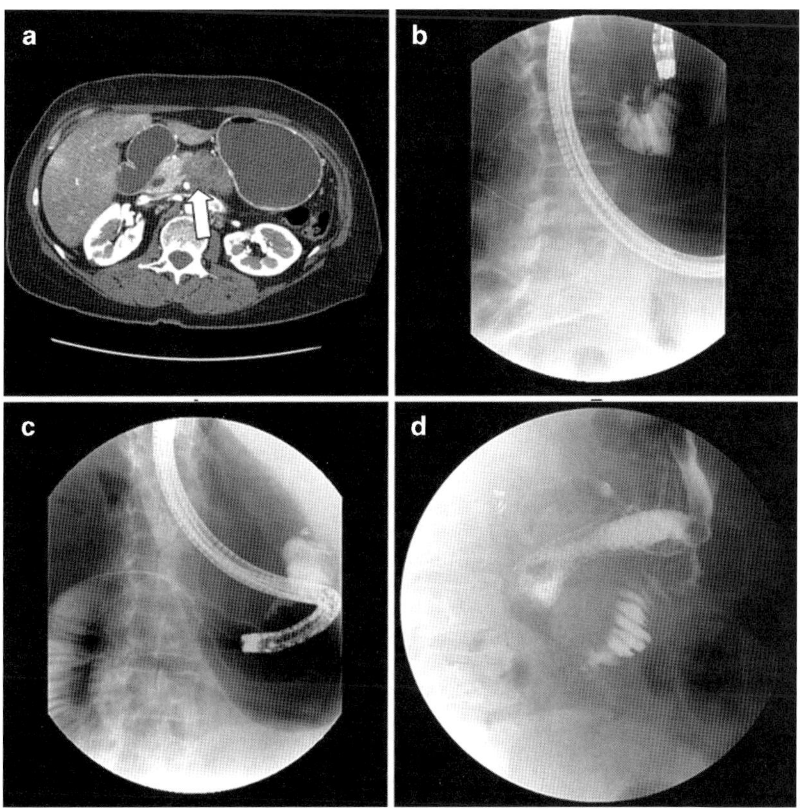

Fig. 2. Abdominal CT scan demonstrating a markedly dilated stomach and large pancreatic mass (*arrow*) (**a**). Contrast was injected following which a guide wire was placed across the stenosis (**b**). Wallflex™ (Boston Scientific, Natick, MA) stent deployment was successful (**c**); an upper GI series performed following stent deployment demonstrates passage of contrast through the stent (**d**) indicating luminal patency.

or injection of contrast into the submucosa at the proximal margin of the stricture may be performed. This allows for visualization of the proximal margin during deployment in the event that stent deployment occurs with the endoscope tip in the stomach (see below).

In cases where the obstructing lesion extends into the duodenal bulb, the proximal end of the stent should be brought through the pylorus and positioned in the stomach. Most early generation self-expanding metal enteral stents contained sharp edges on the proximal and distal ends. Due to the thin-walled duodenum and increased risk of stent-related perforation, trans-pyloric deployment was preferable to leaving the proximal edge of the stent within the duodenal bulb. The design of the latest generation enteral stent (see below) has eliminated the sharp proximal and distal ends making (theoretically) deployment within the duodenal bulb safer, thus potentially obviating trans-pyloric positioning, unless clinically indicated (Gupta and Freeman 2008).

Complications

The major risk of enteral stent placement is intestinal perforation, which has been reported to occur in 0.7% of individuals (Chopita et al. 2007; Dormann et al. 2004). The risk is increased in cases where balloon dilation is performed or when stents are deployed around intestinal angulations, which are relatively "fixed" in position due to obstructing malignant neoplasms. Because most patients in whom enteral stents are placed have an underlying advanced malignancy, surgical repair of stent-related intestinal perforation may be technically difficult or impossible, resulting in peritonitis and death. As such, proper informed consent of patients considered for enteral stent placement is imperative.

The performance of endoscopy in patients with gastric outlet obstruction can lead to aspiration of gastric contents and resultant pneumonia. This risk is increased in cases performed without adequate measures taken to protect the airway or insufficient gastric decompression. Another risk of enteral stent placement within the duodenum is biliary obstruction and precipitation of cholangitis. This complication is not limited to patients with a native papilla. Subclinically occluded biliary stents can become completely occluded by the radial expansive force of the duodenal stent. Accordingly, measurement of liver chemistries and a CT scan of the abdomen are essential parts of preprocedural planning for patients in whom duodenal stents may cross the major papilla. ERCP should be performed prior to duodenal stent placement in patients with evidence of biliary obstruction. However, "prophylactic" biliary stenting is not supported by any clinical evidence to date (Gupta and Freeman 2008).

Other complications of enteral stent placement include stent migration (5%), bleeding (0.5%) (especially with older stent designs) in addition to stent occlusion (18%) (Chopita et al. 2007; Gupta and Freeman 2008; Dormann et al. 2004). Stent migration in malignant disease is rare. Migrated stents may pass spontaneously or, in rare cases, lead to small bowel obstruction or delayed intestinal perforation requiring surgery. Occlusion of enteral stents can be secondary to food bolus impaction, tissue hyperplasia, or tumor in-growth. Food bolus impaction can typically be handled endoscopically, whereas in-growth of tumor and tissue hyperplasia require placement of a second endoprosthesis (Chopita et al. 2007; Gupta and Freeman 2008). Finally, newer-generation enteral stents are fashioned from nitinol (see below). Although superior in terms of radial expansive force, these devices foreshorten. In cases where an adequate "safety" margin of 2–3 cm of stent on either end of the obstruction does not exist, recurrent intestinal obstruction following stent foreshortening can be observed. Stent revision (insertion of a longer stent) is required in such cases.

Postoperative Care

Patients are typically allowed nothing by mouth for the first 24 h following enteral stent placement as most prostheses require this period of time to reach maximum expansion. A liquid diet can be initiated after 24 h, and if tolerated, the diet advanced to a maximum of mechanical soft or puree. An upper GI series (Fig. 2) with small bowel follow-through should be obtained in patients with continued obstructive symptoms following enteral stent placement, in order to rule out early complications such as stent migration, malposition, or more distal intestinal obstruction. Patients with severe pain, fever, or leukocytosis should undergo a CT scan of the abdomen in order to evaluate for intestinal perforation.

Many patients with long-standing gastric or duodenal outlet obstruction will have coexisting gastroparesis. In these cases, enteral stent placement may not provide adequate symptomatic relief and treatment with promotility agents may be required. In patients for whom promotility agents do not provide adequate relief of symptoms, alternative methods of nutrition should be discussed and a decompressive gastrostomy considered.

Clinical Efficacy

Over the past several years, enteral SEMS placement has emerged as an alternative to surgery for the palliation of malignant gastric outlet obstruction. Several uncontrolled case series have demonstrated technical success rates of greater than 90% (Adler and Baron 2002; Dumas et al. 2000; Nassif et al. 2003). Dormann and colleagues (Dormann et al. 2004) performed a systematic review of the published series on the use of SEMS for palliation of gastroduodenal malignancies. Findings included successful stent deployment in 589 of 606 patients (97%) in whom it was attempted. Clinical success, as defined by resumption of oral intake following stent placement, was achieved in 89% of patients in whom stents could be successfully placed with full resolution of symptoms occurring at a mean of 4 days. Procedure-related mortality was zero. Major complications such as bleeding and perforation occurred in 1.2% of patients; stent migration was reported in 5%.

There are now several small series in the literature, which compare SEMS placement to surgical bypass for the treatment of malignant gastroduodenal outlet obstruction (Maetani et al. 2007; Mehta et al. 2006; Fiori et al. 2004; Jeurnink et al. 2007). Most have found high technical success rates for both procedures. However, patients who underwent surgical bypass tended to have an increased duration of hospitalization, a higher rate of postoperative complications, and a longer time interval to restoration of oral intake. A survival benefit has not been demonstrated for either modality. Regardless, in patients with incurable malignancies and anticipated short-term survival, the advantages of SEMS placement may provide for an improved quality of life over surgery (Gupta and Freeman 2008; Lowe et al. 2007).

Available Devices

At present, there are two devices that are approved in the USA for palliation of malignant gastroduodenal obstruction: Wallflex and Wallstent (Boston Scientific, Natick, MA).

Both devices can be deployed either through the endoscope or over a guide wire using fluoroscopic control. The Wallstent is fashioned from Elgiloy and is available in 20 or 22 mm with lengths ranging between 6 and 9 cm.

The Wallflex enteral stent is the latest generation of stents to be introduced in North America. As opposed to the Wallstent, the ends of the Wallflex stent are rounded and not sharp, which, in theory, may decrease the risk of stent-related bowel perforation. Other differences include a less rigid delivery system with a tapered end, which may allow for access to difficult anatomy. The Wallflex stent is fashioned from nitinol and the diameter of the stent body is 22 mm with a proximal "flare" to 27 mm; available lengths are 6, 9, and 12 cm.

Like its esophageal counterpart, the Niti-S Pyloric Stent (Taewoong Medical, Korea) is fashioned from a double-layered nitinol outer core with an inner polyurethane covering. Although this stent is not currently available in the USA, the double-layered design represents important technology, potentially reducing tumor in-growth and resultant stent occlusion, which can require endoscopic re-intervention.

Alternative Treatments

Alternatives to enteral stent placement for the treatment of malignant gastric or duodenal outlet obstruction include surgical gastroenteric anastomosis, placement of an enteric feeding tube combined with a decompressive gastrostomy, in addition to placement of a decompressive gastrostomy with or without parenteral nutrition.

COLONIC STENTING

Indications

Obstructing colorectal neoplasms, namely adenocarcinoma, can lead to significant morbidity and mortality. Not surprisingly, relief of obstruction from intrinsic neoplastic disorders of the large bowel is the leading indication for colonic stent placement (Gupta and Freeman 2008). Colonic stents can be placed to relieve obstruction for extracolonic malignancies, which cause extrinsic compression, leading to colonic obstruction (Gupta and Freeman 2008). Cancers of the prostate, ovary, and cervix can often lead to colonic obstruction due to this mechanism. Colonic stents have also occasionally been placed for benign disease including ischemic colonic strictures, strictures related to diverticular disease, and Crohn's and anastomotic strictures (Forshaw et al. 2006; Small et al. 2008; Suzuki et al. 2004). The focus of the discussion that follows is colonic stenting for malignant obstruction.

In patients with malignant colonic obstruction, stents have been used in two scenarios. The first is in patients who either have metastatic disease at the time of presentation or in those who are poor surgical candidates. In this situation, colonic stenting is palliative. The second is in patients who are good surgical candidates with complete colonic obstruction in whom a bowel preparation is preferred to a diverting colostomy with Hartmann's pouch followed by a second surgery several weeks to months later. If successful in relief of obstruction, colonic stenting in this group of patients allows for a "single-step" operation (Gupta and Freeman 2008).

Contraindications

As for other endoscopic procedures performed under conscious sedation, patients medically unfit for endoscopy should not undergo colonic stent placement. This procedure is also contraindicated in patients with signs or symptoms consistent with intestinal perforation and peritonitis. In some patients, obstructing colonic malignancies can perforate the colon yet not be associated with gross peritonitis. Identification of mesenteric fat at endoscopy should alert the endoscopist to the presence of a perforation and the stent should not be placed. Patients with obstructing colonic lesions approximating the anal verge should not undergo colonic stenting as there may be insufficient clearance for expansion of the distal portion of the stent. In addition, stents placed in this region may cross the dentate line leading to severe discomfort.

Colonic stents should not be placed in patients with uncontrolled coagulopathy or those with life expectancy less than 30 days. Finally, individuals with multiple obstructing colonic lesions are unlikely to benefit from the placement of a single colonic stent.

Procedure

Because patients with acute colonic obstruction cannot undergo full oral bowel preparation, colonic stents are typically placed into the unprepped colon. In patients with obstruction of the rectosigmoid or descending colon, enemas may be used to clear the distal colon. The choice of endoscope depends on the location of the obstruction. Lesions within the left colon up to the splenic flexure can typically be reached using a sigmoidoscope or therapeutic upper endoscope while those in the more proximal colon will require the use of a colonoscope. Patients with acute colonic obstruction should undergo nasogastric suction to decompress the bowel proximal to the stenosis and reduce the risk of aspiration of gastric contents. A gastrografin enema should be performed for planning purposes in all patients with suspected proximal obstruction and in those patients with distal obstruction in whom additional stricture characterization is desired (Gupta and Freeman 2008).

After sedating the patient, the endoscope is advanced through the unprepped colon to the level of the stenosis. Insufflation should be used judiciously as overdistension can lead to proximal bowel perforation. Once the level of the stenosis is reached, a stiff guide wire can be placed through the stricture using an ERCP catheter or balloon catheter. Injection of contrast through the stenosis should be performed to help to define the length of the obstruction (Fig. 3). Passage of the endoscope proximal to the stricture is not mandatory and can lead to colonic perforation. Because visualization may be difficult in the colon and some devices cannot be placed through the endoscope, an endoscopic clip should be placed 1–2 cm below the distal margin of obstruction to allow for fluoroscopic visibility. Alternatively, water- or lipid-soluble contrast material can be injected with a sclerotherapy needle to delineate stricture margins.

The choice of stent should be 3–4 cm longer than the estimated length of the obstruction in order to allow for adequate coverage, especially with stents fashioned from nitinol, which tend to foreshorten as they expand. Stents can be delivered through the working channel (Fig. 3) of the endoscope or over the guide wire alone. In either case, deployment should be performed under fluoroscopic control. Because obstructing colonic neoplasms can often cause acute angulations in the bowel, maintaining proper endoscope position during stent deployment can often require the assistance of a nurse, technician, or additional physician.

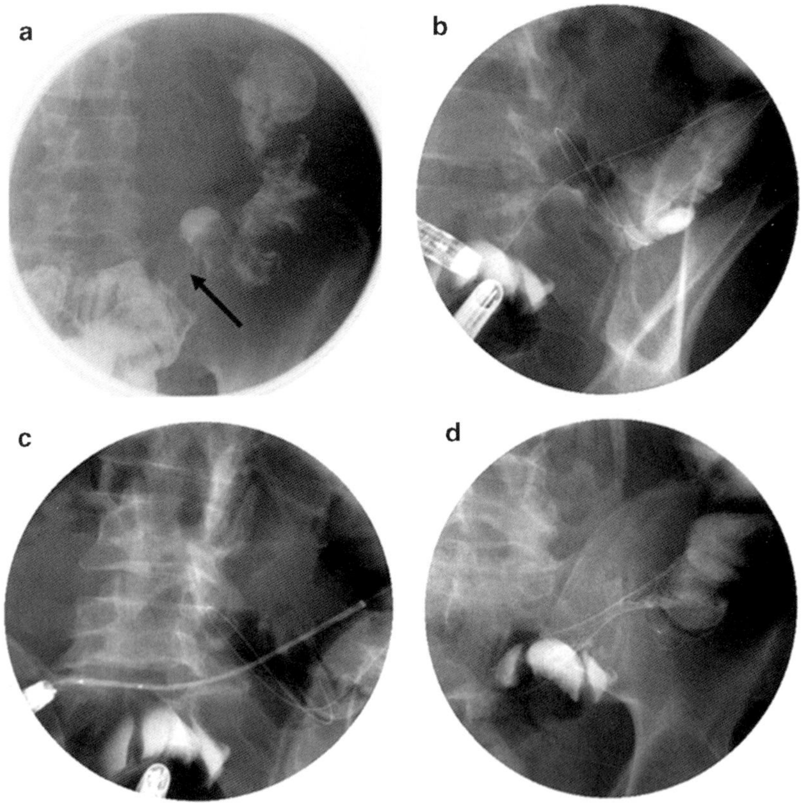

Fig. 3. Barium enema demonstrating a severe stenosis (*arrow*) in the sigmoid colon (**a**). A guide wire was placed beyond the stenosis following injection of contrast (**b**). A through the scope (Wallflex™, Boston Scientific, Natick, MA) stent was positioned across the stenosis over the guide wire, through the scope (**c**) and deployed in satisfactory position (**d**)

Complications

The major complication associated with colonic stent placement is intestinal perforation. This occurs in up to 4.5% of cases (Watt et al. 2007). Many cases of colonic perforation are encountered when stents are placed around acute angulations in the colon. This is due to straightening of the bowel, which occurs with expansion of the stent. Prompt recognition, administration of broad spectrum antibiotics, and surgical consultation are essential in cases where perforation occurs.

Other complications related to colonic stent placement include bleeding, stent migration (11.8%), and occlusion (7.3%) (Watt et al. 2007). Like other enteral stents, occlusion is typically due to in-growth of tumor or bolus impaction. In the case of tumor-related occlusion, revision with a second stent typically leads to clinical improvement. Migrated stents may pass spontaneously or require endoscopic removal if they become lodged at the anal verge.

Postoperative Care

Most patients who undergo successful colonic stent placement experience immediate relief of symptoms. A clear liquid diet can be initiated after 24 h and if surgery is planned, a full bowel prep can be administered. In patients undergoing palliative stenting, diet can be advanced as tolerated.

Patients who do not experience colonic decompression following stent placement should undergo an abdominal radiograph to determine whether the stent has migrated or is malpositioned (Gupta and Freeman 2008). If the stent appears in good position with full expansion, repeat endoscopy can be considered to determine the reason for stent dysfunction or whether a second, upstream obstruction exists (more common in extrinsic malignancy). Alternatively, a water-soluble contrast study can be obtained initially. Patients with signs and symptoms of peritonitis following stent placement should undergo an urgent abdominal CT scan to evaluate for colonic perforation.

Clinical Data

Several case series and pooled analyses have now demonstrated the efficacy of colonic stent placement (Watt et al. 2007; Repici et al. 2007; Siddiqui et al. 2007b). In a comprehensive review of available data, Sebastian and colleagues (Sebastian et al. 2004) reported a technical success rate of more than 93% for stent placement on the first attempt. Clinical success rates, as defined by colonic decompression (either clinically or radiographically), were found to be greater than 88%. Compared to surgery, SEMS placement in the colon was associated with a shorter duration of hospitalization, lower rates of complications, and a decrease in the need for colostomy (Tilney et al. 2007; Ng et al. 2006). The limited available evidence also suggests that initial SEMS placement for malignant colonic obstruction is a cost-effective strategy when compared to surgery (Singh et al. 2006; Targownik et al. 2004). In many centers, an attempt at SEMS placement is now the preferred strategy for the initial management of acute colonic obstruction secondary to malignancy (Kozarek 2008).

Available Devices

There are currently four SEMS approved by the U.S. Food and Drug Administration for the palliation of malignant colonic obstruction. The colonic Wallstent, Wallflex, and Ultraflex Precision are all manufactured by Boston Scientific (Natick, MA). The colonic Wallstent is fashioned from Elgiloy and, like the duodenal version, is available in a 20 or 22 mm diameter and lengths of 6 and 9 cm. The delivery system is 10 Fr, with a working length of 230 cm. The colonic Wallflex is fashioned from nitinol. However, as opposed to the Wallstent, the ends of the stent are interwoven, which may potentially decrease the risk of perforation. The Wallflex colonic stent is available in diameters ranging from 22 to 25 mm and has a 27 or 30 mm proximal flare. Lengths are 6, 9, and 12 cm, and they are inserted using a 10 Fr delivery system with a working length of either 135 or 230 cm. Finally, the Ultraflex Precision colonic stent is fashioned from nitinol, has a central diameter of 25 mm and a 30 mm proximal flare. This device can only be inserted over an endoscopically or fluoroscopically positioned guide wire using a 105-cm long delivery catheter.

The colonic Z stent (Cook Medical) is a stainless steel stent, which is available in lengths of 4, 6, 8, 10, and 12 cm. The stent can only be placed over a guide wire under fluoroscopic control as the delivery catheter is 10 mm. All the stents are 25 mm in shaft diameter with a 35 mm proximal flare. The introducer is 40 cm in length and its use is, therefore, limited to the left colon.

Alternative Procedures

Alternatives to colonic stenting for acute colonic obstruction include a diverting colostomy or, in patients who are not surgical candidates, placement of a trans-rectal colonic decompression tube.

SUMMARY OF KEY POINTS

- Self-expandable stent are utilized for the treatment of two benign diseases of the esophagus: perforation and anastomotic leaks in addition to refractory benign esophageal strictures.
- Tumors located in the mid- to upper esophagus raise the theoretical risk of causing airway obstruction.
- The risk of stent migration is typically lowest in patients with intrinsic strictures of the esophagus.
- For most malignant lesions, a partially or fully covered SEMS is preferable to an uncovered stent in order to prevent the tumor in-growth.
- The major drawback to partially or fully covered stents is the increased risk of stent migration.
- Stents placed in this location obliterate the natural reflux barrier and patients almost invariably develop reflux of gastric contents into the proximal esophagus or oropharynx; specifically designed "antireflux" stents may help to decrease symptoms.
- Because endoscopic measurements may be slightly inaccurate, it is best to err on the side of a longer (rather than shorter) stent in order to decrease the risk of failing to palliate the obstructing lesion.

REFERENCES

Adler DG, Baron TH. Endoscopic palliation of malignant gastric outlet obstruction using self-expanding metal stents: experience in 36 patients. Am J Gastroenterol. 2002;97:72–8.

Alam TA, Baines M, Parker MC. The management of gastric outlet obstruction secondary to inoperable cancer. Surg Endosc. 2003;17:320–3.

Baron TH. Minimizing endoscopic complications: endoluminal stents. Gastrointest Endosc Clin N Am. 2007; 17:83–104. vii.

Bartelsman JF et al. Palliation of patients with esophagogastric neoplasms by insertion of a covered expandable modified Gianturco-Z endoprosthesis: experiences in 153 patients. Gastrointest Endosc. 2000;51:134–8.

Bethge N, Sommer A, Vakil N. Palliation of malignant esophageal obstruction due to intrinsic and extrinsic lesions with expandable metal stents. Am J Gastroenterol. 1998;93:1829–32.

Chopita N, Landoni N, Ross A, Villaverde A. Malignant gastroenteric obstruction: therapeutic options. Gastrointest Endosc Clin N Am. 2007;17:533–44. vi-vii.

Christie NA et al. Results of expandable metal stents for malignant esophageal obstruction in 100 patients: short-term and long-term follow-up. Ann Thorac Surg. 2001;71:1797–801. discussion 1801–2.

Conigliaro R et al. Polyflex stents for malignant oesophageal and oesophagogastric stricture: a prospective, multicentric study. Eur J Gastroenterol Hepatol. 2007;19:195–203.

Conio M et al. A randomized prospective comparison of self-expandable plastic stents and partially covered self-expandable metal stents in the palliation of malignant esophageal dysphagia. Am J Gastroenterol. 2007;102:2667–77.

Cook TA, Dehn TC. Use of covered expandable metal stents in the treatment of oesophageal carcinoma and tracheo-oesophageal fistula. Br J Surg. 1996;83:1417–8.

Cordero Jr JA, Moores DW. Self-expanding esophageal metallic stents in the treatment of esophageal obstruction. Am Surg. 2000;66:956–8. discussion 958–9.

Costamagna G, Marchese M, Iacopini F. Self-expanding stents in oesophageal cancer. Eur J Gastroenterol Hepatol. 2006;18:1177–80.
Dasgupta A et al. Airway complications of esophageal self-expandable metallic stent. Gastrointest Endosc. 1998;47:532–5.
De Olabozal J, Roberts J, Hoeltgen T, Berkelhammer C. Double stenting to prevent airway compression in proximal malignant esophageal strictures. Am J Gastroenterol. 2001;96:2800–1.
De Palma GD et al. Self-expanding metal stents for palliation of inoperable carcinoma of the esophagus and gastroesophageal junction. Am J Gastroenterol. 1995;90:2140–2.
De Palma GD et al. Plastic prosthesis versus expandable metal stents for palliation of inoperable esophageal thoracic carcinoma: a controlled prospective study. Gastrointest Endosc. 1996;43:78–82.
De Palma GD et al. Impact on the quality of remaining life of treatment with self-expandable metal prostheses in patients with inoperable esophago-cardial cancer. Results of a study of 107 consecutive patients treated with Ultraflex-type prostheses. Minerva Gastroenterol Dietol. 1999;45:95–106.
Domschke W, Foerster EC, Matek W, Rodl W. Self-expanding mesh stent for esophageal cancer stenosis. Endoscopy. 1990;22:134–6.
Dormann A, Meisner S, Verin N, Wenk Lang A. Self-expanding metal stents for gastroduodenal malignancies: systematic review of their clinical effectiveness. Endoscopy. 2004;36:543–50.
Dua KS. Stents for palliating malignant dysphagia and fistula: is the paradigm shifting? Gastrointest Endosc. 2007;65:77–81.
Dumas R et al. Palliative endoscopic treatment of malignant duodenal stenosis by metal prosthesis. Gastroentérol Clin Biol. 2000;24:714–8.
Eickhoff A et al. Self-expanding metal stents versus plastic prostheses in the palliation of malignant dysphagia: long-term outcome of 153 consecutive patients. J Clin Gastroenterol. 2005;39:877–85.
Elton E. Esophageal cancer. Dis Mon. 2005;51:664–84.
Enzinger PC, Mayer RJ. Esophageal cancer. N Engl J Med. 2003;349:2241–52.
Farivar AS, Vallieres E, Kowdley KV, Wood DE, Mulligan MS. Airway obstruction complicating esophageal stent placement in two post-pneumonectomy patients. Ann Thorac Surg. 2004;78:e22–3.
Fiori E et al. Palliative management of malignant antro-pyloric strictures. Gastroenterostomy vs. endoscopic stenting. A randomized prospective trial. Anticancer Res. 2004;24:269–71.
Fiorini AB et al. Expandable metal coil stent for treatment of broncho-esophageal fistula. Gastrointest Endosc. 1995;42:81–3.
Fleischer DE, Bull-Henry K. A new coated self-expanding metal stent for malignant esophageal strictures. Gastrointest Endosc. 1992;38:494–6.
Forshaw MJ, Sankararajah D, Stewart M, Parker MC. Self-expanding metallic stents in the treatment of benign colorectal disease: indications and outcomes. Colorectal Dis. 2006;8:102–11.
Freeman RK, Van Woerkom JM, Ascioti AJ. Esophageal stent placement for the treatment of iatrogenic intrathoracic esophageal perforation. Ann Thorac Surg. 2007a;83:2003–7. discussion 2007–8.
Freeman RK, Ascioti AJ, Wozniak TC. Postoperative esophageal leak management with the Polyflex esophageal stent. J Thorac Cardiovasc Surg. 2007b;133:333–8.
Frimberger E. Expanding spiral-a new type of prosthesis for the palliative treatment of malignant esophageal stenoses. Endoscopy. 1983;15 Suppl 1:213–4.
Ginsberg GG. Palliation of malignant esophageal Dysphagia: would you like plastic or metal? Am J Gastroenterol. 2007;102:2678–9.
Gupta K, Freeman M. Enteral and colonic self-expanding metallic stents. Rev Gastroenterol Disord. 2008;8:83–97.
Holm AN, de la Mora Levy JG, Gostout CJ, Topazian MD, Baron TH. Self-expanding plastic stents in treatment of benign esophageal conditions. Gastrointest Endosc. 2008;67:20–5.
Homs MY et al. Prior radiation and/or chemotherapy has no effect on the outcome of metal stent placement for oesophagogastric carcinoma. Eur J Gastroenterol Hepatol. 2004a;16:163–70.
Homs MY et al. Single-dose brachytherapy versus metal stent placement for the palliation of dysphagia from oesophageal cancer: multicentre randomised trial. Lancet. 2004b;364:1497–504.
Hunerbein M, Stroszczynski C, Moesta KT, Schlag PM. Treatment of thoracic anastomotic leaks after esophagectomy with self-expanding plastic stents. Ann Surg. 2004;240:801–7.
Jeurnink SM et al. Gastrojejunostomy versus stent placement in patients with malignant gastric outlet obstruction: a comparison in 95 patients. J Surg Oncol. 2007;96:389–96.

Johnson E et al. Survival and complications after insertion of self-expandable metal stents for malignant oesophageal stenosis. Scand J Gastroenterol. 2006;41:252–6.

Kauer WK, Stein HJ, Dittler HJ, Siewert JR. Stent implantation as a treatment option in patients with thoracic anastomotic leaks after esophagectomy. Surg Endosc. 2008;22:50–3.

Kawasaki R, Sano A, Matsumoto S. Long-term outcomes and complications of metallic stents for malignant esophageal stenoses. Kobe J Med Sci. 2003;49:133–42.

Kiernan PD, Sheridan MJ, Hettrick V, Vaughan B, Graling P. Thoracic esophageal perforation: one surgeon's experience. Dis Esophagus. 2006;19:24–30.

Kinsman KJ et al. Prior radiation and chemotherapy increase the risk of life-threatening complications after insertion of metallic stents for esophagogastric malignancy. Gastrointest Endosc. 1996;43:196–203.

Kostopoulos PP et al. Are metal stents effective for palliation of malignant dysphagia and fistulas? Dig Liver Dis. 2003;35:275–82.

Kotsis L, Zubovits K, Vadasz P. Management of malignant tracheoesophageal fistulas with a cuffed funnel tube. Ann Thorac Surg. 1997;64:355–8.

Kozarek R. Making sense out of colonic stents. Gastrointest Endosc. 2008;67:85–7.

Kozarek RA et al. Use of the 25 mm flanged esophageal Z stent for malignant dysphagia: a prospective multicenter trial. Gastrointest Endosc. 1997;46:156–60.

Lam YH et al. Self-expandable metal stents for malignant dysphagia. Aust N Z J Surg. 1999;69:668–71.

Langer FB et al. Management of postoperative esophageal leaks with the Polyflex self-expanding covered plastic stent. Ann Thorac Surg. 2005;79:398–403. discussion 404.

Lowe AS et al. Self-expandable metal stent placement for the palliation of malignant gastroduodenal obstruction: experience in a large, single, UK centre. Clin Radiol. 2007;62:738–44.

Maetani I et al. Self-expandable metallic stent placement for palliation in gastric outlet obstructions caused by gastric cancer: a comparison with surgical gastrojejunostomy. J Gastroenterol. 2007;40:932–7.

McGrath JP, Browne M, Riordan C, Ravi N, Reynolds JV. Expandable metal stents in the palliation of malignant dysphagia and oesophageal-respiratory fistulae. Ir Med J. 2001;94:270–2.

Mehta S et al. Prospective randomized trial of laparoscopic gastrojejunostomy versus duodenal stenting for malignant gastric outflow obstruction. Surg Endosc. 2006;20:239–42.

Moores DW, Ilves R. Treatment of esophageal obstruction with covered, self-expanding esophageal Wallstents. Ann Thorac Surg. 1996;62:963–7.

Nagy A, Brosseuk D, Hemming A, Scudamore C, Mamazza J. Laparoscopic gastroenterostomy for duodenal obstruction. Am J Surg. 1995;169:539–42.

Nassif T et al. Endoscopic palliation of malignant gastric outlet obstruction using self-expandable metallic stents: results of a multicenter study. Endoscopy. 2003;35:483–9.

Ng KC et al. Self-expanding metallic stent as a bridge to surgery versus emergency resection for obstructing left-sided colorectal cancer: a case-matched study. J Gastrointest Surg. 2006;10:798–803.

Papachristou GI, Baron TH. Use of stents in benign and malignant esophageal disease. Rev Gastroenterol Disord. 2007;7:74–88.

Profili S et al. Effective management of intrathoracic anastomotic leak with covered self-expandable metal stents. Report on three cases. Emerg Radiol. 2008;15:57–60.

Radecke K, Lang H, Frilling A, Gerken G, Treichel U. Successful sealing of benign esophageal leaks after temporary placement of a self-expanding plastic stent without fluoroscopic guidance. Z Gastroenterol. 2006;44:1031–8.

Radiology., B.S.o.I. ROST: Registry if Iesophageal Stenting, first report 2004. (Hanley-on-Thames: Dendrite Clinical Systems, 2004).

Raijman I, Lynch P. Coated expandable esophageal stents in the treatment of digestive-respiratory fistulas. Am J Gastroenterol. 1997;92:2188–91.

Raijman I et al. Expandable esophageal stents: initial experience with a new nitinol stent. Gastrointest Endosc. 1994;40:614–21.

Raijman I, Siddique I, Ajani J, Lynch P. Palliation of malignant dysphagia and fistulae with coated expandable metal stents: experience with 101 patients. Gastrointest Endosc. 1998;48:172–9.

Razzaq R, Laasch HU, England R, Marriott A, Martin D. Expandable metal stents for the palliation of malignant gastroduodenal obstruction. Cardiovasc Interv Radiol. 2001;24:313–8.

Repici A et al. Temporary placement of an expandable polyester silicone-covered stent for treatment of refractory benign esophageal strictures. Gastrointest Endosc. 2004;60:513–9.

Repici A et al. Stenting of the proximal colon in patients with malignant large bowel obstruction: techniques and outcomes. Gastrointest Endosc. 2007;66:940–4.

Rhodes M, Nathanson L, Fielding G. Laparoscopic biliary and gastric bypass: a useful adjunct in the treatment of carcinoma of the pancreas. Gut. 1995;36:778–80.

Rollhauser C, Fleischer DE. Late migration of a self-expandable metal stent and successful endoscopic management. Gastrointest Endosc. 1999;49:541–4.

Schubert D et al. Endoscopic treatment of thoracic esophageal anastomotic leaks by using silicone-covered, self-expanding polyester stents. Gastrointest Endosc. 2005;61:891–6.

Sebastian S, Johnston S, Geoghegan T, Torreggiani W, Buckley M. Pooled analysis of the efficacy and safety of self-expanding metal stenting in malignant colorectal obstruction. Am J Gastroenterol. 2004;99:2051–7.

Siddiqui AA, Loren D, Dudnick R, Kowalski T. Expandable polyester silicon-covered stent for malignant esophageal strictures before neoadjuvant chemoradiation: a pilot study. Dig Dis Sci. 2007a;52:823–9.

Siddiqui A, Khandelwal N, Anthony T, Huerta S. Colonic stent versus surgery for the management of acute malignant colonic obstruction: a decision analysis. Aliment Pharmacol Ther. 2007b;26:1379–86.

Siersema PD. New developments in palliative therapy. Best Pract Res Clin Gastroenterol. 2006;20:959–78.

Siersema PD, Hop WC, Dees J, Tilanus HW, van Blankenstein M. Coated self-expanding metal stents versus latex prostheses for esophagogastric cancer with special reference to prior radiation and chemotherapy: a controlled, prospective study. Gastrointest Endosc. 1998;47:113–20.

Siersema PD, Homs MY, Haringsma J, Tilanus HW, Kuipers EJ. Use of large-diameter metallic stents to seal traumatic nonmalignant perforations of the esophagus. Gastrointest Endosc. 2003;58:356–61.

Singh H, Latosinsky S, Spiegel BM, Targownik LE. The cost-effectiveness of colonic stenting as a bridge to curative surgery in patients with acute left-sided malignant colonic obstruction: a Canadian perspective. Can J Gastroenterol. 2006;20:779–85.

Small AJ, Young-Fadok TM, Baron TH. Expandable metal stent placement for benign colorectal obstruction: outcomes for 23 cases. Surg Endosc. 2008;22:454–62.

Song HY et al. Covered, expandable esophageal metallic stent tubes: experiences in 119 patients. Radiology. 1994;193:689–95.

Sundelof M et al. Palliative treatment of malignant dysphagia with self-expanding metal stents: a 12-year experience. Scand J Gastroenterol. 2007;42:11–6.

Suzuki N et al. Colorectal stenting for malignant and benign disease: outcomes in colorectal stenting. Dis Colon Rectum. 2004;47:1201–7.

Targownik LE et al. Colonic stent vs. emergency surgery for management of acute left-sided malignant colonic obstruction: a decision analysis. Gastrointest Endosc. 2004;60:865–74.

Tilney HS et al. Comparison of colonic stenting and open surgery for malignant large bowel obstruction. Surg Endosc. 2007;21:225–33.

Toikkanen VJ et al. Expandable metallic stents in the management of malignant oesophageal obstruction. Ann Chir Gynaecol. 2000;89:20–3.

Tuebergen D et al. Treatment of thoracic esophageal anastomotic leaks and esophageal perforations with endoluminal stents: efficacy and current limitations. J Gastrointest Surg. 2008;12:1168–76.

Vakil N et al. A prospective, randomized, controlled trial of covered expandable metal stents in the palliation of malignant esophageal obstruction at the gastroesophageal junction. Am J Gastroenterol. 2001;96:1791–6.

Verschuur EM et al. A new esophageal stent design (Niti-S stent) for the prevention of migration: a prospective study in 42 patients. Gastrointest Endosc. 2006;63:134–40.

Watt AM, Faragher IG, Griffin TT, Rieger NA, Maddern GJ. Self-expanding metallic stents for relieving malignant colorectal obstruction: a systematic review. Ann Surg. 2007;246:24–30.

Xinopoulos D et al. Palliative treatment of advanced esophageal cancer with metal-covered expandable stents. A cost-effectiveness and quality of life study. J BUON. 2005;10:523–8.

Yano F, Mittal SK. Post-operative esophageal leak treated with removable silicone-covered polyester stent. Dis Esophagus. 2007;20:535–7.

Yano F, El Sherif A, Filipi CJ, Mittal SK. Use of temporary esophageal stent in management of perforations after benign esophageal surgery. Surg Laparosc Endosc Percutan Tech. 2008;18:283–5.

Zwischenberger JB, Savage C, Bidani A. Surgical aspects of esophageal disease: perforation and caustic injury. Am J Respir Crit Care Med. 2002;165:1037–40.

4 Endoscopic Management of Nonvariceal Upper Gastrointestinal Bleeding

Fadi Rahhal, M.D. and Subbaramiah Sridhar

CONTENTS

Keywords: Endoscopic Management of Non-Variceal Upper Gastrointestinal Bleeding

INTRODUCTION

Acute upper GI bleeding (UGIB) is a common medical emergency with an annual rate of 150–200 hospitalizations per 100,000 population and a 5–10% mortality rate. It is the result of bleeding from any part of the GI tract proximal to the ligament of Treitz (Lewis et al. 2002).

Patients with acute UGIB can present with one or more of the following: coffee ground vomiting, hematemesis, melena, and/or hematochezia. The determining factor for the way these patients present is directly related to the rate and severity of bleeding; the slower the bleeding, the darker the appearance of the blood and vice versa.

Melena indicates blood that has been present in the GI tract for at least 14 h and it is more likely to be the result of an upper bleeding source. However, 5–10% of melena can be due to a very slow bleeding from a lower GI source. Hematochezia on the other hand, which is mostly the result of lower GI bleeding, can be a manifestation of an upper GI bleeding lesion in around 15% of the instances when the blood loss is more than 1 L and transit time is less than 4 h in association with hemodynamic instability.

From: *Clinical Gastroenterology: Diagnostic and Therapeutic Procedures in Gastroenterology*,
Edited by: G. Y. Wu, S. Sridhar, DOI 10.1007/978-1-59745-044-7_4,

Nasogastric (NG) lavage can be helpful in confirming the upper source of the bleeding when blood or coffee ground colored contents are aspirated. However, a non-bloody aspirate does not rule it out. NG lavage can be negative in up to 16% of patients with UGIB, especially those with duodenal source. Endoscopy then remains the mainstay modality for finding the exact source.

CAUSES OF UGIB

Multiple endoscopic studies evaluating patients with UGIB have revealed different causes with varying degrees of incidence.

A prospective series evaluating 1,000 cases with UGIB showed the following (Jutabha and Jensen 1996):

1. Peptic ulcer disease was the most common cause, accounting for about 55% of the cases. *H. pylori* infection and nonsteroidal antiinflammatory drugs were the major culprits in addition to stress and gastrin hypersecretion. Rare infections such as *Herpes simplex* and cytomegalovirus can lead to ulcers in immunosuppressed patients.
2. Varices including esophageal or gastric in patients with cirrhosis or mesenteric veins thrombosis accounted for about 14%.
3. Arteriovenous malformation, 6%.
4. Mallory–Weiss tears, 5%.
5. Tumors and erosions, 4% each: benign tumors include leiomyoma, lipomas, or polyps while malignant ones include adenocarcinoma, lymphoma, Kaposi sarcoma, carcinoid, or melanoma.
6. Dieulafoy's lesions, which consist of protruding vessels without the presence of ulcers, accounted for about 1%.
7. Other rare causes, 11%: gastric antral vascular ectasia, radiation-induced telangiectasia, blue rubber bleb nevus syndrome, aortoenteric fistula, and postsurgical conditions.

Another larger database study focusing on 243,428 upper endoscopies performed between 2000 and 2004 showed that ulcers were the most common endoscopic findings in patients with UGIB accounting for 33% of the cases, followed by erosions which accounted for 19%. Gastric ulcers were more common than duodenal ulcers, 55% versus 37%. Patients with variceal bleeding were excluded from the analysis (Enestvedt et al. 2008).

In this chapter, we have concentrated only on the endoscopic management of peptic ulcer bleeding.

Initial Evaluation of Patients with UGI Bleeding

Stability of the patients' vital signs and hemodynamics is crucial to obtain prior to any kind of endoscopic intervention. Patients develop orthostatic hypotension after losing approximately 20% of their total blood volume, and develop shock after more than 40% loss. Intravenous fluid resuscitation and blood transfusion are very important initial interventions to ensure patients' stability.

Once the patient has become hemodynamically stable, upper endoscopy can be performed to provide diagnosis and further prognostic information, both of which will dictate subsequent management.

Several risk factors influence the outcome of an acute UGIB with regard to rebleeding and mortality. A prospective multicenter population-based study including almost 4,000 patients has shown that age, shock, and comorbidity prior to endoscopy, diagnosis, and

Table 1
Numerical score for independent predictors of mortality

	Score			
Variable	0	1	2	3
Age	<60	60–79	>80	
Shock	No shock SBP≥100 HR<100	Tachycardia HR≥100 SBP≥100	Hypotension SBP<100	
Comorbidities	No major comorbidities		CHF CAD	Renal failure, liver failure, disseminated malignancy
Diagnosis	MWT No lesion No SRH	All other diagnosis	Malignant upper GI tract	
Major SRH	None or dark spot only		Blood in the upper tract, adherent clot, visible or spurting vessel	

stigmata of recent hemorrhage (SRH) postendoscopy are all independent predictors of mortality. A numerical score using these parameters was then formulated and validated to predict outcomes in such patients (Table 1) (Rockall et al. 1996).

An initial risk score of 0 predicts a 0.2% mortality in contrast to 50% mortality with a maximum score of 7. A complete risk score of 0 predicts no mortality versus more than 40% with a score of 8 or higher (maximum 11). Both mortality and rebleeding rates increased in a stepwise fashion as the score goes up. This scoring system can be very helpful in identifying patients who are at low risk of rebleeding and negligible risk of death and hence might be considered for early discharge or outpatient treatment with consequent resource savings (Rockall et al. 1996).

Anatomy of a Bleeding Ulcer

Peptic ulcers usually bleed because of erosion into an underlying medium-sized arteriole in the submucosal plexus of vessels. Posterior wall duodenal bulb ulcers and lesser curve gastric ulcers usually bleed because of erosion into larger caliber arterioles and, therefore, fall into high-risk group of ulcers. Endoscopic therapy usually stops the bleeding if the underlying vessel is smaller than 1 mm in size (Swain et al. 1986).

Timing of Endoscopy

The timing of endoscopy has been a subject of debate in patients who are supposedly "stable." It is known that about 80% of the patients stop bleeding with no therapy and, therefore, it has been debated whether endoscopy in those patients makes any difference to their outcome. A subgroup of patients may have risk factors for recurrent bleeding and, therefore, endoscopic examination may provide important information for appropriate and effective therapy. Spiegel et al. investigated the optimal timing of endoscopy after presentation in patients with gastrointestinal bleeding. Twenty-three studies were reviewed. The largest randomized trial of high-risk patients showed no mortality benefit, but a significant decrease in transfusion requirements with early endoscopy. Seven of the eight studies, examining the effect of early endoscopy on the length of stay as a measure of resource utilization, demonstrated a significant reduction in cost compared with that of delayed endoscopy (Spiegel et al. 2001). The definition of urgent endoscopy is performing procedure between 2 to 24 hours after presentation with bleeding. The National Institute of Health and the American Society of Gastrointestinal Endoscopy recommends urgent endoscopy for patients who present with active bleeding or those considered as "high-risk" patient for rebleeding (Consensus Development Panel 1989; Standards of Practice Committee 1992).

Administration of proton pump inhibitors (PPI) before endoscopy have been studied by Lau et al. for a preemptive effect on the need for endoscopic therapy. It was shown that high-dose omeprazole, 80 mg IV bolus followed by continuous infusion of 8 mg/h before endoscopy accelerated the resolution of signs of bleeding in ulcers and reduced the need for endoscopic therapy (Lau et al. 2007).

ENDOSCOPIC THERAPY OF BLEEDING PEPTIC ULCERS

Peptic ulcers are the most common causes of UGIB accounting for about half of the cases. Gastric or duodenal ulcers can be classified endoscopically according to Forrest classification as shown in Table 2 and Fig. 1:

Rebleeding rates and mortality of each of the above ulcers with and without endoscopic interventions are shown in Table 3 (Laine et al. 1996; Jensen 1999).

Class I and II ulcers do clearly benefit from endoscopic therapy as discussed below.

Patient Monitoring

It is important to maintain adequate oxygenation of the patient as arterial desaturation can occur during the procedure. Pulse oxymetry and blood pressures should be continually recorded. Pressurized infusion bags and resuscitation equipment should be readily available. Competent assistants and nurses should be monitoring the patient and assisting the endoscopist.

Table 2
Forrest classification

Active bleeding	
Class Ia	Ulcer with arterial spurting
Class Ib	Ulcer with active oozing
Signs of recent hemorrhage	
Class IIa	Ulcer with nonbleeding visible vessel
Class IIb	Ulcer with adherent clot
Class IIc	Ulcer with hematin cover
No signs of recent hemorrhage	
Class III	Ulcer with clean base

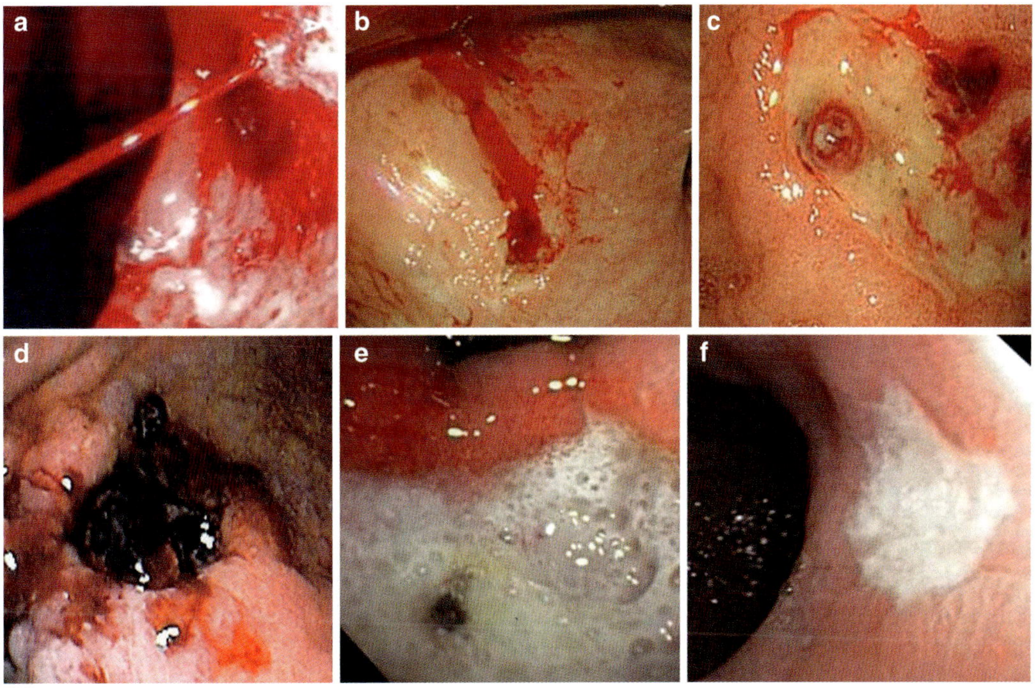

Fig. 1. Forrest classification (**a**) Class Ia ulcer; (**b**) Class Ib ulcer; (**c**) Class IIa ulcer; (**d**) Class IIb ulcer; (**e**) Class IIc ulcer; (**f**) Class III ulcer.

Table 3
Rebleeding rates and mortality of ulcers with and without endoscopic interventions

Findings	*% Rebleeding without endoscopic treatment*	*% Mortality*	*Rebleeding after endoscopic therapy*
Active arterial spurting	90	11	15–30
Visible vessel	50	11	15–30
Adherent clot	12–33	7	5
Oozing without stigmata	10–27	?	N/A
Flat pigment spot	7	3	N/A
Clean based	<5	2	N/A

Patient Position

The left lateral position is generally preferred. In this position, blood in the stomach gravitates towards the fundus and the greater curve of the body of the stomach. Occasionally, the patient is rolled to the right lateral decubitus position and occasionally the head of the bed is elevated into a sitting position so that the cardia of the stomach can be well examined as shown in Fig. 2.

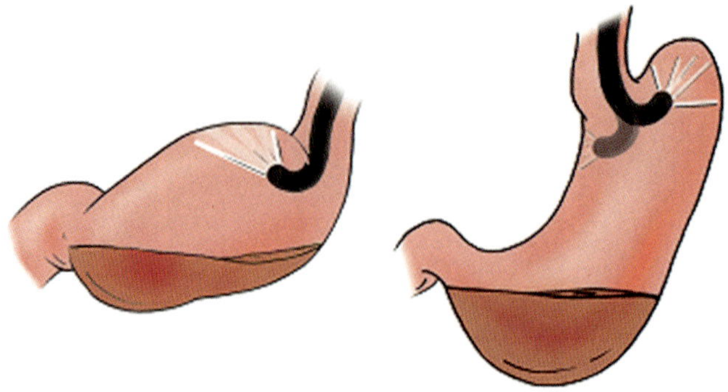

Fig. 2. Patient positions.

GASTRIC LAVAGE

Gastric lavage is usually unnecessary as the majority of the bleeding lesions are located in the duodenum, antrum, or lesser curvature while most of the blood tends to pool in the fundus when the patient is lying in the left lateral decubitus position. However, if lavage is still needed, an overtube can be placed to protect the airway while repeated intubation for lavage is performed.

ENDOSCOPIC TREATMENT

Endoscopy can be performed using a diagnostic or a therapeutic endoscope. Each has its own advantages and disadvantages. The diagnostic endoscope is more flexible and easy to manipulate, but it has a smaller 2.8 mm instrument channel that limits irrigation and suctioning in addition to only accommodating a 7 French multipolar or heater probe. On the other hand, the therapeutic scope has two channels, a 2.8 mm and a 3.7 mm one. One channel can be used for irrigation and/or suctioning while the other can be used to introduce an injection needle or a 10 Fr probe. However, the therapeutic endoscope has a larger external diameter, is less flexible and, therefore, harder to manipulate.

Endoscopic therapeutic interventions include thermal and nonthermal techniques. The thermal techniques can be divided into electrocoagulation and nonelectrocoagulation, while the nonthermal ones include needle injection, tissue glue, and endoclip placement (Table 4).

Thermal Therapy

Electrothermocoagulation

This thermal method uses direct heat therapy in combination with mechanical compression to produce a strong sealing of the bleeding vessel. Several types of probes are available for endoscopic therapy; they can be applied directly or with an acute angle and most of them have built in irrigation channel to help wash away blood and clots. The three currently available methods are the monopolar, liquid monopolar, and the multipolar

Table 4
Agents and devices for the treatment of GI bleeding

Accessories needed
Therapeutic endoscope (preferred)
Injection needle
Multipolar or heat probe
Endoclips
Epinephrine
Sclerosing agent

electrocoagulation. In monopolar electrocoagulation, the current flows through the patient and exits via a ground plate. However, the depth of coagulation and tissue adherance is unpredictable, thus rendering this method less popular for use. The liquid monopolar or electrohydrothermal method allows the application of a film of water or normal saline to the tip of the probe to reduce tissue stickiness, but does not solve the problem of lack of predictability of the depth of tissue injury. The multipolar probe is made of three pairs of electrodes arranged in a linear array at the tip connected to a power generator. Patient grounding is not needed since the flow of the electrical current is limited to between the electrodes on the probe where tissue can be heated up to 100°C on contact. The depth of the injury is shallow compared to the previously mentioned two methods, with less risk for transmural damage and capability to coagulate vessels of up to 2 mm in diameter. Seven Fr and ten Fr probes are available. The latter requires a therapeutic scope with 3.7 mm inner channel diameter.

The Technique

The probe should be pushed firmly against the blood vessel while delivering the heat to achieve good foot-printing and, hence, more lasting homeostasis. Here, the larger (10 Fr) probe is preferred. A low current setting is recommended (15 and 25 W) and a sustained period of probe application is used (10–14, 2-s pulses).

Nonelectrothermocoagulation

This includes heat probe and microwave coagulation. A heat probe consists of a metal tip covered with Teflon that is heated by a computer-controlled coil to a temperature of 250°C in order to deliver 15–30 joules of energy. The probe should be pushed firmly against the vessel while delivering the energy for about 8 s of contact time followed by extensive irrigation prior to retrieval of the probe in order to minimize tissue shearing and immediate rebleeding. On the other hand, microwave coagulation uses microwave energy directed to tissue via a 2.7 mm diameter coaxial cable, the terminal portion of which ends in a needle-like electrode, which projects about 2–3 mm. The bleeding lesion is penetrated by the electrode and microwave energy is delivered to be absorbed by water-rich tissue that results in thermal coagulation. Vessels up to 3 mm in size can be coagulated.

The Technique

Here, a larger probe is preferred (10 Fr) and a firm pressure is applied over the bleeding point using 3–4, 30 J pulses before changing the position. A "probe print or cavitation" at the site of the bleeding point is considered a good endpoint.

INJECTION THERAPY

Agents Used

This is a nonthermal technique that uses epinephrine or sclerosants such as 1% polidocanol, 5% ethanolamine, absolute alcohol, 1.5% sodium tetradecyl sulfate, hypertonic saline, and 50% dextrose solution (Table 5). Epinephrine is the most commonly established and widely used agent for homeostasis of ulcers. Injection therapy can be used with standard endoscope using a disposable 23 or 25 Ga sclerotherapy needle Epinephrine or sclerosants are injected into and around the bleeding point at the base of the ulcer to raise submucosal blebs followed by cessation of bleeding.

The mechanism of action of epinephrine is believed to be prolonged vasoconstriction for up to 2 h, platelet activation and aggregation, and activation of the coagulation cascade (Chung et al. 1990; ÓBrien 1963). With large volumes, it also exerts a local temponade effect on the vessel (Leung et al. 1994). It is metabolized on a first pass by the liver and hence, up to 20 mL can be injected safely in patient with good liver function. More care and smaller volumes should be used in patients with hepatic dysfunction because of the risk for systemic side effects, the most common of which is tachycardia (Sung et al. 1993). Epinephrine has a low tissue-damaging potential and does not cause ulcers, necrosis, or perforation. It can be injected blindly into the pool of blood in active bleeding patients in order to slow the bleeding and localize the lesion for further direct interventions (Leung et al. 1994).

Sclerosants, on the other hand, cause bowel wall spasm and early edema with subsequent inflammation and thrombosis of the vessel. Absolute alcohol causes rapid dehydration and rapid fixation of the tissue leading to obliteration of the bleeding vessel. The degree of tissue damage is directly related to the volume of the sclerosant injected with higher volumes carrying higher risk for ulceration and perforation.

Table 5
Agents for the treatment of GI bleeding

Sclerosing agents
Polidocanol, 1%
Ethanolamine, 5%
Absolute alcohol
Sodium tetradecyl sulfate, 1.5%
Hypertonic saline
Dextrose solution, 50%

Thrombin/Fibrin Glue

Injection of a solution of thrombin and fibrinogen via a standard injection needle can obliterate and compress the bleeding point. Thrombin promotes the conversion of fibrinogen to fibrin leading to the production of a local fibrin clot without any potential for tissue injury or necrosis. However, the potential complications include thrombosis, embolization, viral transmission, and anaphylactic reaction; it is still not FDA approved for endoscopic use.

The Technique

An injection needle with a retractable tip is used. Generally, 1:10,000 concentration of epinephrine is used. We use smaller volumes of the solution in aliquots of 1–2 mL. We recommend injecting, if possible, all the four quadrants at least 3–4 mm away from the bleeding point. The assistant should be instructed to retract the needle after each aliquot of injection. Generally, mucosal paleness is noted after injection of epinephrine. The nursing assistant may encounter resistance in injecting the solution. We usually inject the mucosa distal to the bleeding point first, which may raise the mucosa and tilt the bleeding point towards the endoscope. Whether the use of smaller or larger volumes of epinephrine is preferable is a matter of debate. Lin and his group have proposed larger volumes of epinephrine (mean 16.5 mL) as the rebleeding risk was lower in this group when compared with smaller volumes, 15.4% versus 30.8%, with a mean of 8 mL (Lin et al. 2002a).

MECHANICAL CLIPS

Hemoclip application is a mechanical method of homeostasis. The clips can control large-sized arterioles. The clips can be cumbersome and difficult to deploy in difficult locations and especially in the retroflexed position. Clip application is not for diffuse bleeding with no identifiable vessel. Four types of endoclips are currently available on the market: The Rotating clip, the QuickClip, the TriClip, and the Resolution clip. Specifications of each of these devices are summarized in Table 6.

Before starting the procedure, the Rotating clip is loaded onto an applicator and kept ready for use. The applicator can be reused after sterilization. Although this device is cheaper compared to the other clips that are disposable, a major drawback is the need to reload the device with a clip in the middle of the procedure. This can be easily overcome by preloading two or three clip applicators before the start of the procedure and keeping them ready to use. QuickClip is a single-use device that comes preloaded on a disposable applicator in a sterile package. The TriClip is a three-pronged single-use device with a flushing mechanism. An advantage of the Resolution clip is that it can be opened and closed up to five times to achieve a satisfactory position prior to deployment (Fig. 3). Although not specifically designed to be rotated, it can be rotated counterclockwise with minimal effort, if needed.

Table 6
Types of clips and their specifications (Modified from Kaltenbach et al. 2006)

Company Product Name	*Olympus*			*Boston Scientific*	*Wilson Cook*	
	Rotating Clip	QuickClip 2	QuickClip 2 Long	Resolution Clip	TriClip	TriClip
Catalog number	HX-LR/QR-1 HX-6UR-1	HX-201LR/ UR-135	HX-201LR/UR-135 L	M005226XX	TC-8–12	TC-7–12
Ready-to-use	No	Yes	Yes	Yes	Yes	Yes
Clip size	>2.8 mm (5LR/ QR) >3.2 mm (6UR)	>2.8 mm	>2.8 mm	>2.8 mm	>3.2 mm	>2.8 mm
Working length	230 cm (6U), 195 cm (5Q) and 165 cm (5 L)	240 cm (UR) and 165 cm (LR)	240 cm (UR), 165cm (LR)	235 cm 155 cm	205 cm	207 cm
Maximum Clip length (initial)	Various Max 17 mm	15 mm	17 mm	20 mm	18.5 mm	18.5 mm
Maximum Clip length (deployed)	Various Max 13 mm	11 mm	13 mm	15.5 mm	14.5 mm	14.5 mm
Maximum opening width	Various Max 11 mm	9.5 mm	11 mm	11 mm	12 mm	12 mm
Rotatability	Rotatable	Rotatable	Rotatable	Not Rotatable	Not rotatable	Not rotatable
Flushing	No	No	No	No	Yes	No
Re-opening capability	None	None	None	Up to five times	None	None
Clip material	Stainless steel	Stainless steel	Stainless steel	Stainless steel	Stainless steel	Stainless steel
Radiopacity	Radiopaque	Radiopaque	Radiopaque	Radiopaque	Radiopaque	Radiopaque

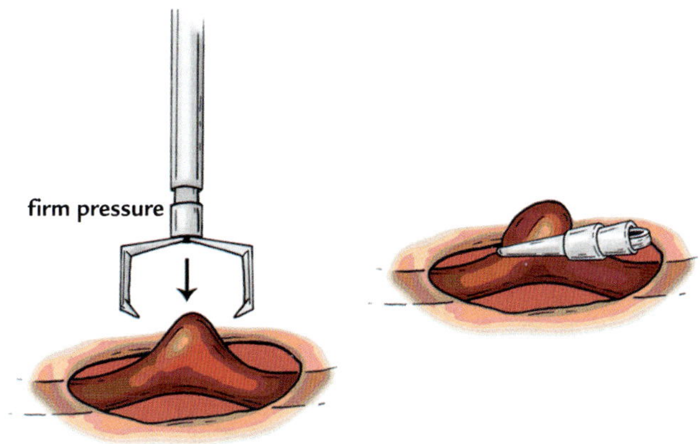

Fig. 3. Clip application.

The Technique

The operator and the assistant should be familiar with the type of clip being used and the method of clip application. It is also very important to have a rough idea of the direction of blood flow in the underlying arteriole. The clip applicator exits the endoscope at the 8 o'clock position of the endoscopic field and therefore any lesion at this position is easier to be targeted. It is also important to rotate the shaft of the endoscope to bring the bleeding vessel to this position. First, the outer sheath should be pulled back to barely expose the tip of the clip prior to insertion into the channel. The device is then inserted into the channel of the endoscope. Once the tip is visualized on the screen, the outer sheath should be pulled further for full exposure of the clip. The clip is then opened to its "maximum" width, rotated to the desired angle (only for rotatable clips), placed over the target, closed, and deployed (note that only the resolution clip may be reopened if position is not satisfactory). The handles of different clips vary slightly in the direction of forces applied to perform each of the prementioned steps. The direction of the course of the underlying arteriole is important. We try to apply the first clip proximal to the bleeding point and the second clip distal to it on the bleeding vessel. By using this method, we achieve clipping of both sides of the underlying arteriole (Figs. 4 and 5).

CHOICE OF TECHNIQUES

Three therapies are currently considered to be standard with respect to endoscopic management of nonvariceal UGIB, mainly bleeding ulcers. This includes epinephrine injection, thermal contact devices (multipolar or heat probe), and endoclip placement.

Multiple studies of epinephrine injection vs. thermal therapy have shown no significant difference between the two modalities. But, other randomized trials have shown that the addition of thermal or sclerosant therapy to epinephrine injection was superior to epinephrine injection alone, especially in patients with actively bleeding vessels. On the other hand, other data showed that epinephrine followed by thermal therapy provided better efficacy than thermal therapy alone (Bianco et al. 2004). However, a recent meta-analysis of 20 studies showed that dual endoscopic therapy proved significantly superior to

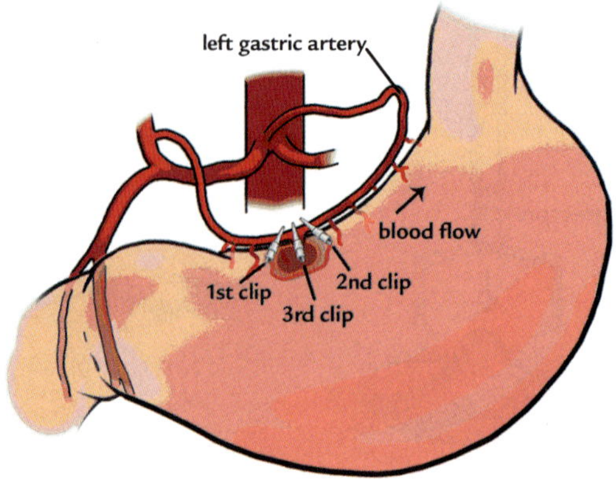

Fig. 4. Clip application with respect to blood flow.

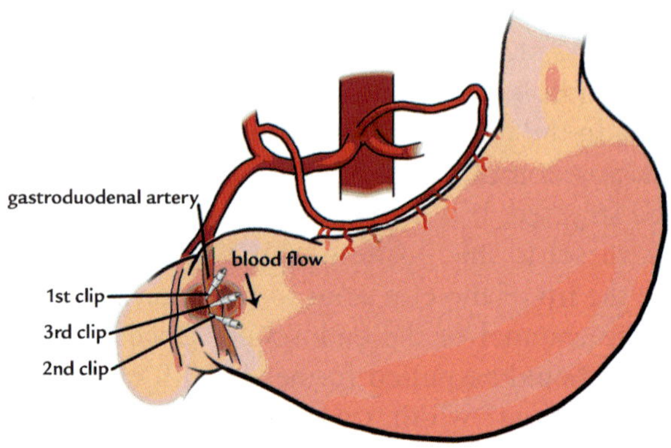

Fig. 5. Clip application with respect to blood flow.

epinephrine injection alone, but had no advantage over thermal or mechanical monotherapy in improving the outcome of patients with high-risk patients with peptic disease (Marmo et al. 2007). Even after endoscopic therapy, rebleeding rates remained around 20%.

With respect to hemoclips, several randomized trials are available. One study by Cipolletta et al. evaluated hemoclip versus heater probe in 113 patients with major stigmata of ulcer hemorrhage and showed that hemoclip was safe and effective in treatment of severe ulcer bleeding and was superior to heater probe in preventing early recurrent bleeding (Cipolletta et al. 2001). On the other hand, Gevers et al. evaluated sclerosant injection versus hemoclip application versus combination of the two in 105 patients with non-bleeding or actively bleeding visible vessels. The use of hemoclips alone appeared to fail because of difficulty with hemoclip placements and incomplete vessel compressions and the mechanical therapy was inferior to injection therapy (Gevers et al. 2002). A randomized trial by Lin et al. studied the effectiveness of hemoclip versus heater probe in 80 patients with actively bleeding or nonbleeding visible vessels. Heater probe was shown to be superior to hemoclip in control of bleeding, with initial homeostasis achieved in 85% of the patients in the hemoclip group versus 100% in the heater probe group (Lin et al. 2002b).

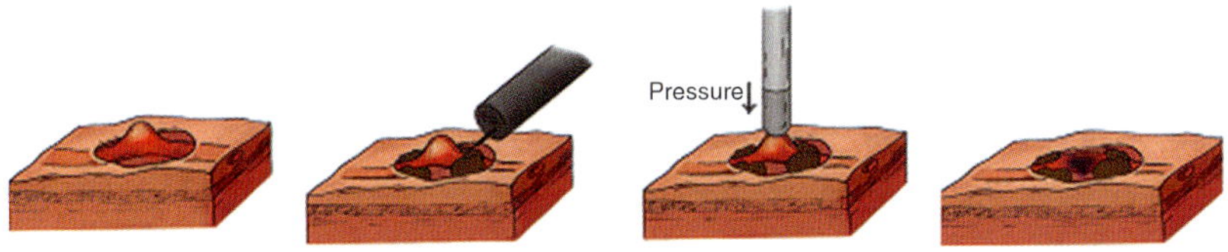

Fig. 6. Needle injection followed by thermal therapy.

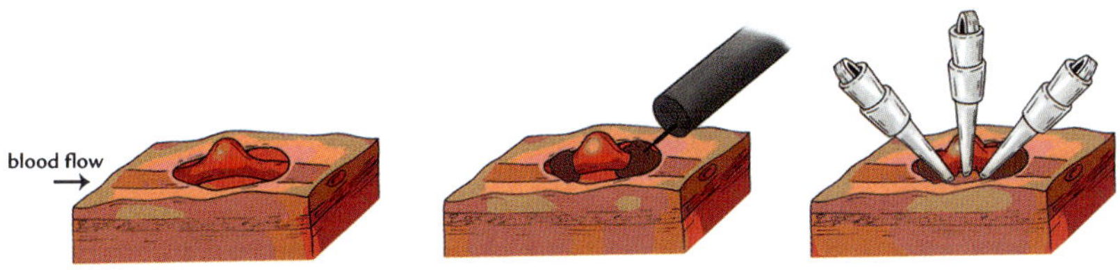

Fig. 7. Needle injection followed by clip placement.

The variability of these results suggested that the effectiveness of mechanical therapy could be operator-dependent.

The choice of endoscopic treatment (Figs. 6 and 7) also depends on the stigmata of the underlying ulcer at the time of endoscopy (Table 7).

Forrest Class Ia and Ib (Actively Bleeding Ulcers)

For these types of ulcers, the authors prefer injecting smaller volumes of 1:10,000 epinephrine, up to a total of 15–20 mL, in four quadrants within 2–4 mm of the bleeding point, followed by either mechanical clip application or thermal therapy using a large probe. The probe is applied with firm pressure, using 20–25 W power, setting 10 s. with 10 s pulses. This is followed by irrigation and removal of the probe. The same method is repeated if necessary until a good probe print is visible. If clip application is chosen based on the site of the ulcer and the rough anatomical course of the underlying arteriole, then a resolution clip is applied first proximally to the bleeding point, then distal to the bleeding point, and finally directly on the bleeding point (Chung et al. 1997; Jensen et al. 1994).

Forrest Class IIa (Ulcer with Nonbleeding Visible Vessel)

For this type of ulcer, we use either a combination of epinephrine plus thermal therapy or epinephrine plus clip application or thermal therapy alone. The method is the same as described above for Forrest types Ia and Ib.

Forrest Class IIb (Ulcer with Adherent Clot)

For this type of ulcer, our approach is to irrigate the clot with a jet of water followed by injection of aliquots of 1:10,000 epinephrine as described above. We use a snare (without current) to trim the clot very carefully, as shown in Fig. 8 (Jensen et al. 1996). Extra care

Table 7
Endoscopic therapy recommendations and end points

	Forrest class Ia (spurting)	*Forrest class Ib (oozing)*	*Forrest II a (visible vessel)*	*Forrest IIb (adherent clot)*
Epinephrine	Yes	Yes	Yes	Yes
Probe size	Large	Large	Large	Large
Probe pressure	Firm	Firm	Firm	Firm
Power setting	15–20 W	15–20 W	15–20 W	15–20 W
Pulse duration	8–10 s	8–10 s	8–10 s	8–10 s
Clip	Yes	Yes	Yes	Yes
End point	Bleeding stops	Oozing stops	Vessel flattens or successful clipping	Vessel flattens or successful clipping

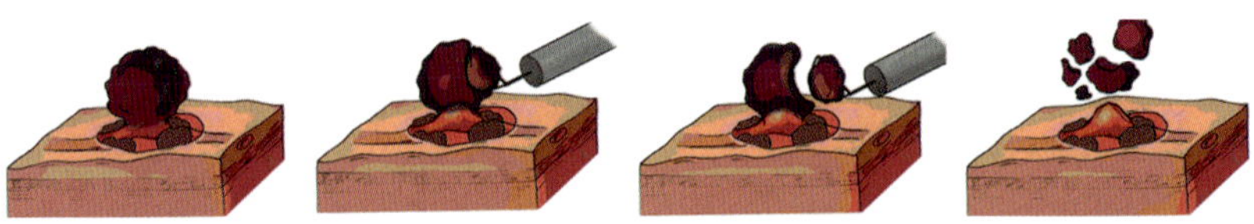

Fig. 8. Clot removal.

should be taken not to guillotine the clot entirely from the base. This may shear off the underlying arteriole and precipitate bleeding. If the underlying vessel is exposed well, then we use the method as described for Forrest IIa ulcers.

Forrest IIc and III types of ulcers generally do not require endoscopic therapy.

Post-endoscopic Therapy

Although endoscopic therapy is effective for bleeding peptic ulcers, bleeding does recur in up to 15–20% of patients (Lau et al. 2000). Most of the rebleeding occurs within the first 3 days and the mortality rate in these patients is high. In vitro studies have shown that a high intragastric pH can facilitate platelet aggregation, suggesting that inhibition of gastric acid secretion to maintain a neutral PH should stabilize clots and prevent recurrent bleeding (O'Brien et al. 1963). IV proton pump inhibitor (PPI) infusion after endoscopic homeostasis (80 mg IV bolus followed by 8 mg per h) for 72 h was studied in 240 patients and was shown to decrease the percent for rebleeding to around 7% (Lau et al. 2000).

Lau et al. compared endoscopic retreatment to surgery in patients who rebled. Bleeding was considered to have recurred in the event of any one of the following: vomiting of fresh blood, hypotension and melena, or a requirement of more than four units of blood in the 72-h period after endoscopy. Forty-eight patients with rebleeding were assigned to endoscopic retreatment and 44 were assigned to surgery. Of the 48 patients, 35 had long-term control of bleeding while the other 13 had undergone salvage surgery, 11 because retreatment failed, and two because of perforation. Five patients in the endoscopy retreatment group died within 30 days compared to eight patients in the surgery group ($P=0.37$). Seven patients in the endoscopy group (including six who underwent salvage surgery) had complications compared to 16 in the surgery group ($P=0.03$). It was concluded that endoscopic retreatment reduced the need for surgery without increasing the risk of death, and was associated with fewer complications (Lau et al. 1999).

Mallory–Weiss Tears

Mallory–Weiss tears usually occur on the gastric side of the gastroesophageal junction. Bleeding stops spontaneously in 80–90% of patients and recurs only in 0–5%. Endoscopic therapy is effective for actively bleeding patients, but is not needed if no active bleeding is seen.

Second-Look Endoscopy

Second-look endoscopy is usually not necessary after successful endoscopic therapy unless rebleeding occurs. However, in patients with gastric ulcers, relook endoscopy in 6–8 weeks should be performed to confirm complete healing of the ulcers while the patient is on PPI therapy and off nonsteroidal antiinflammatory drugs. Further investigations should be performed for nonhealing ulcers.

CONCLUSIONS

Endoscopic management of acute UGIB has evolved greatly over the years. The techniques should be carefully chosen depending on the severity of the bleeding, ulcer location, availability of equipment and, most importantly, the experience of the endoscopist.

SUMMARY OF KEY POINTS

- Acute upper GI bleeding (UGIB) is a common medical emergency with an annual rate of 150–200 hospitalizations per 100,000 population and a 5–10% mortality rate.
- Nasogastric (NG) lavage can be helpful in confirming the upper source of the bleeding when blood or coffee ground colored contents are aspirated. However, a non-bloody aspirate does not rule it out. NG lavage can be negative in up to 16% of patients with UGIB, especially those with duodenal source.
- Patients develop orthostatic hypotension after losing approximately 20% of their total blood volume, and develop shock after more than 40% loss.
- The National Institute of Health and the American Society of Gastrointestinal Endoscopy recommends urgent endoscopy for patients who present with active bleeding or those patients considered as "high-risk" for rebleeding.
- Administration of proton pump inhibitors (PPI) before endoscopy accelerated the resolution of signs of bleeding in ulcers and reduced the need for endoscopic therapy.
- Endoscopic therapeutic interventions include thermal and nonthermal techniques.
- The techniques should be carefully chosen depending on the severity of the bleeding, ulcer location, availability of equipment, and the experience of the endoscopist.

ACKNOWLEDGMENTS

I respectfully acknowledge Dr. Dharma Thiruvaiyaru, Ph.D., Dept. of Mathematics, Statistics and Computer Sciences, Augusta State University, Augusta, Georgia, for critically reviewing the chapter.

REFERENCES

Bianco MA, Rotondano G, Marmo R, Piscopo R, Orsini L, Cipolletta L. Combined epinephrine and bipolar probe coagulation vs. bipolar probe coagulation alone for bleeding peptic ulcer: a randomized controlled trial. Gastrointest Endosc. 2004;60:910–5.

Chung SCS, Leung JWC, Leung FW. Effect of submucosal epinephrine injection on local gastric blood flow: a study using laser doppler flowmetry and reflectance spectrophotometry. Dig Dis Sci. 1990;35:1008–11.

Chung SS, Lau JY, Sung JJ, Chan AC, Lai CW, Ng EK, et al. Randomised comparison between adrenaline injection alone or adrenaline injection plus heat probe treatment for actively bleeding ulcers. Br Med J. 1997;314:1307–11.

Cipolletta L, Bianco MA, Marmo R, Rotondano G, Piscopo R, Vingiani AM, et al. Endoclips versus heater probe in preventing early recurrent bleeding from peptic ulcer: a prospective and randomized trial. Gastrointest Endosc. 2001;53:147–51.

Consensus Development Panel. Therapeutic endoscopy and bleeding ulcers. J Am Med Assoc. 1989;262:1369–72.

Enestvedt BK, Gralnek IM, Mattek N, Lieberman DA, Eisen G. An evaluation of endoscopic indications and findings related to nonvariceal upper-GI hemorrhage in a large multicenter consortium. Gastrointest Endosc. 2008;67:422–9.

Gevers AM, De Goede E, Simoens M, Hiele M, Rutgeerts P. A randomized trial comparing injection therapy with hemoclip and with injection combined with hemoclip for bleeding ulcers. Gastrointest Endosc. 2002;55:466–9.

Jensen DM. Endoscopic control of nonvariceal upper gastrointestinal hemorrhage. In: Yamada T, Alpers DH, Laine L, Owyang C, Powell DW, editors. Textbook of Gastroenterology. 3rd ed. Philadelphia: Lippincott Williams & Wilkins; 1999. p. 2857–79.

Jensen DM, Kovacs TO, Randall GM, et al. Prospective study of thermal coagulation (Gold probe) versus combination injection and thermal treatment of high risk patients with severe ulcer or Mallory Weiss bleeding. Gastrointest Endosc. 1994;40:25.

Jensen DM, Kovacs TOG, Jutabha R, Savides T, Cheng S, Jensen ME, et al. Initial results of a multicenter, randomized controlled trial of medical versus combination endoscopic therapy for prevention of recurrent severe ulcer hemorrhage from non-bleeding adherent clots. Gastrointest Endosc. 1996;43:352.

Jutabha R, Jensen DM. Management of severe upper gastrointestinal bleeding in the patient with liver disease. Med Clin North Am. 1996;80:1035–68.

Kaltenbach T, Friedland S, Barro J, Soetikno R. Clipping for upper gastrointestinal bleeding. Am J Gastroenterol. 2006;101:915–8.

Laine L, Stein C, Sharma V. A prospective outcome study of patients with clot in an ulcer and the effect of irrigation. Gastrointest Endosc. 1996;43:107–10.199.

Lau JY, Sung JJ, Lam YH, Chan AC, Ng EK, Lee DW, et al. Endoscopic retreatment compared with surgery in patients with recurrent bleeding after initial endoscopic control of bleeding ulcers. N Engl J Med. 1999;340:751–6.

Lau JY, Sung JJ, Lee KK, Yung MY, Wong SK, Wu JC, et al. Effect of intravenous omeprazole on recurrent bleeding after endoscopic treatment of bleeding peptic ulcers. N Engl J Med. 2000;343:310–6.

Lau JY, Leung WK, Wu JCY, Chan FKL, Wong VWS, Chiu PWY, et al. Omeprazole before endoscopy in patients with gastrointestinal bleeding. N Engl J Med. 2007;356:1631–40.

Leung JW, Chung SCS. Practical management of nonvariceal upper gastrointestinal bleeding. In: Tytgat GNJ, Classen M, editors. Practice of therapeutic endoscopy. New York: Longman group; 1994. p. 1–16.

Lewis JD, Bilker WB, Farrar JT, Strom BL. Hospitalization and mortality rates from peptic ulcer disease and GI bleeding in the 1990s: relationship to sales of nonsteroidal anti-inflammatory drugs and acid suppression medications. Am J Gastroenterol. 2002;97:2540–9.

Lin HJ, Hsieh YH, Tseng GY, Perng CL, Chang FY, Lee SD. A prospective, randomized trial of large-versus small-volume endoscopic injection of epinephrine for peptic ulcer bleeding. Gastrointest Endosc. 2002;55:615–9.

Lin HJ, Hsieh YH, Tseng GY. A prospective, randomized trial of endoscopic hemoclip versus heater probe thermocoagulation for peptic ulcer disease. Am J Gastroenterol. 2002 Sep; 97(9):2250–4.

Marmo R, Marmo R, Rotondano G, Piscopo R, Bianco MA, D'Angella R, et al. Dual therapy versus monotherapy in the endoscopic treatment of high-risk bleeding ulcers: a meta-analysis of controlled trials. Am J Gastroenterol. 2007;102:279–89.

O'Brien JR. Some effects of adrenaline and anti-adrenaline compounds on platelets in vitro and in vivo. Nature. 1963;200:763–4.

Rockall TA, Logan RFA, Devlin HB, Northfield TC. Risk assessment after acute gastrointestinal haemorrhage. Gut. 1996;38:316–21.

Spiegel BM, Vakil NB, Ofman JJ. Endoscopy for acute nonvariceal upper gastrointestinal tract hemorrhage: is sooner better? A systematic review. Arch Intern Med. 2001;161:1393–404.

Standards of Practice Committee. The role of endoscopy in the management of non-variceal acute upper gastrointestinal bleeding. Guidelines for clinical application. Gastrointest Endosc. 1992;38:760–4.

Sung JY, Chung SCS, Low JM, Cocks R, Ip SM, Tan P, et al. Systemic absorption of epinephrine after endoscopic submucosal injection in patients with bleeding peptic ulcers. Gastrointest Endosc. 1993;39:20–2.

Swain CP, Storey DW, Bown SG, Heath J, Mills TN, Salmon PR, et al. Nature of the bleeding vessel in recurrently bleeding gastric ulcers. Gastroenterology. 1986;90:595–608.

5 Endoscopic Management of Varices and Variceal Hemorrhage

Joshua Hall and Subbaramiah Sridhar

CONTENTS

Keywords: Endoscopic, Management, Varices, Variceal, Hemorrhage

INTRODUCTION

Acute variceal hemorrhage is a medical emergency. Approximately 40% of patients with cirrhosis are found to have esophageal varices on endoscopic evaluation (Bosch et al. 2003), and approximately one third of patients will experience variceal hemorrhage (Kleber et al. 1991; The North Italian Endoscopic Club for the Study and Treatment of Esophageal Varices 1988). The mortality of an initial variceal hemorrhage has been found to be as high as 30% (The North Italian Endoscopic Club for the Study and Treatment of Esophageal Varices 1988). The risk of variceal hemorrhage is increased in large varices and in those that demonstrate red wale markings, as well as in patients with high Child's scores, those with previous episodes of variceal hemorrhage, and in patients who continue to ingest alcohol (The North Italian Endoscopic Club for the Study and Treatment of Esophageal Varices 1988). The size of the varix is the single most important predictor of bleeding risk. Primary prophylaxis of varices should be considered in varices larger than 5 mm (de Franchis and Primignani 2001). Esophageal varices are graded according to size and appearance. Grade 1 varices are small, straight, and flatten with distention of the esophagus (Fig. 1). Grade 2 varices are tortuous, comprise less than one third of the lumen,

From: *Clinical Gastroenterology: Diagnostic and Therapeutic Procedures in Gastroenterology*,
Edited by: G. Y. Wu, S. Sridhar, DOI 10.1007/978-1-59745-044-7_5,

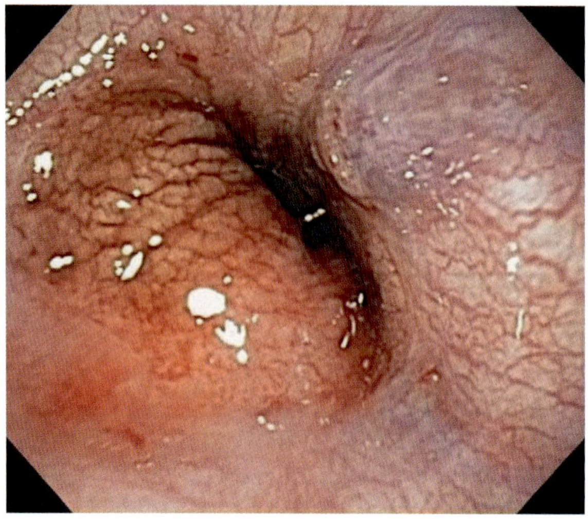

Fig. 1. An endoscopic view of grade 1 esophageal varices.

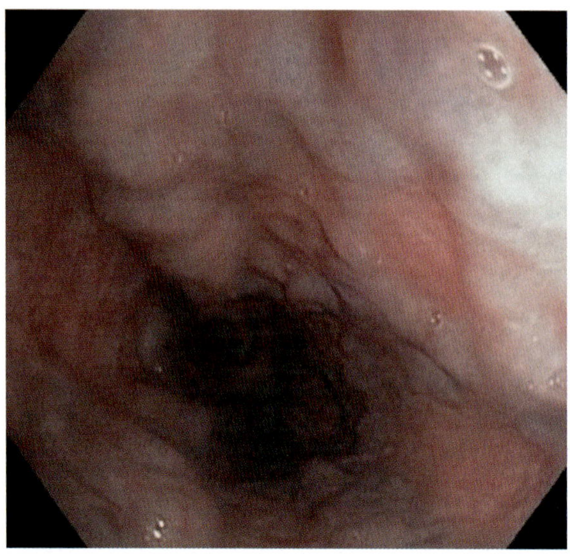

Fig. 2. An endoscopic view of grade 2 esophageal varices.

and do not disappear with distention (Fig. 2). Grade 3 varices are tortuous and comprise greater than one third of the lumen (Figs. 3 and 4).

RISK ASSESSMENT OF PATIENTS

Assessing the risk of variceal hemorrhage is essential to the proper treatment of esophageal varices. The treatment of varices should be considered in terms of primary prophylaxis, secondary prophylaxis, and treatment of acute hemorrhage. Primary prophylaxis is the treatment of varices prior to a bleeding episode, while secondary prophylaxis encompasses treatment after one or more bleeding episodes.

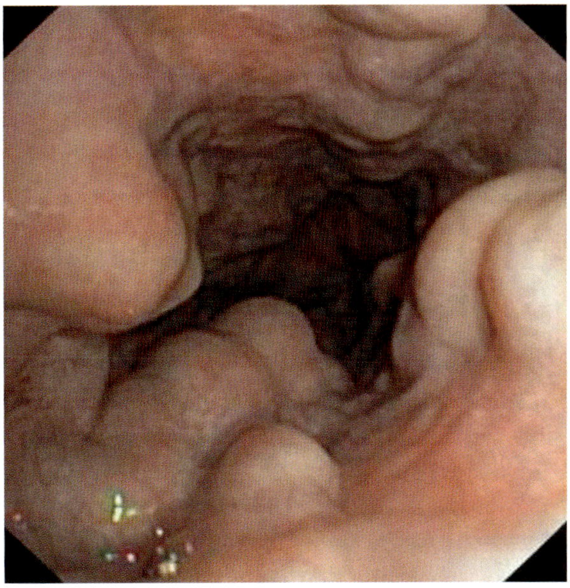

Fig. 3. An endoscopic view of grade 3 esophageal varices without stigmata of recent bleeding.

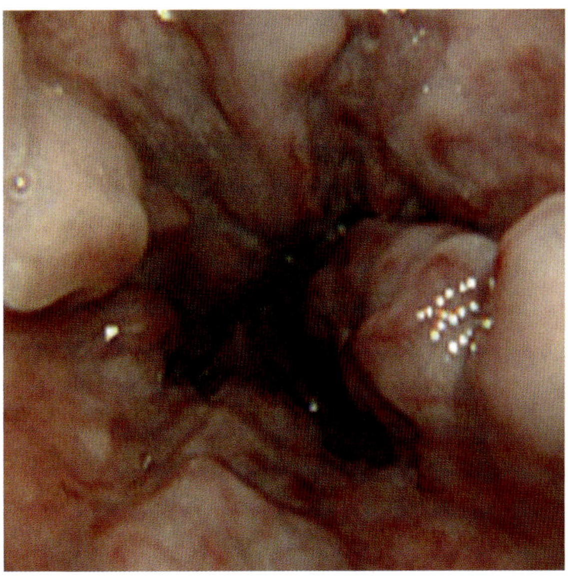

Fig. 4. An endoscopic view of grade 3 esophageal varices with stigmata of recent bleeding.

Primary Prophylaxis

Ideally, the risk of hemorrhage in a patient with cirrhosis could be established by calculating the hepatic venous pressure gradient (HVPG), as bleeding is unlikely to occur at a pressure gradient less than 12 mm Hg. However, this procedure is invasive, costly, and not routinely performed. Clinical parameters such as platelet count and Child–Pugh score can be used to predict which patients will have large varices (Chalasani et al. 1999; Schepsis et al. 2001).

However, it is generally recommended that all patients with cirrhosis undergo screening endoscopy.

Patients should have a recent laboratory evaluation including hemoglobin, platelet count, and prothrombin time prior to endoscopic evaluation. Adequate intravenous access should be established, and the procedure should be performed by an endoscopist experienced in assessment and ligation of varices. The size of the varices along with the presence of stigmata dictates the need for intervention. Varices <5 mm can be monitored with surveillance endoscopy, while those >5 mm are at higher risk of hemorrhage, and should be considered for ligation and/or medical management. Stigmata such as red wales or pigmented spots should also be considered to be signs of high risk for hemorrhage, and ligation should be considered.

A reduction of the HVPG by >20% or to less than 12 mm Hg can significantly reduce the incidence of an initial variceal hemorrhage (D'Amico et al. 2006). More importantly, a reduction by >20% also reduces mortality in patients with esophageal varices (D'Amico et al. 2006; Groszmann et al. 1990). Non-selective beta blockers such as propranolol and nadolol (nadolol has fewer systemic side effects than propranolol) lower HVPG, and are the primary therapeutic interventions used for this purpose. These medications act by reducing splanchnic blood flow and portal pressure. Beta blockers are initiated at a low dose, and then slowly titrated to increasing doses in order to achieve a 25% reduction in resting heart rate. The vast majority of patients will experience some level of portal venous pressure reduction, but only 35% will attain the desired reduction of >20% (Feu et al. 1995). Primary prophylaxis with non-selective beta blockers results in a reduction in the risk of bleeding by approximately 40% (D'Amico et al. 1999; Pagliaro et al. 1992).

High-risk esophageal varices, such as those greater than 5 mm in diameter or those demonstrating stigmata, should be considered for band ligation during endoscopy. This technique involves the use of a banding device, which attaches to the tip of an upper endoscope, and works by aspirating the varix into the banding chamber, where a rubber band is deployed around the vessel. This results in ligation or thrombosis of the vessel. Some studies have shown that band ligation is superior to beta-blockers in the prevention of hemorrhage (Triantos et al. 2006; Sarin et al. 1999). However, a more recent meta-analysis, which only used trials with adequate bias control, showed no difference in bleeding rates or mortality between those groups that underwent band ligation versus those treated with beta-blockers (Gluud et al. 2007). Band ligation often requires multiple endoscopic therapy sessions as patients must return every 2–4 weeks for repeat banding until the varices have been completely ligated. Thereafter, the patients will require continued surveillance as their varices frequently recur.

Sclerotherapy utilizing agents such as ethanol, sodium morrhuate, ethanolamine oleate, or sodium tetradecyl sulfate, a previously preferred endoscopic technique for variceal ablation, has been supplanted by band ligation because ligation has a better safety profile, and results in less long-term bleeding episodes. The overall benefit of sclerotherapy for treatment of esophageal varices has not been clearly demonstrated (Teres et al. 1993). In fact, although sclerotherapy lowers subsequent bleeding episodes, it has been shown to increase mortality (The Veterans Affairs Cooperative Variceal Sclerotherapy Group 1991). Thus, the band ligation should be favored over sclerotherapy for primary prophylaxis.

Secondary Prophylaxis

Secondary prophylaxis refers to treatment of varices following an episode of hemorrhage. Treatment in this group of patients is essential, as two-thirds will have a second episode of hemorrhage within 1 year (D'Amico, 2004). As mentioned previously, large varix size, the presence of stigmata of recent bleeding, and severity of liver disease, all increase rebleeding risk. A reduction of the HVPG by >20% results in a significant reduction in the recurrence of bleeding. Non-selective beta-blockers have been shown to decrease recurrent bleeding and improve survival at 2 years when used for secondary prophylaxis (Bernard et al. 1997). Similar to primary prophylaxis, the heart rate should be reduced by 25% or to a resting rate of 55. Long acting nitrates may be added to beta-blocker therapy as they can further decrease portal venous pressure. However, these agents have not been shown to reduce mortality when used as monotherapy, and can add to the side effect profile of medical management causing reduced patient compliance. One study showed a reduced incidence of rebleeding when medical management was compared to band ligation performed every 2–3 weeks, especially for those patients who had achieved >20% reduction in HVPG (Villanueva et al. 2001; Chalasani and Boyer 2005). The risk of complications for medical management remains lower than that of endoscopic management. However, other studies have found differing results when comparing endoscopic versus medical management, especially when treating patients with non-cirrhosis-related portal hypertension (Sarin et al. 2005). More importantly, the combination of endoscopic ligation with medical management has recently been shown to decrease rebleeding rates when compared to single modality therapy (De la Peña et al. 2005; Gonzalez et al. 2008). Sclerotherapy with sodium morrhuate or ethanolamine has been shown to be as effective as band ligation in controlling the initial bleeding episode. But, these agents were not shown to be as effective at preventing rebleeding episodes and had a much higher risk of complications (Laine et al. 1993). Therefore, sclerotherapy should be avoided for secondary prophylaxis of hemorrhage. Variceal band ligation is performed every 2–3 weeks until obliteration of the varices is complete. This usually requires three to four sessions with subsequent surveillance endoscopy for the recurrence of varices, which commonly occurs.

INITIAL MANAGEMENT OF ACUTE VARICEAL HEMORRHAGE

Presentation of variceal hemorrhage is seldom subtle, as patients often present with massive hematemesis with resulting tachycardia and hypotension (Fig. 5). Patients may also demonstrate signs of hepatic encephalopathy on presentation. Initial management should involve stabilization of the patient including preserving hemodynamic stability and airway patency. Adequate intravenous access should be established, and resuscitation with intravenous fluids and blood products should be initiated. Coagulation studies and platelet count must be obtained as soon as possible. Fresh frozen plasma transfusion may be considered for patients with elevated prothrombin times. Central venous pressure monitoring may assist in the management of fluid administration. Overenthusiastic fluid administration should be avoided, especially with normal saline as this may raise portal pressure and increase the risk of subsequent bleeding. Patients should be managed in an intensive care setting if possible. Endotracheal intubation should be strongly considered for airway protection as patients are at risk for aspiration in the setting of large volume bleeding, agitation, and the risk of the ensuing endoscopy. Pharmacologic therapy is integral for the cessation of hemorrhage. Somatostatin analogues such as octreotide reduce portal pressure by

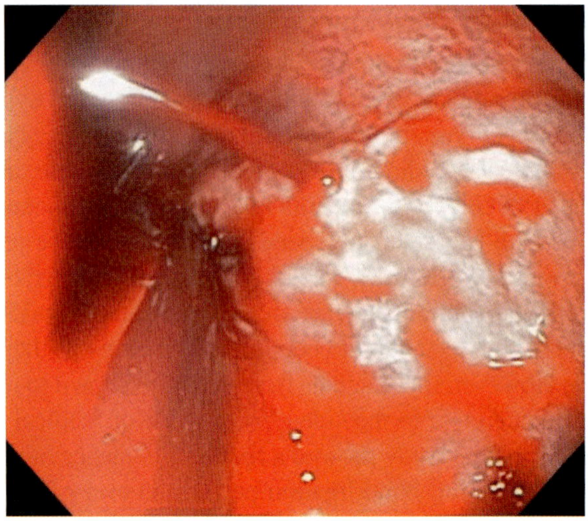

Fig. 5. An endoscopic view of active variceal hemorrhage in the esophagus.

inhibiting release of glucagon and inducing splanchnic vasoconstriction. Pharmacologic therapy should be initiated in the emergency department. These agents control bleeding in up to 85% of patients and may be equivalent to endoscopic therapy for this purpose (Jenkins et al. 1997; Sung et al. 1993; D'Amico et al. 2003). Therapy with octreotide can be continued for several days. However, the majority of the benefit is obtained within the first 24 h of treatment. Terlipressin, a vasopressin analogue with fewer systemic side effects than vasopressin, has been shown to be as effective as the somatostatin analogues in the control of active variceal hemorrhage (Ioannou et al. 2001). Unfortunately, terlipressin is not available in the USA. Intravenous administration of a proton pump inhibitor is often utilized in order to raise the intragastric and intraesophageal pH, and optimize coagulation capability. Antibiotic use (fluoroquinolone or third-generation cephalosporin) should be initiated on admission as this intervention has been shown to decrease infection risk, including the risk of spontaneous bacterial peritonitis as well as urinary tract infections and pneumonia, and reduce mortality (Blaise et al. 1994; Bernard et al. 1999). Early antibiotic use has also been shown to decrease the risk of future rebleeding (Jun et al. 2006).

Following interventions to achieve hemodynamic stabilization and management with octreotide, proton pump inhibitor, and antibiotics, more definitive therapy should be initiated with endoscopy, especially in those patients that continue to demonstrate evidence of continued bleeding. Endoscopy should be performed by an endoscopist experienced in management of variceal bleeding, and in a controlled setting such as the intensive care unit. The patient must have adequate IV access prior to the procedure. Endoscopic therapy is effective in hemorrhage control in approximately 90% of cases. Variceal band ligation and sclerotherapy are equally efficacious in controlling variceal hemorrhage. However, band ligation is preferred as it causes fewer complications and has a lower incidence of rebleeding (Lo et al. 1997). Unfortunately, the banding mechanism can interfere with visualization of an actively spurting vessel, necessitating the use of sclerotherapy, which allows the operator a full-field of vision.

In some situations, medical management and endoscopic techniques are unsuccessful in controlling variceal hemorrhage. This situation generally necessitates the placement of a

Sengstaken–Blakemore or Minnesota tube to control bleeding while a more definitive approach is pursued. The Sengstaken–Blakemore tube has two balloons, one that inflates in the stomach and another that inflates in the esophagus. It has four lumens, one each for inflating the esophageal and gastric balloons, one for aspirating the stomach, and one for suctioning secretions in the esophagus. Prior to placement of a tamponade balloon, the patient should undergo endotracheal intubation if that has not already been performed. The physician managing the bleeding patient must confirm functioning balloons and suction ports prior to insertion. Following intubation, the tube is inserted, and the position is confirmed by auscultation while air is insufflated into the gastric port. The position can also be established via endoscopic visualization. The gastric balloon is then inflated with 50–100 mL of air and the position of the balloon is then confirmed radiographically. Once confirmation has been obtained, the balloon is then inflated with a total of 300–350 mL of air, and the apparatus is pulled upward and may be placed in traction. It is this external, upward traction that tamponades the bleeding varices. The position of the tube exiting the nostril (our preferred method) or the mouth should be marked for future reference. If bleeding is not controlled with this intervention, then the esophageal balloon should be inflated to approximately 25–35 mm Hg. Both the gastric and the esophageal balloons must be periodically deflated to avoid pressure necrosis of the mucosa. Balloon tamponade is very effective in hemorrhage control. But, unfortunately it can cause severe complications, including ulceration, esophageal or gastric perforation, and aspiration. The tube should be considered only as a bridge to more definitive treatment and should be removed within 12–24 h of placement.

The transjugular intrahepatic portosystemic shunt (TIPS) procedure should be considered in the remaining 10% of patients in whom endoscopic control of variceal hemorrhage is not possible. In this procedure, a shunt is created by an interventional radiologist between the hepatic and portal vein with an expandable metal stent through the liver parenchyma, under fluoroscopic guidance. TIPS is effective in controlling hemorrhage from both esophageal and gastric varices. It has a lower short-term mortality rate than surgical shunts and provides equally efficacious portal decompression. Unfortunately, approximately one quarter of patients develop hepatic encephalopathy following placement of TIPS. The procedure also markedly increases the 30-day mortality of patients with elevated Child–Pugh scores or advanced MELD (Model For End-Stage Liver Disease) scores (Chalasani et al. 2000). Surgical shunts are also a consideration in situations where TIPS is not feasible or not available. Surgical shunting should also be considered when definitive therapy is sought for treatment of varices nonamenable to endoscopic therapy in patients who are not liver transplant candidates (Table 1).

Table 1
Initial management of acute variceal hemorrhage

- Initial resuscitation of bleeding patient.
- Correction of coagulation and platelet count.
- Avoid over-enthusiastic fluid administration.
- Management should be in the intensive care unit.
- IV octreotide, proton pump inhibitor, antibiotic.
- Low threshold for intubation and ventilation.

Several endoscopic therapies are available for the management of acute variceal hemorrhage:

Endoscopic variceal band ligation (EVL), injection sclerotherapy, argon plasma coagulation, detachable endoloops and snares

ENDOSCOPIC VARICEAL BAND LIGATION

The basic principle of ligation of varices is that elastic bands are used to strangulate a varix, causing thrombosis, inflammation, and necrosis and finally sloughing of the overlying mucosa. There are some drawbacks to this technique. The endoscope has to be withdrawn and loaded with a banding cylinder, which obviously takes several minutes, and can be costly in the setting of acute hemorrhage. Second, although the cylinder is transparent, it can reduce the viewing field, which makes visualization of the bleeding site difficult, especially with a vigorously bleeding vessel. Therefore, it is important to survey the upper gastrointestinal tract initially for the presence and the grade of varices and exclude any other cause for bleeding prior to attaching the cylinder to the endoscope (Fig. 6). When the decision has been made to pursue EVL, the endoscope is withdrawn and the banding device is affixed to the end of the endoscope before reintubation of the endoscope.

Technique

The banding device consists of a transparent cylinder preloaded with elastic bands, which can be attached to the tip of the endoscope. Trigger threads traverse through the biopsy channel and wind around the trigger wheel. The endoscope is advanced and positioned in such a way that the tip of the endoscope faces tangentially to the varix, as close to the gastroesophageal junction or the most distal point of the variceal column as possible. It is better to treat the varix below, (a location in the esophagus distal) to the bleeding point. The suction should be turned to "maximum or high." The varix is then suctioned into the banding chamber, which gives rise to "complete red out or blue out" (Fig. 7). Once the varix has completely filled the chamber during suctioning (Fig. 8) a single band (or possibly two) is fired using the trigger wheel. Successful deployment of the band on to the varix causes a knuckle in the varix (Fig. 9). The band, left in this location (Fig. 10) will then cause thrombosis and ligation of the vessel. The endoscopist should proceed with

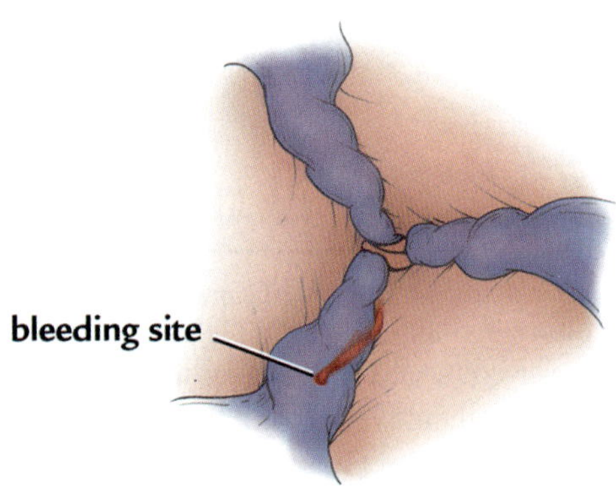

Fig. 6. An artist's depiction of a bleeding esophageal varix.

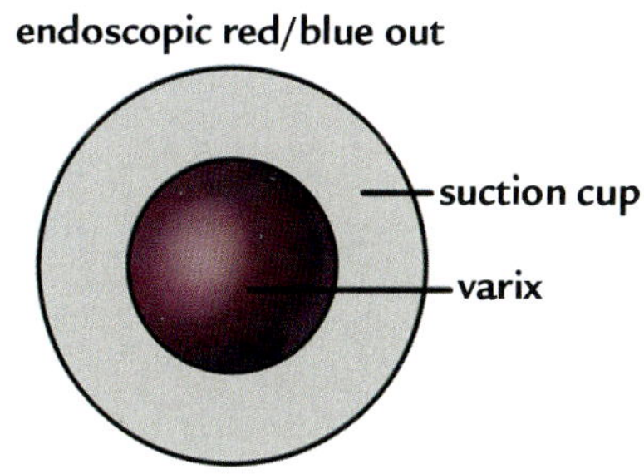

Fig. 7. "Blue-out" during band ligation of an esophageal varix.

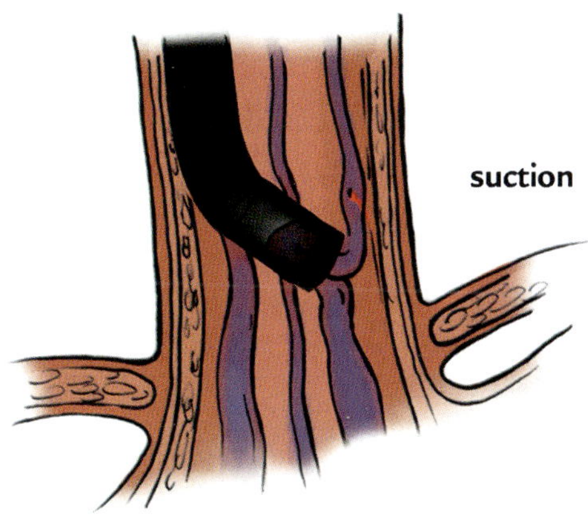

Fig. 8. An artist's depiction of suction of an esophageal varix into the cap of a band ligator.

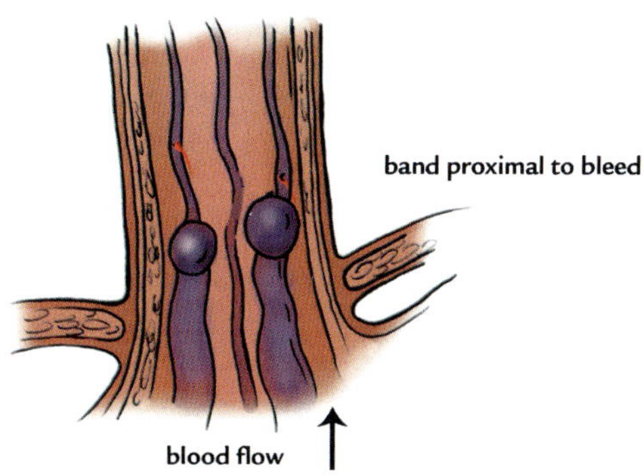

Fig. 9. An artist's depiction of a successful banding of esophageal varices.

banding of other varices in a spiral fashion. With regard to prophylactic banding, one study demonstrated that applying more than 6 bands per session prolonged endoscopy time and did not reduce the total number of sessions required to obliterate visible varices (Ramirez et al. 2007). Thus, prophylactic banding should generally be limited to 6 or fewer band ligations per session. The complications associated with band ligation include ulceration and stricture formation (Table 2).

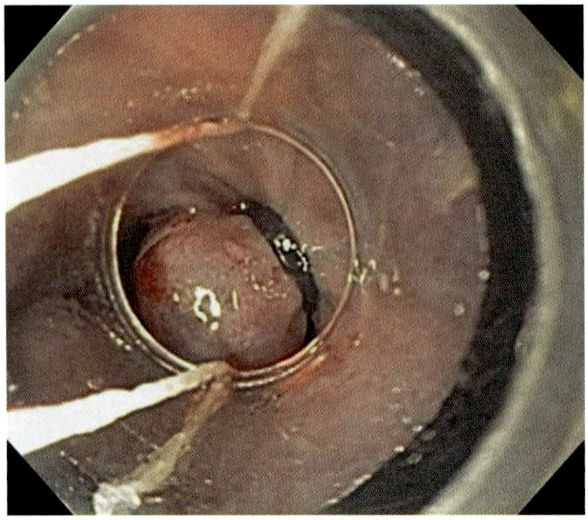

Fig. 10. An endoscopic view of band just placed on an esophageal varix using a band ligator.

Table 2
Items to be present for endoscopic banding

- Banding kit
  1. Transparent cylinder loads with 4, 6, or 10 bands
  2. Trigger cord
  3. Trigger wheel
  4. Loading catheter
  5. Irrigation adapter
- Suction turned to maximum or high prior to suctioning the varix into the cylinder.

Injection Therapy

The sclerosants of choice are generally either 5% ethanolamine oleate or 5% sodium morrhuate. It is always advisable to keep a tamponade balloon readily available (Sengstaken–Blakemore) during sclerotherapy.

Technique

All injection devices consist of a fine needle with a beveled edge at the tip of a plastic tube, the proximal end of which has a luer lock. It may help to orientate oneself within the esophagus and to grade the varices before therapy. It is advisable to inject the most distal varices first so that bleeding will not obscure the field of view of more proximal uninjected varices.

With the patient lying in the left lateral position, a drop of water or sclerosant from the tip of the needle or the catheter protruding from the biopsy channel will fall "down" to the left. If this point is considered to be 6 o' clock on a clock-face, then the varices can be recorded around the clock. Similarly, a small pool of secretions may also serve the same purpose. We generally record the varices and their grades just above the gastroesophageal junction and approximately 5 cm proximally. The lower 5 cm is the most common site of bleeding and, therefore, it is here that the injections should be placed. This area is also rich in large perforating vessels, which feed the varices from the periesophageal plexus of veins (McCormack et al. 1983). "Red blebs" are very thin areas, which are prone to bleeding and, therefore, should not be injected directly. No attempt should be made to inject ulcers and thrombosed varices on follow-up endoscopy as further ulceration and bleeding may occur.

Various techniques for injection have been endorsed throughout the literature. While some investigators advocate intravariceal injection, others advocate paravariceal injection, in order to cause fibrosis around the vessel and avoid systemic complications from the sclerosant. Others advocate a combination approach. It is difficult to determine which approach is most effective as many "intravariceal" injections may result in paravariceal injections.

Intravariceal Injection

Large varices are easier to inject and, therefore, it is reasonable to choose the largest varix nearest to the 6 o' clock position, just above the gastroesophageal junction. The injector with its needle properly retracted is advanced through the biopsy channel and is advanced into the field of view. The needle is then pushed out and positioned between 30° and 45°. This is achieved by manipulating the tip of the endoscope. The injector is then inserted into the varix, and the sclerosant is injected (Fig. 11). Bulging and blanching are the signs of extravasation, which should be avoided. An experienced nurse can detect an intravariceal injection from the lower resistance felt on compressing the syringe plunger. In spite of taking extreme caution, extravasation may still go undetected and, therefore, it is advisable that no more than 2 mL of sclerosant be injected at any one site. On withdrawal of the needle, a little bleeding may occur. Our practice is to insert the needle into the variceal column followed by injection of the sclerosant. After the injection, we maintain sufficient pressure on the varix for at least 15 s, and then gradually withdraw the needle while maintaining pressure with the catheter tip for at least another 15 s. The catheter is gradually released watching for any evidence of

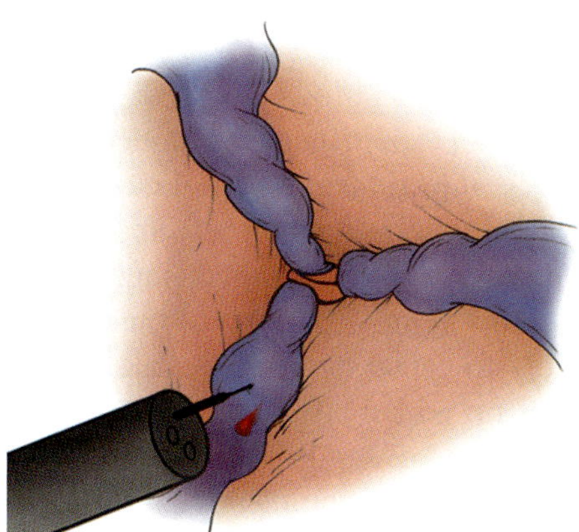

Fig. 11. An artist's depiction of intravariceal injection of sclerosant into an esophageal varix.

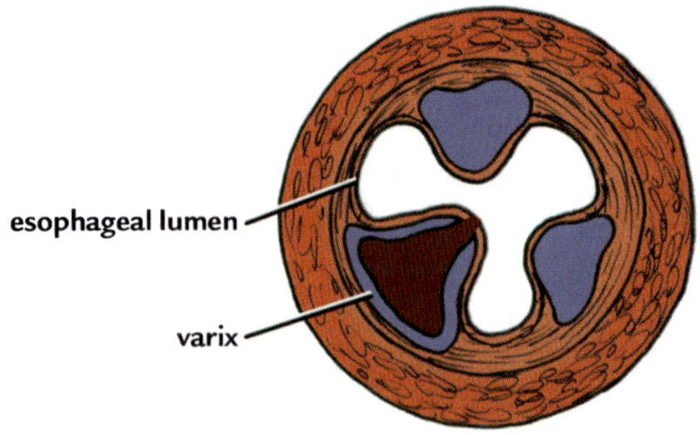

Fig. 12. An artist's depiction of an esophageal varix immediately after intravariceal injection of a sclerosant.

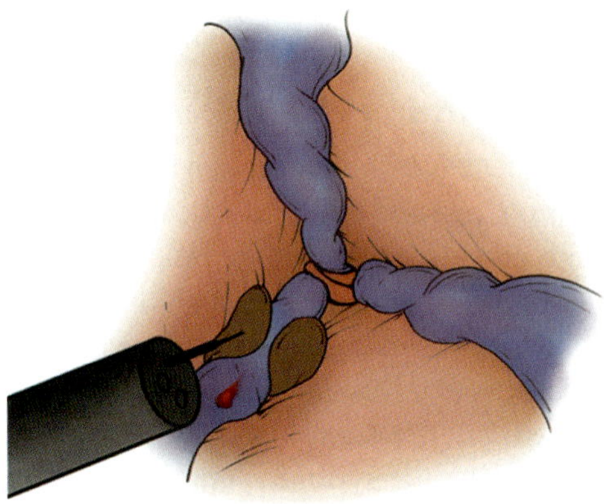

Fig. 13. An artist's depiction of an esophageal varix immediately after paravariceal injection of a sclerosant.

bleeding (Fig. 12). If any signs of bleeding appear, the catheter is firmly applied to the varix and it is re-injected. If the varices are large, further, more distal injections within a 5-cm zone may be required. The needle is carefully withdrawn into the sheath before removing the injection catheter from the biopsy channel.

Paravariceal Injection

Paravariceal injections of sclerosants produce fibrosis without ulceration or thrombosis of the varices. Small volumes of sclerosants are injected superficially adjacent to the variceal columns (Fig. 13). The injections are done more obliquely and superficially than for variceal thrombosis. Injections should begin just above the gastroesophageal junction and proceed in a spiral manner, up the esophagus, causing a uniform edematous sheath surrounding the variceal columns in the distal part of the esophagus (Fig. 14). Some endoscopists inject into the varices to cause thrombosis, and make injections adjacent to and over the surface of the varices for added effect.

Endoscopic sessions are repeated every 1–3 weeks, and it may require six to eight sessions before obliteration of the varices is complete. Sclerotherapy has been associated with ulceration, esophageal perforation, esophageal stricture, portal vein thrombosis, and pulmonary embolism.

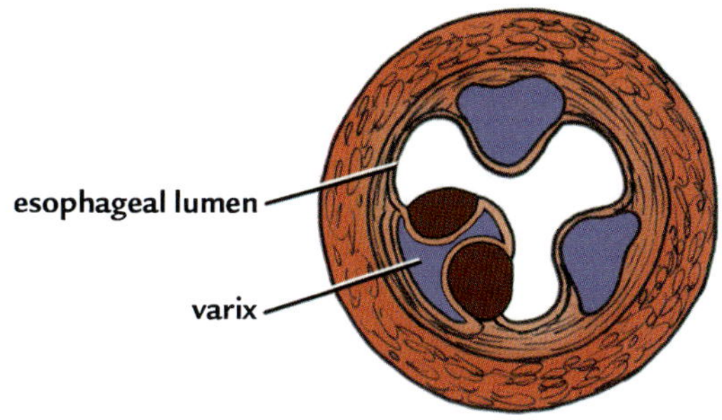

Fig. 14. An artist's depiction of a cross-sectional view of an esophageal varix immediately after paravariceal injection of a sclerosant.

Table 3
Items to be present for endoscopic injection

• Injector
• Sclerosant
• Syringes
• Goggles
• Experienced nurse
• Sengstaken-Blakemore tube

COMBINATION OF BAND LIGATION AND SCLEROTHERAPY

Combination treatment may hasten variceal eradication. Some endoscopists inject smaller volumes of sclerotherapy agents immediately after banding just proximal to the band ligation sites. Venous stasis above the banded site may enhance the effect of therapy. Others prefer injecting the sclerosant between the banded sites. It should be remembered that these approaches may not be superior to band ligation alone (Laine et al. 1996; Saeed et al. 1997; Djurdjevic et al. 1999; Garg et al. 1999) (Table 3).

Argon Plasma Coagulation

Argon Plasma Coagulation (APC) utilizes argon gas to conduct a high-frequency electrical current to produce coagulation that is only a few millimeters deep, without tissue contact by the probe. Several studies have demonstrated that APC may reduce the rebleeding rate of esophageal varices following effective band ligation therapy (Nakamura et al. 2001; Furukawa et al. 2002). Further studies should be performed before this procedure is performed in routine practice.

Gastric Varices

Gastric varices are found with advanced portal hypertension, and are the source of hemorrhage in approximately 10% of patients with variceal bleeding. Gastric varices (GOV)

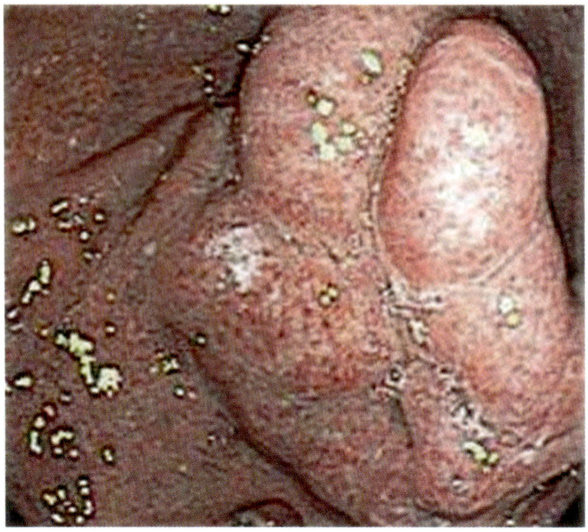

Fig. 15. An endoscopic view of gastric varices.

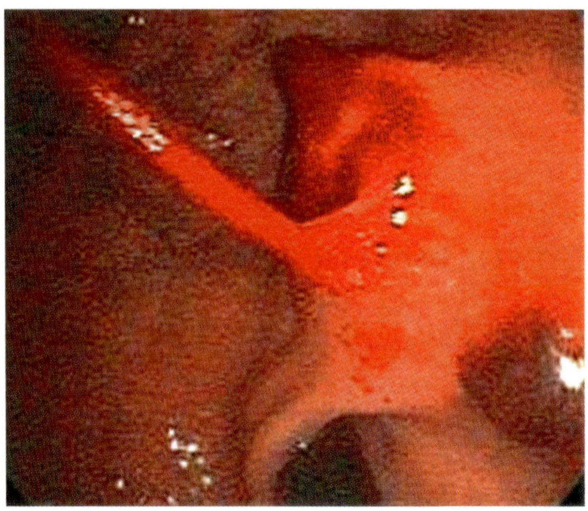

Fig. 16. An endoscopic view of an actively bleeding gastric varix.

are classified according to location and continuity with esophageal varices. GOV1 extend from the esophagus a short distance past the GE junction. GOV2 are in continuity with esophageal varices and extend into the fundus. IGV1 are isolated varices in the fundus, and IGV2 are isolated varices that occur in the body or antrum of the stomach. Gastric fundal varices are less likely to bleed than those found in other locations but the magnitude of blood loss is comparatively more severe to esophageal variceal hemorrhage (Figs. 15 and 16) (Sarin et al. 1992).

The initial management of gastric variceal bleeding is similar to that of esophageal variceal bleeding, and should include hemodynamic stabilization, adequate IV access, central venous pressure monitoring, consideration of endotracheal intubation, and intravenous administration of octreotide, a proton pump inhibitor, and antibiotics (either a fluoroquinolone or a third-generation cephalosporin). Unfortunately, large randomized controlled trials pertaining to endoscopic management of gastric varices do not exist. Band ligation in the stomach can be complicated by large ulcerations because of the mucosa overlying the vessel being banded. Sclerotherapy utilizing ethanolamine oleate or sodium morrhuate for gastric varices is often ineffective, and because it requires larger amounts of sclerosants than esophageal sclerotherapy, can often lead to complications. Treatment with cyanoacrylate has been shown to effectively control bleeding. However, this treatment has been shown to cause ulceration, bacteremia, and embolic disease. Cyanoacrylate is not currently approved for treatment in the USA and, therefore, is not discussed in detail here. Thrombin injections (approximately 1,000 IU) have also been shown in small trials to effectively control bleeding from gastric varices in up to 90% of patients, and decrease rebleeding rates to 20% at 6 weeks follow-up, without any reported adverse effects (Ramesh et al. 2008; Yang et al. 2002; Przemioslo et al. 1999 Apr). Several sessions of therapy are generally required. The use of a detachable snare with simultaneous sclerotherapy and O-ring ligation was recently reported in the literature to achieve hemostasis of gastric variceal hemorrhage in 8 out of 8 patients with a 97% resolution of gastric varices in 35 patients for whom it was used for primary or secondary prophylaxis of bleeding (Yoshida et al. 1999). A Linton–Nachlas tube can temporarily halt bleeding while a more definitive treatment is pursued in those patients who continue to bleed. The Linton–Nachlas tube has a larger gastric balloon than the Sengstaken–Blakemore tube and, thus, causes more effective tamponade of gastric variceal bleeding. TIPS or surgical shunting are highly effective in controlling gastric variceal bleeding. Devascularization, as described by Sugiura and Futagawa, is a final option for control of bleeding varices. As with esophageal varices, nonselective beta blockers should be considered for primary and secondary prophylaxis in order to decrease the HVPG (Fig. 17).

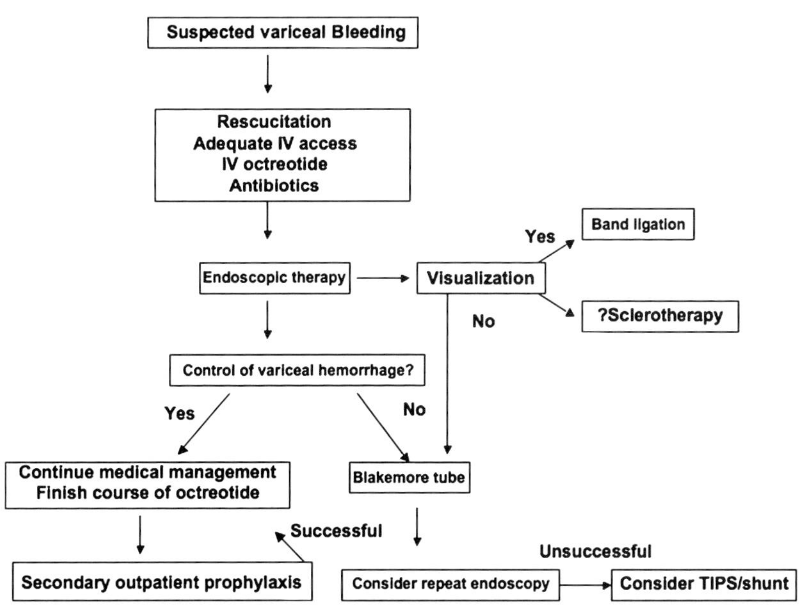

Fig. 17. An algorithm for the management of variceal hemorrhage.

Follow-up

Following endoscopic therapy, patients will require close follow-up as complications are a well-known aspect of current therapy. Patients undergoing sclerotherapy are at risk for ulceration, bleeding, chest pain, and perforation. Band ligation can induce ulcers, bleeding, and strictures. Patients who undergo obliteration of varices for primary or secondary prophylaxis will need endoscopic sessions every 2–4 weeks, until obliteration is complete, and then subsequent surveillance endoscopies to monitor for recurrence of disease. Patients who are initiated on nonselective beta-blockers will need to gradually increase their dose every 5 days in order to achieve a 25% reduction from baseline heart rate or a resting heart rate of 55/min. Patients will need to be monitored for bradycardia and hypotension, and should be counseled on compliance, as these agents can cause unpleasant side effects such as fatigue, wheezing, gastrointestinal symptoms, and impotence.

It is beyond the scope of this chapter to discuss the relative costs of various treatment modalities; however, with increasing cost-constraints, physicians dealing with variceal hemorrhage should be aware of the cost-effectiveness of different treatments with consideration of their level of expertise and the availability of different therapeutic options.

SUMMARY OF KEY POINTS

- The management of varices can be categorized into primary prophylaxis, secondary prophylaxis, and management of acute hemorrhage.
- Current therapeutic endoscopic modalities now offer outcomes superior to previous treatment methods, and new options for prophylaxis and management of acute hemorrhage appear imminent.
- Regardless of technological advances, the foundation of hemorrhage management remains rooted in the medical stabilization of the patient prior to endoscopic therapy.

REFERENCES

Bosch J, Abraldes JG, Groszmann R. Current management of portal hypertension. J Hepatol. 2003;38:S54.

Kleber G, Sauerbruch T, Ansari H, Paumgartner G. Prediction of variceal hemorrhage in cirrhosis: a prospective follow-up study. Gastroenterology. 1991;100:1332–7.

The North Italian Endoscopic Club for the Study and Treatment of Esophageal Varices. Prediction of the first variceal hemorrhage in patients with cirrhosis of the liver and esophageal varices. N Engl J Med. 1988;319:983–9.

de Franchis R, Primignani M. Natural history of portal hypertension in patients with cirrhosis. Clin Liver Dis. 2001;5:645.

Chalasani N, Imperiale TF, Ismail A, et al. Predictors of large esophageal varices in patients with cirrhosis. Am J Gastroenterol. 1999;94:3285–91.

Schepsis F, Camma C, Niceforo D, et al. Which patients with cirrhosis should undergo endoscopic screening for esophageal varices detection? Hepatology. 2001;33:333–8.

D'Amico G, JC Garcia-Pagan, Luca A, Bosch J. Hepatic vein pressure gradient reduction and prevention of variceal bleeding in cirrhosis: a systematic review. Gastroenterology. 2006;131:1611–24.

Groszmann RJ, Bosch J, Grace ND, et al. Hemodynamic events in a prospective randomized trial of propranolol versus placebo in the prevention of a first variceal hemorrhage. Gastroenterology. 1990;99:1401–7.

Feu F, JC Garcia-Pagan, Bosch J, et al. Relation between portal pressure response to pharmacotherapy and risk of recurrent variceal haemorrhage in patients with cirrhosis. Lancet. 1995;346:1056–9.

D'Amico G, Pagliaro L, Bosch J. Pharmacological treatment of portal hypertension: an evidence-based approach. Semin Liver Dis. 1999;19:475–505.
Pagliaro L, D'Amico G, Sorensen TI, et al. Prevention of first bleeding in cirrhosis. A meta-analysis of randomized trials of nonsurgical treatment. Ann Intern Med. 1992;117:59–70.
Triantos C, Vlachogiannakos J, Manolakopoulos S, et al. Is banding ligation for primary prevention of variceal bleeding as effective as beta-blockers, ad is it safe? Hepatology. 2006;43:196–7.
Sarin SK, Lamba GS, Kumar M, Misra A, Murthy NS. Compaison of endoscopic ligation and propranolol for the primary prevention of variceal bleeding. N Engl J Med. 1999;340:988–93.
Gluud LL, Klingenberg S, Nikolova D, Gluud C. Banding ligation versus beta-blockers as primary prophylaxis in esophageal varices: systematic review of randomized trials. Am J Gastroenterol. 2007;102:2842–8.
Teres J, Bosch J, Bordas JM, et al. Propranolol versus sclerotherapy in preventing variceal rebleeding: a randomized controlled trial. Gastroenterolgy. 1993;105:1508–14.
The Veterans Affairs Cooperative Variceal Sclerotherapy Group. Prophylactic sclerotherapy for esophageal varices in men with alcoholic liver disease: a randomized, single-blind, multicenter clinical trial. N Engl J Med. 1991;324:1779–84.
D'Amico G. Esophageal varices: from appearance to rupture; natural history and prognostic indicators. In: Portal hypertension in the 21st century. Netherlands, Kluwer: 2004.
Bernard B, Lebrec D, Mathurin P, Opolon P, Poynard T. Beta-adrenergic antagonists in the prevention of gastrointestinal rebleeding in patients with cirrhosis: a meta-analysis. Hepatology. 1997;25:63–70.
Villanueva C, Minana J, Ortiz J, et al. Endoscopic ligation compared with combined treatment with nadolol and isosorbide mononitrate to prevent recurrent variceal bleeding. N Engl J Med. 2001;345:647–55.
Chalasani N, Boyer TD. Primary prophylaxis against variceal bleeding: beta-blockers, endoscopic ligation, or both? Am J Gastroenterol. 2005;100:805–7.
Sarin SK, Wadhawan M, Gupta R, Shahi H. Evaluation of endoscopic variceal ligation (EVL) versus propanolol plus isosorbide mononitrate/nadolol (ISMN) in the prevention of variceal rebleeding: comparison of cirrhotic and noncirrhotic patients. Dig Dis Sci. 2005;50:1538–47.
De la Peña J, Brullet E, Sanchez-Hernández E, Rivero M, Vergara M, Martin-Lorente JL, et al. Variceal ligation plus nadolol compared with ligation for prophylaxis of variceal rebleeding: a multicenter trial. Hepatology. 2005;41:572–8.
Gonzalez R, Zamora J, Gomez-Camarero J, Molinero LM, Bañares R, Albillos A. Meta-analysis: Combination endoscopic and drug therapy to prevent variceal rebleeding in cirrhosis. Ann Intern Med. 2008;149:109–22.
Laine L, El-Newihi HM, Migikovsky B, Sloane R, Garcia F. Endoscopic ligation compared with sclerotherapy for the treatment of bleeding esophageal varices. Ann Intern Med. 1993;119:1–7.
Jenkins SA, Shields R, Davies M, Elias E, Turnbull AJ, Bassendine MF, et al. A multicentre randomised trial comparing octreotide and injection sclerotherapy in the management and outcome of acute variceal haemorrhage. Gut. 1997;41:526–33.
Sung JJ, Chung SC, Lai CW, Chan FK, Leung JW, Yung MY, et al. Octreotide infusion or emergency sclerotherapy for variceal haemorrhage. Lancet. 1993;342:637–41.
D'Amico G, Pietrosi G, Tarantino I, Pagliaro L. Emergency sclerotherapy versus vasoactive drugs for variceal bleeding in cirrhosis: a Cochrane meta-analysis. Gastroenterology. 2003;124:1277–91.
Ioannou G, Doust J, Rockey DC. Terlipressin for acute esophageal variceal hemorrhage. Cochrane Database Syst Rev. 2001;(1):CD002147.
Blaise M, Pateron D, Trinchet JC, Levacher S, Beaugrand M, Pourriat JL. Systemic antibiotic therapy prevents bacterial infection in cirrhotic patients with gastrointestinal hemorrhage. Hepatology. 1994;20:34–8.
Bernard B, Grangé JD, Khac EN, Amiot X, Opolon P, Poynard T. Antibiotic prophylaxis for the prevention of bacterial infections in cirrhotic patients with gastrointestinal bleeding: a meta-analysis. Hepatology. 1999;29:1655–61.
Jun CH, Park CH, Lee WS, Joo YE, Kim HS, Choi SK, et al. Antibiotic prophylaxis using third generation cephalosporins can reduce the risk of early rebleeding in the first acute gastroesophageal variceal hemorrhage: a prospective randomized study. J Korean Med Sci. 2006;21:883–90.
Lo GH, Lai KH, Cheng JS, Lin CK, Huang JS, Hsu PI, et al. Emergency banding ligation versus sclerotherapy for the control of active bleeding from esophageal varices. Hepatology. 1997;25:1101–4.

Chalasani N, Clark WS, Martin LG, Kamean J, Khan MA, Patel NH, et al. Determinants of mortality in patients with advanced cirrhosis after transjugular intrahepatic portosystemic shunting. Gastroenterology. 2000;118:138–44.

Ramirez FC, Colon VJ, Landan D, Grade AJ, Evanich E. The effects of the number of rubber bands placed at each endoscopic session upon variceal outcomes: a prospective, randomized study. Am J Gastroenterol. 2007;102:1372–6. Epub 2007 Apr 16.

McCormack TT, Rose JD, Smith PM, Johnson AG. Perforating veins and blood flow in oesophageal varices. Lancet. 1983;2:1442–4.

Laine L, Stein C, Sharma V. Randomized comparison of ligation versus ligation plus sclerothreapy in patients with bleeding esophageal varices. Gastroenterology. 1996;110:529–33.

Saeed ZA, Stiegmann GV, Ramirez FC, et al. Endoscopic variceal ligation is superior to combined ligation and sclerotherapy for esophageal varices: a multicenter prospective randomized trial. Hepatology. 1997;25:71–4.

Djurdjevic D, Janosevic S, Dapcevic B, et al. Combined ligation and sclerotherapy versus ligation alone for eradication of bleeding esophageal varices: a randomized and prospective trial. Endoscopy. 1999;31:286–90.

Garg PJK, Joshi YK, Tabndon RK. Comparison of endoscopic variceal sclerotherapy with sequential endoscopic band ligation plus low-dose sclerotherapy for secondary prophylaxix of variceal hemorrhage: a prospective randomized study. Gastrointest Endosc. 1999;50:369–73.

Nakamura S, Mitsunaga A, Murata Y, Suzuki S, Hayashi N. Endoscopic induction of mucosal fibrosis by argon plasma coagulation (APC) for esophageal varices: a prospective randomized trial of ligation plus APC vs. ligation alone. Endoscopy. 2001;33:210–5.

Furukawa K, Aoyagi Y, Harada T, Enomoto H. The usefulness of prevention consolidation therapy of esophageal varices using an argon plasma coagulation technique. Hepatol Res. 2002;23:220–5.

Sarin SK, Lahoti D, Saxena SP, Murthy NS, Makwana UK. Prevalence, classification and natural history of gastric varices: a long-term follow–up study in 568 portal hypertension patients. Hepatology. 1992;16:1343–9.

Ramesh J, Limdi JK, Sharma V, Makin AJ. The use of thrombin injections in the management of bleeding gastric varices: a single-center experience. Gastrointest Endosc. 2008;68:883–6.

Yang WL, Tripathi D, Therapondos G, Todd A, Hayes PC. Endoscopic use of human thrombin in bleeding gastric varices. Am J Gastroenterol. 2002;97:1381–5.

Przemioslo RT, McNair A, Williams R. Thrombin is effective in arresting bleeding from gastric variceal hemorrhage. Dig Dis Sci. 1999 Apr;44(4):778–81.

Yoshida T, Harada T, Shigemitsu T, Takeo Y, Miyazaki S, Okita K. Endoscopic management of gastric varices using a detachable snare and simultaneous endoscopic sclerotherapy and O-ring ligation. J Gastroenterol Hepatol. 1999;14:730–5.

6 Argon Plasma Coagulation

John W. Birk and Antarpreet Kaur

CONTENTS

Keywords: Argon, Plasma, Coagulation, Hemostasis, Ablation

INTRODUCTION

Argon plasma coagulation (APC) is an electrosurgical procedure in which electrical energy in the form of ionized argon gas is transferred to target tissue. The APC device uses non-contact thermal energy in the form of ionized gas or plasma for coagulation of the tissue. This technique was first used in open surgical and laparoscopic procedures nearly 2 decades ago. With the development of flexible probes and special electrical waveforms in 1990s, APC has been adopted for use in flexible endoscopy for the treatment of various gastrointestinal conditions. APC is an efficacious, safe, and easy-to-use method of hemostasis and devitalization of tissues. This chapter will discuss the indications and contraindications for APC, provide a detailed step-by-step description of the procedure, and an evidence-based review of the procedure.

INDICATIONS

The main indications for APC can be divided into two broad categories, hemostasis and ablation.

From: *Clinical Gastroenterology: Diagnostic and Therapeutic Procedures in Gastroenterology*,
Edited by: G. Y. Wu, S. Sridhar, DOI 10.1007/978-1-59745-044-7_6,

Hemostasis

This includes its use for gastric antral vascular ectasia, cecal A-V malformations, radiation proctitis, and occasionally bleeding peptic ulcer disease.

In gastric antral vascular ectasia syndrome or watermelon stomach, patients usually present with transfusion-dependent iron deficiency anemia. It commonly affects patients with cirrhosis, but patients with a variety of other chronic diseases such as kidney failure are predisposed. The treatment duration with APC is usually more than one session (average 2.4) and the efficacy has been shown to be more than 80% in various retrospective studies (Wahab et al. 1997; Leclaire et al. 2008; Probst et al. 2001).

For cecal A-V malformations, the success rate for APC in stopping transfusion requirement has been reported to be 65% (Vargo 2004).

For radiation proctitis, APC has been reported to successfully ameliorate rectal bleeding in more than 90% cases (Hendrik 2008). Symptomatic treatment is usually achieved after two treatment sessions, and transfusion dependency is improved in 95% of cases (Wahab et al. 1997; Sydney et al. 2006).

Arteriovenous malformations (AVM) of the stomach, small bowel, and the colon have been successfully treated with APC. A combination of anesthetic infusion followed by an APC application has been used to treat the vascular lesions of Osler–Weber–Rendu disease. Dieulafoy's lesions can also be treated.

Endoscopic treatment of ulcer bleeding with active spurting or non-bleeding visible vessels is usually accomplished with epinephrine injection and/or thermal tamponade techniques. However, APC has been used as a thermal tamponade agent (Morris and Tucker 2009). Limited data are available to evaluate the utility of APC in esophageal varices either as a primary modality or in conjunction with other modalities.

Ablation

Ablation literally means removing abnormal growths or harmful material by mechanical means. The applications of APC for ablation therapy include gastrointestinal tumor palliation, stent placement, trimming in resected lesions, and non-dysplastic Barrett's esophagus.

Controversy surrounds the use of APC in ablative therapy for Barrett's epithelium. The possibility of residual nests of metaplastic cells underneath the layer of neosquamous epithelium remains a concern (Wahab et al. 1997; Hendrik 2008). Strictures can also occur, making it a less-than-ideal therapy.

APC is used alone or in concert with other treatment modalities in the palliation of esophageal, gastric, and rectal malignancies. It is useful to both maintain luminal patency and control bleeding. APC has efficacy equal to or better than other non-surgical ablation techniques in tumor palliation (Wahab et al. 1997). More than 95% patients have been shown to have improvement in their tumor-related symptoms, and the recurrence rate of symptoms was shown to be low at 6% (Eickoff et al. 2007). However, in contrast to endoscopic or surgical resection, no tissue diagnosis can be made with APC.

Devitalization of adenoma remnants after polypectomy or endoscopic mucosal resection (EMR) of adenomatous lesions often leaves tissue remnants along the edge of the resected area, particularly after piecemeal resection. APC has been shown to be well tolerated and 78% successful in treating such lesions (Vargo 2004; Dekovich 2009).

An interesting use of APC has been in the treatment of Zenker's diverticulum, where it has been shown to be effective and safer than open surgical procedures (Rabenstein et al. 2007).

An unusual use of APC has been to shorten previously placed biliary, esophageal, or colonic metallic stents in treatment of stent-induced ulceration, and to allow for the placement of plastic stents after occlusion (Vargo 2004).

CONTRAINDICATIONS

All conditions that contraindicate endoscopy as well as those that may jeopardize the safe operation of the APC device are included among the contraindications. International Normalized ratios (INR) of greater than 1.6, platelet count of less than 50,000, and recent antiplatelet drug usage are contraindications. In addition, an inability to clearly visualize or reach the target lesion precludes the APC use.

Relative contraindications include the need for curative therapy in ablation of dysplastic lesion as in residual neoplastic islands because of the associated high rate of recurrence.

PROCEDURE DESCRIPTION

The Plasma Coagulator Device

Components of the plasma coagulator include an argon-compatible, high-frequency monopolar electrosurgical generator, APC unit, argon gas source, foot activation switch, flexible delivery catheters (probes), grounding pads, and accessories (filter membrane, connector hose). The disposable probes are available in 1.5 mm, 2.3 mm (the most commonly used size), and 3.2 mm diameters. The 2.3 mm or 7 Fr probe is the size regularly used in endoscopy due to its ability to be used universally in almost all endoscopes. Standard probes are 220 cm long. But, 300 cm probes can be used for push enteroscopy. The most commonly used APC device and endoscopic catheters are manufactured by ERBE Elektromedizin (Tubingen, Germany) (Fig. 1). Different types of nozzle orientations can be used depending on the lesion to be ablated. Side-firing tips are helpful in ablating tangential, hard-to-reach lesions. Front-firing tips are used for flat lesions, and circumferential tips for ablating polyps and tumors (Figs. 2 and 3). The current generators can deliver between 5,000 and 6,500 V. Power adjustments can be made between 0 and 155 W (Vargo 2004).

The Circuit: Monopolar Versus Bipolar

Both monopolar and bipolar accessories are used in endoscopy. The terms refer to the manner in which the circuit is completed. With monopolar accessories, the circuit is completed via a remote return electrode (grounding pad). The energy leaving the active electrode (e.g., polypectomy snare) travels in paths of least resistance through the patient's body to be collected over the grounding pad and returned to the generator to complete the circuit. Grounding pads are usually placed close to the treatment site to keep the circuit as short as possible (Morris and Tucker 2009). APC uses a monopolar circuit.

In bipolar devices, grounding pads are not needed. These devices have both the active and return electrodes closely spaced into the working tip of the probe. Energy travels from the active electrode to the return electrode though a very small portion of tissue in contact with the probe's tip (Morris and Tucker 2009).

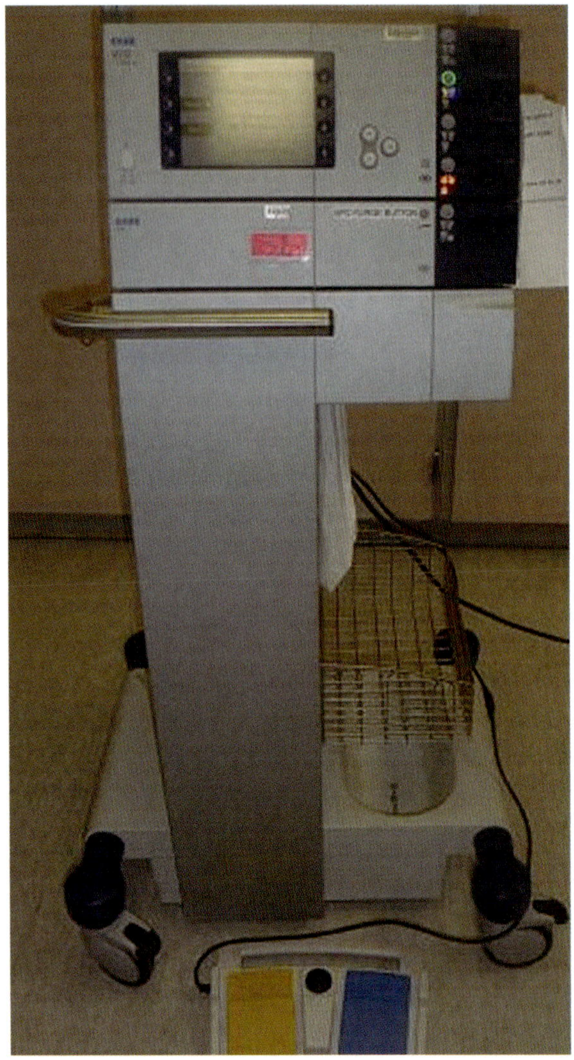

Fig. 1. An illustration of the ERBE APC device.

Mechanics

In endoscopy, disposable APC probes are designed to operate through the working channel of flexible endoscopes. These probes are available in a variety of nozzle orientations along with different diameters. The probes are made of Teflon and contain a recessed tungsten electrode at the distal tip. The electrical current and argon gas travel through the flexible probe and become ionized at the point of contact with the electrode. It is this ionized argon plasma that allows electrical current to flow between the probe and the tissue without any direct contact. The application of this energy causes coagulation of tissue (Vargo 2004).

The plasma beam follows the path of least electrical resistance. This phenomenon permits the argon plasma to be applied both en-face and tangentially, allowing the treatment of regions that are difficult to access. The depth of the tissue destruction is limited due to increased resistance and diminished current flow through the coagulated tissue.

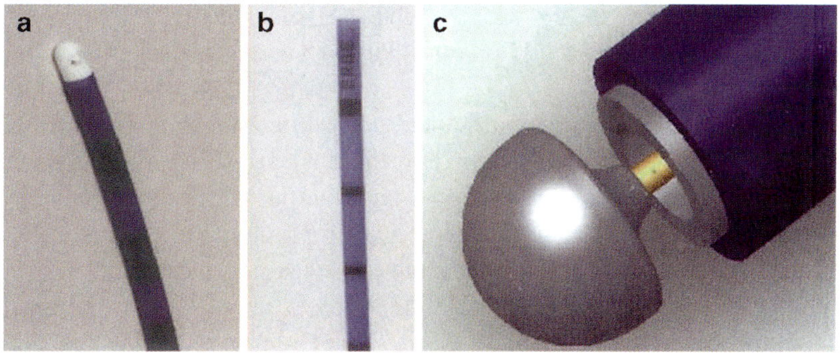

Fig. 2. Photographs of APC probes: (**a**) side firing; (**b**) front firing, and (**c**) circumferential (magnified) tips.

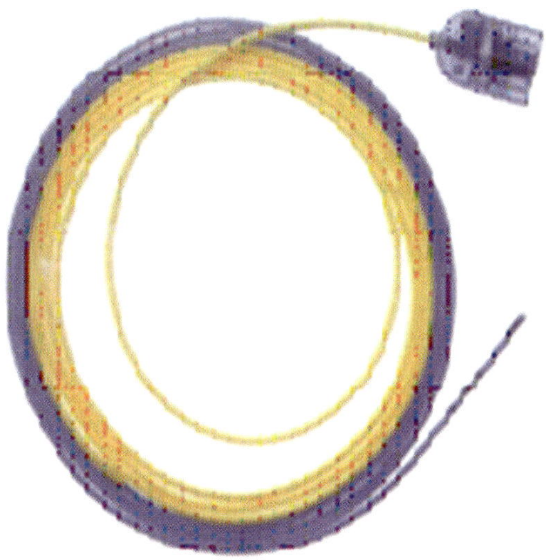

Fig. 3. A photograph of an APC probe/integrated filter and probe.

Generally, the zone of coagulation is 1–3 mm. This is a key advantage APC has over other modalities including NdYAG Laser, Bicap, and thermal probe as this unique property of limited penetration decreases the risk of perforation that is associated with direct contact application of a probe.

The three important factors influencing the thermal impact of APC are the duration of the application, the power setting, and the probe to tissue distance. Flow rate also influences the outcomes of the APC application. Three zones of tissue effect are encountered. The desiccation zone is located at the point of current contact with the incident tissue; deeper layers of the tissue effect include a coagulation zone and devitalization zone.

First- and Second-Generation APCs

Recently, second-generation APCs with new modes or waveforms have been introduced into endoscopy. The overall efficiency of the device has been improved by 30–50%, so lower power settings can be used to produce the same thermal effect, and the same power settings can be used for deeper and more extensive tissue injury than expected previously. The second-generation APC modes, "Forced," "Pulsed," and "Precise" have different coagulation effects (Hendrik 2008).

Forced APC provides continuous output and corresponds to settings on the earlier first-generation systems. Pulsed APC provides intermittent current with two options: Effect 1 pulses approximately 1 per second with high-energy output with each impulse, while Effect 2 pulses approx. 16 times per second with lower energy output per impulse. The latter may be preferred when superficial treatment of large surface areas is desired.

Precise APC utilizes an integrated regulation system to control argon plasma flow. This results in a more superficial depth of injury when compared with the other settings (Rabenstein et al. 2007).

Technique

The patient is kept fasting the night prior to the procedure, and for colonoscopy a full bowel preparation. Also, antiplatelet and anticoagulation drugs should be stopped if possible. When the lesion is identified on endoscopy, the grounding pad is placed in proximity, and argon is turned on usually at a flow rate of 0.5–1.5 L/min. The power settings are based on the location of the lesions with usual power settings between 20 and 100 W. Lower settings in the range of 20 W are used in cecum and small bowel lesions because of the relative thinness of the bowel wall at those locations. Higher power, 40–80 W, is used for tumor ablations of the esophagus and rectum.

The probe is passed via the endoscope so that the tip hovers over the target tissue. The tip of the probe needs to be within 1 cm of the target tissue in order for the ionized plasma to reach the target tissue. Since APC causes different penetrations depending on the site, the lesion, and the individual patient, calibration with the first impulse is done. This is done by intentionally firing a pulse when the probe is too far away from the tissue to deliver any coagulation, and continuing to fire pulses while gradually moving the probe closer to the tissue until the first coagulation occurs. It is important not to fire too close or while touching the tissue, as that can cause a deeper injury, similar to electrocautery.

Occasionally, the probe must be retrieved to clean the probe and remove debris and ablated tissue. Intermittent suction serves to clear the field of smoke and prevents excessive insufflation of the bowel. Care is taken to release the hot gas in open air as it can burst the canisters if entrapped.

COMPLICATIONS

The complications are usually divided into major and minor categories. Major complications are relatively rare, less than 0.3%.

Minor Complications

Submucosal emphysema is the most commonly encountered benign complication of APC occurring in up to 10% of cases. This usually results in no serious implications, but its resolution should be monitored. No treatment is usually required.

GI tract distention can occur during argon gas introduction leading to patient discomfort. Repeated aspiration of the gas can reduce strain on the bowel wall and, hence, reduce this complication (Hendrik 2008).

Rectal pain and tenesmus is usually observed in rectal manipulations, especially if the procedure is done near the dentate line (Silva et al. 1999).

Neuromuscular stimulation is a muscular contraction reflexively triggered by electrical stimulation of the nerves innervating the muscle and may cause pain (Hendrik 2008).

Major Complications

Perforation of the bowel is a rare, but life-threatening complication that can occur when there is direct contact of the probe with the mucosa. One third of the perforations require surgical management while the rest can be managed conservatively with bowel rest, antibiotics, and clipping. Rectovaginal fistula formation has been described in case reports (Silva et al. 1999).

Infections ranging from local involvement causing only pain and fever to bacteremia have been described, prompting some to advocate the use of preprocedure antibiotics, although no guidelines recommend this at present (Tam et al. 2000).

Stricture formation at the site of the APC application has been observed in non-dysplastic Barrett's ablation of the esophagus and in the rectum after the treatment of proctitis.

Gas explosions have been reported as a result of ignition of inflammable gases due to inadequate bowel cleansing (Numberg et al. 2007).

Cardiology clearance should be obtained in patients with implanted devices to avoid as APC-induced arrhythmias from interference with implanted cardiac devices (Hendrik 2008).

POSTOPERATIVE CARE

The extent of postoperative care depends on the indication for APC, the underlying pathology, and the general condition of the patient. Most elective hemostatic procedures are outpatient-based and thus, the postoperative care is limited to observing patients closely for 6 h in a recovery room, and monitoring vital signs closely. Sicker patients with active bleeding or patients requiring palliation of tumors might need to be admitted for observation.

ALTERNATIVE PROCEDURES

Thermal coagulation with heater probes is still used for hemostasis, but not as commonly in cancer ablation due to higher recurrence rates. Heater probes have higher perforation rates than alternatives.

Bipolar electrocautery is a useful technology for hemostasis and is sometimes used for endoscopic ablation. Its usefulness in tissue ablation is limited by its small treatment field. It is still considered in patients with implanted pacemakers (Dumot and Greenwald 2008).

Laser NdYAG laser, KTP (potassium titanyl phosphate) laser and argon lasers have been used for tumor ablation, and for treating vascular lesions. KTP with a wavelength better absorbed by hemoglobin is more helpful in hemostasis while NdYAG helps to ablate deeper tissue (Dumot and Greenwald 2008). All of these require the use of bulky expensive equipment and some require special certification for use.

Cryotherapy is the application of extremely cold temperatures for medical treatment. It is widely used in various skin and mucosal cancers and in ablation of non-dysplastic lesions. The immune reaction created by cryotreatment is a unique feature of this therapy (Dumot and Greenwald 2008).

Limited access to the equipment is a major reason why it has never been fully adopted to use with endoscopy.

Photodynamic therapy with porfimer as a photosensitizer has been used in Barrett's esophagus as an alternative to APC with similar efficacy and complication rates (Siersema 2005).

Radiofrequency ablation is the use of thermal energy indirectly for destroying malignant cells. HALO is now considered the treatment of choice for Barrett's esophagus as shown in recent studies (Nicholas et al. 2009).

COSTS

The cost of an APC cart, which includes a coagulator, generator, and cart, is approximately $26,000, which is greater than the cost of a standard electrosurgical generator used for electrocoagulation and considerably less than the cost of a laser. The probes cost $198.00 per unit. The costs and billing codes are shown in Tables 1 and 2.

SUMMARY OF KEY POINTS

- APC is an electrosurgical endoscopic procedure indicated for hemostasis and devitalization of tissues.
- APC has been used with great success in radiation proctitis, bleeding arterio-venous malformations, removal of large adenomatous polyps and gastrointestinal tumor palliation.

Table 1
APC costs

Item	*Cost*
ERBE APC Probe	$198
Professional charge	$408
Room charges (our institution)	$758
Recovery charge (our institution)	$240

Table 2
APC RVU and billing code

RVU	10.74
CPT code (Medicare)	43258

- Advantages include noncontact mode, axial, radial, and retrograde application, controllable depth of coagulation, and low cost of purchase and maintenance.
- APC has a lower rate of perforation when compared with other modalities due to noncontact coagulation of the tissue. But, the lack of tissue sampling is a disadvantage in its use for removal of suspicious lesions.
- When performed correctly, APC is an effective, safe, and easy endoscopic procedure.

REFERENCES

Wahab PJ, Mudler CJJ, Den Harog G, Thies JE. Argon plasma coagulation in flexible gastrointestinal endoscopy: pilot experiences. Endoscopy. 1997;29:176–81.

Leclaire S et al. Bleeding vascular ectasia treated by argon plasma coagulation: a comparison between patients with and without cirrhosis. Gastrointest Endosc. 2008;67:218–25.

Probst A, Schuebel R, Wienbeck M. Treatment of watermelon stomach (GAVE syndrome) by means of endoscopic argon plasma coagulation: long term outcome. Z Gastrol. 2001;39:447–52.

Vargo J. Clinical applications of argon plasma coagulator. Am Soc Gastrointest Endosc. 2004;59:1.

Hendrik M. Argon plasma coagulation therapy. Curr Opin Gastroenterol. 2008;24:612–6.

Sydney W, Rex D, et al. Endoscopic treatment of chronic radiation proctopathy. Curr Opin Gastroenterol. 2006;22:536–40.

Morris M, Tucker R. Electrosurgery in gastrointestinal endoscopy: principles to practice. Am J Gastroenterol. 2009;10:1563–74.

Eickoff A, Jakobs R, Schilling D, et al. Prospective nonrandomized comparison of two modes of argon beamer (APC) tumor desobstruction: effectiveness of the new pulsed APC versus forced APC. Endoscopy. 2007;39:637–42.

Dekovich A. Endoscopic treatment of colonic obstruction. Curr Opin Gastroenterol. 2009;25:50–4.

Rabenstein T, May A, Michel J, et al. Argon plasmacoagulation for flexible endoscopic Zenker's diverticulotomy. Endoscopy. 2007;39:141–5.

Silva RA, Correia AJ, Dias LM, Viana HL. Argon plasma coagulation therapy for treatment of symptomatic radiation induced procto-sigmoiditis. Gastrointest Endosc. 1999;50:221–4.

Tam W, Moore J, Schoeman M. Treatment of radiation proctitis with argon plasma coagulation. Endoscopy. 2000;32:667–72.

Numberg D, Pannwitz H, et al. Gas explosion caused by argon plasma coagulation of colonic angiodysplasias. Endoscopy. 2007;9:E182.

Dumot J, Greenwald B. Argon plasma coagulation bipolar cautery and cryotherapy: ABC's of ablative techniques. Endoscopy. 2008;40:1026–32.

Siersema P. Endoscopic therapeutic esophageal interventions: what is new? What needs further study? What can we forget? Curr Opin Gastroenterol. 2005;21:490–7.

Nicholas J, Sharma P, et al. Radiofrequency ablation in Barrett's esophagus with Dysplasia. NEJM. 2009;360:2277–88.

7 Endoscopic Mucosal Resection

Frances Tse

Contents

Keywords: Endoscopic, Mucosal, Resection, Tumor, Lesions

INTRODUCTION

Endoscopic mucosal resection (EMR) is an advanced endoscopic technique used to resect sessile or flat lesions confined to the superficial layers of the gastrointestinal (GI) tract, which cannot be resected by conventional endoscopic techniques. It is increasingly being recognized as a highly effective and minimally invasive alternative to surgery in the management of superficial early GI cancers. By resection through the middle or deeper part of the submucosal layer, EMR allows complete and curative resection of the diseased mucosa. This can be accomplished with minimal cost, morbidity, and mortality, and with the potential of improving the long-term quality of life of patients. Although EMR is primarily a treatment procedure, it can also be used to obtain larger and deeper tissue biopsies for diagnosis.

In Western countries, surgical resection of the lesion and any potentially involved regional lymph nodes has been considered the standard treatment for early GI cancers. In Japan, however, EMR has been widely accepted as a first-line treatment for early GI cancers

From: *Clinical Gastroenterology: Diagnostic and Therapeutic Procedures in Gastroenterology*,
Edited by: G. Y. Wu, S. Sridhar, DOI 10.1007/978-1-59745-044-7_7,

without lymph node metastasis. Since the first case report of EMR for early gastric cancer in 1984 by Tada et al. (1984), the indications for EMR are continuing to expand. This technique is now gaining acceptance worldwide and has been used both diagnostically and therapeutically in both the upper and lower GI tracts. EMR is most commonly used to treat early esophageal dysplasia or cancer, gastric cancer, large flat colorectal polyps, and colorectal cancer.

This review will describe the indications, contraindications, techniques, complications, postoperative care, clinical effectiveness compared to alternative techniques and cost of EMR.

INDICATIONS

Most GI cancers are diagnosed at an advanced stage as a result of symptoms such as abdominal pain, bleeding, and obstruction. Unfortunately, the survival rate for these advanced cancers remains poor, despite treatment including surgery and adjuvant therapy. To improve the prognosis for these patients, one of the strategies is to detect cancer at an early stage through screening programs.

Early GI cancers are defined by their confinement to the mucosa and the submucosa, regardless of their size or the presence of regional lymph node metastasis. The extremely low incidence of lymph node metastasis in these superficial GI cancers means that cure can be effectively achieved by local endoscopic treatment such as EMR in selected cases. The intent is to remove all known submucosal extension of a lesion and to obtain a clear margin for either therapeutic or diagnostic purposes. Currently, EMR is indicated for resection of early superficial GI cancers limited to the mucosa without any regional lymph node metastasis or distant metastasis. EMR is also indicated for removal of premalignant or potentially malignant lesions. In cases in which the etiology of the lesion is still unclear after conventional endoscopic forceps biopsies or the pathological abnormality is suspected to be located in deep mucosa or submucosa (e.g., submucosal tumor, lymphoma, and Menetrier's disease), EMR can be considered to obtain larger biopsy specimens for diagnosis. Indications for EMR in early GI lesions are shown in Table 1.

Before performing EMR, patients must be evaluated for eligibility based on histology, location, lateral margins, and depth of invasion of the lesion.

DEFINING THE LATERAL MARGINS OF THE LESION

Most early cancers are detected during screening of high-risk patients (such as patients with Barrett's esophagus (BE), family history of gastric cancer or colorectal cancer, or history of colonic polyps) or incidentally during endoscopic procedures performed for other unrelated reasons. Unfortunately, the endoscopic appearances of these early lesions are often very subtle, making detection and evaluation quite difficult. To facilitate recognition of these lesions, additional techniques such as chromoendoscopy, magnification endoscopy, and narrow band imaging (NBI) may be used.

Chromoendoscopy, performed by spraying dyes on the mucosa to improve characterization and localization of mucosal abnormalities during endoscopy or colonoscopy, has been reported to improve detection of dysplasia or early cancer (Davila 2009). Any suspicious area identified during routine endoscopy or colonoscopy can be further evaluated with

Table 1
Indications for EMR in early GI lesions

Esophagus
Benign polyps (hyperplastic, adenomatous, metaplastic, and inflammatory)
Well or moderately differentiated squamous cell carcinoma or adenocarcinoma
High-grade dysplasia or intramucosal carcinoma in Barrett's esophagus
Confined to the mucosa
No evidence of lymphovascular involvement
<2 cm in Type IIa, IIb, and IIc lesions
Less than one third of the circumference (stricture formation)
Stomach
Benign polyps (hyperplastic, adenomatous, metaplastic, and inflammatory)
Well or moderately differentiated adenocarcinoma or papillary carcinoma
No evidence of ulcer or ulcer scar on endoscopy and/or pathology (Type III)
Confined to the mucosa
No evidence of lymphovascular involvement
<2 cm in Type IIa lesions or <1 cm in IIb or IIc lesions
Colon
Benign polyps (hyperplastic and adenomatous)
Well or moderately differentiated adenocarcinoma
Confined to mucosa
<2 cm in Type IIa lesions or <1 cm in Type IIb or IIc lesions
Laterally spreading superficial adenoma/carcinoma

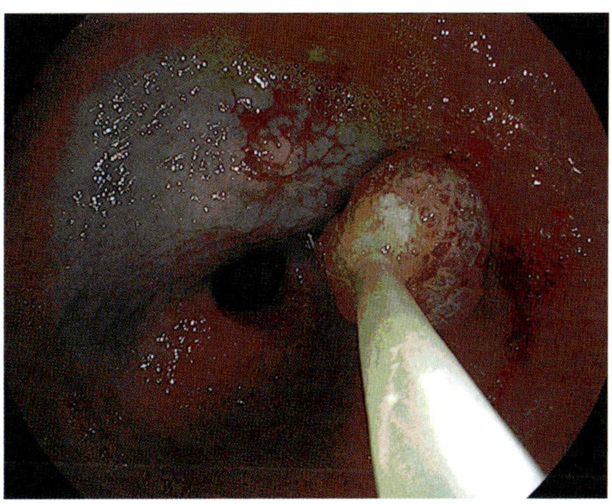

Fig. 1. Methylene blue has been used to highlight a dysplastic lesion in the antrum of the stomach of this patient for resection.

chromoendoscopy to enhance visualization of the lesion and to define the lateral margins to guide resection (Fig. 1). A variety of dyes has been used, including Lugol's iodine (1.5–2.0%) for the evaluation of squamous cell esophageal cancer (Dubuc et al. 2006; Moschler et al. 2006; Inoue et al. 2001), indigo carmine for the evaluation of lesions in the stomach and colon (Kawahara et al. 2009), and methylene blue (0.5–1.0%) for the detection of high-grade dysplasia and early cancer in Barrett's esophagus (Ngamruengphong et al. 2009). Chromoendoscopy with magnification endoscopy may further improve visualization of mucosal detail (Connor and Sharma 2004; Hurlstone and Fujii 2005; Tischendorf et al. 2010). NBI uses optical filters for red–green–blue sequential illumination and narrows the bandwidth of spectral transmittance to enhance mucosal structures and capillaries, and may help in detecting neoplastic changes (Mannath et al. 2010; Muto et al. 2009). These various endoscopic techniques can help improve detection of dysplastic lesions and further delineate the margins of the lesion, and can lead to curative endoscopic resection of these lesions.

DETERMINING THE DEPTH OF TUMOR INVASION

It is well known that lymph node metastasis is a predictor of tumor recurrence post-resection. Estimating the depth of tumor invasion is crucial as the risk of lymph node metastasis increases with depth of tumor invasion into the submucosa. For example, the risk of lymph node metastasis in squamous cell esophageal cancer confined to the mucosa was 4% (Endo and Yoshino 1991). However, once the squamous cell cancer invaded the submucosa, the risk of lymph node metastasis increased to 35%, and the 5-year survival fell from 85% to 60% (Tajima et al. 2000). Similarly, the risk of lymph node metastasis in early gastric cancer confined to the mucosa is 0–5% but the risk increased to 10–20% in tumors extending deep into the submucosa (Kurihara et al. 1998). The risk of nodal metastases for colon cancers deeply invading the submucosa has been reported to be 8–12% compared to 2–3% for those cancers invading the submucosa superficially (Wilcox et al. 1986). Since EMR is completely ineffective in lesions with lymph node metastasis, a superficial lesion with no or low risk for lymph node metastasis is a prerequisite for curative resection.

The depth of tumor invasion can be estimated by endoscopic appearances, but can be improved by the use of endoscopic ultrasound (EUS).

ENDOSCOPIC APPEARANCES

The endoscopic appearances of superficial early cancers were first described in Japan. The Japanese Gastric Cancer Association described three main types of superficial lesions: type I polypoid, type II non-polypoid and non-excavated, and type III non-polypoid with an ulcer (Fig. 2) (Japanese Gastric Cancer Association 1998). Type I is further divided as pedunculated lesions (Ip) and sessile lesions (Is), while type II is subdivided into slightly elevated lesions (IIa), completely flat lesions (IIb), and slightly depressed lesions (IIc). This classification has been applied to describe superficial lesions at other sites.

The depth of invasion can be predicted by the endoscopic appearance of a superficial lesion. For type I lesions, the risk of submucosal invasion increases with the diameter. For type II lesions, invasion of the submucosa is more frequent in IIc depressed lesions (more than 20%) than in other subtypes. A type III lesion should not be resected, as the risk of submucosal invasion is very high.

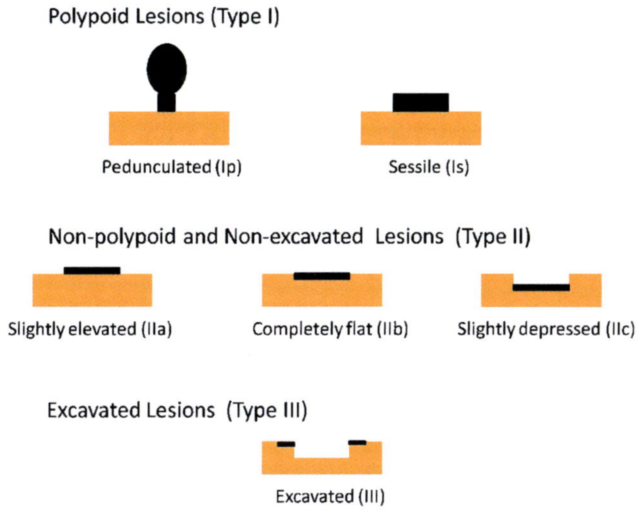

Fig. 2. The endoscopic appearances of superficial lesions as classified by the Japanese Gastric Cancer Association.

ENDOSCOPIC ULTRASOUND

EUS is often recommended for locoregional staging prior to EMR to exclude regional lymph node metastasis and to ascertain the depth of tumor invasion. In particular, high-frequency miniprobe (frequency, 20–30 MHz) may distinguish nine layers within the wall of the GI tract, thus providing better images in assessing tumor penetration. The diagnostic accuracy of the miniprobe in assessing depth of tumor invasion in the esophagus, stomach, and colon ranges from 74% to 92% (Murata et al. 2003; Saitoh et al. 1996; Akahoshi et al. 1998). This high variability in diagnostic accuracy may reflect differences in the frequencies of the probes used, patient populations, and operator expertise. The main limitation of EUS is its tendency to overstage early lesions.

Because of the limitations in these various staging techniques, it has been suggested that EMR is indicated for any superficial lesion as long as the lesion can be safely removed in its entirety. Furthermore, the most important predictor of lymph node metastasis is the degree of differentiation in the deepest portion of the lesion and the presence of lymphovascular invasion. This information can be precisely established by histological analysis of the EMR specimens, thereby allowing stratification and refinement of further treatment.

CONTRAINDICATIONS

EMR should not be performed if there is obvious tumor infiltration into the submucosa or deeper layers of the GI wall according to endoscopic appearances and/or EUS findings. The presence of lymph node metastasis based on EUS ± FNA or CT findings also contraindicates EMR. EMR should not be attempted for lesions that do not "lift" during submucosal injection because "nonlifting" of the lesion is a predictor of deep invasion, and that the lesion is not amenable to EMR. Finally, EMR is contraindicated in patients with uncorrectable coagulopathy or in patients on anticoagulant therapy, but may be performed after stopping the treatment.

PROCEDURE DESCRIPTION

Define the Margins of the Lesion for Resection

Before performing EMR, the lateral margins of the lesion should be identified with the help of chromoendoscopy and marked with electrocautery using, for example, a needle knife, heater probe, or argon plasma coagulator.

Submucosal Injection

The lesion is then injected with saline or other agents into the submucosal space creating a "cushion." This "cushion" allows for safe resection of flat mucosal lesions without causing mechanical or electrocautery damage to the deeper layers of the bowel wall and, thus, may reduce the risk of perforation and bleeding. Submucosal injection can also help in assessing the depth of tumor penetration. If the lesion is easily lifted with elevation of the overlying mucosa, it means that there is no deep submucosal invasion. On the other hand, the "non-lifting sign" has been found to have 100% sensitivity, 99% specificity, and 83% positive predictive value for invasive carcinoma (Uno and Munakata 1994).

There exists no standardization of the type of injection solution. A mixture of saline with epinephrine is the most widely used. However, injected saline dissipates within minutes. Other injectables that dissipate more slowly have been used including 50% dextrose, glycerol (10% glycerol/5% fructose), and hyaluronic acid. A small amount of dye such as methylene blue is often added in the injectable to help demarcate the resection margins. The volume of injected solution varies from 5 to 50 mL depending on the size of the lesion.

Resection Techniques

In general, resection techniques can be classified as (1) injection assisted EMR; (2) cap-assisted EMR (EMR-C); and (3) ligation-assisted EMR (EMR-L).

Injection-Assisted EMR

After submucosal injection of the lesion, a polypectomy snare is placed around the lesion, which is then resected using electrocautery. As a variation of this technique, a forceps can be passed down a double-channel endoscope to grasp and lift the lesion, which is then resected by using a polypectomy snare (Fig. 3).

Cap-Assisted EMR

This technique uses a special transparent cap fitted to the tip of the endoscope (Fig. 4). After submucosal injection to lift the target lesion, a small electrocautery snare is inserted through the channel of the endoscope and is then opened and positioned within the rim of the cap. After the lesion is suctioned into the cap, the lesion is snared and resected by using electrocautery.

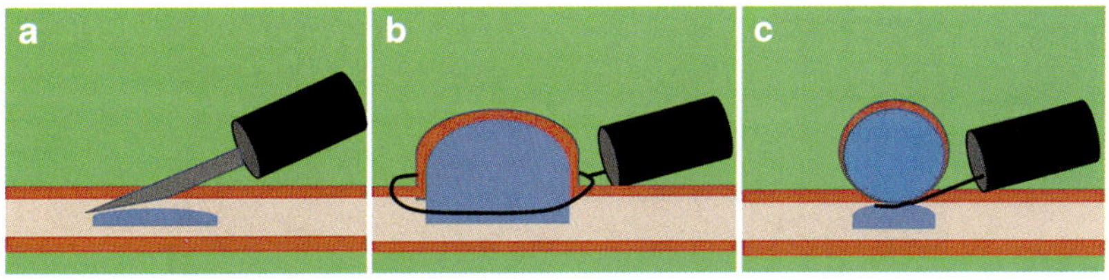

Fig. 3. Injection-assisted EMR. (**a**) Submucosal injection of a flat lesion. (**b**) A snare is placed around the elevated lesion. (**c**) Lesion is resected using electrocautery.

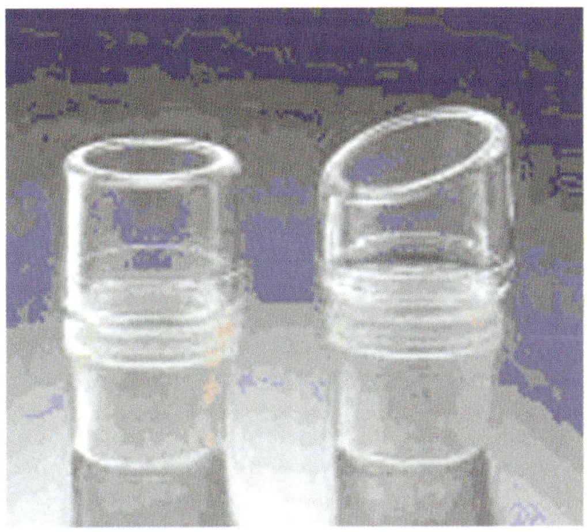

Fig. 4. Transparent caps for cap-assisted EMR (K-001, Olympus America Inc., Melville, NY) (Courtesy of Olympus America, Inc.).

Ligation-Assisted EMR

This technique uses a standard endoscopic variceal ligation device that is fitted on an endoscope (Fig. 5). The lesion is first suctioned and ligated with a rubber band without prior submucosal injection. A standard electrocautery snare is then used to resect the lesion above or below the level of the rubber band (Fig. 6). A recently introduced multibanding mucosectomy (MBM) kit uses a specially designed 6-band ligator that permits insertion of a snare without removal of the banding apparatus (Duette, Cook, Medical, Winston-Salem, NC). Up to six resections can be carried out without the need of removing the scope. This technique is faster and easier to perform than the EMR-C technique. However, the visibility through the ligation cap is inferior to that of the cap of EMR-C, which makes it difficult to target focal lesions. In addition, the resected specimen is smaller with this system compared with the EMR-C.

Because of the size of the snare, cap, and ligation device, the above EMR techniques cannot be used to remove lesions larger than 2 cm in one piece. This limitation prevents accurate pathologic staging in some cases and increases the risk of cancer recurrence. A newer technique termed endoscopic submucosal dissection (ESD), using specially developed endoscopic knives, has been developed in Japan for *en bloc* resection of large lesions (Gotoda et al. 2006).

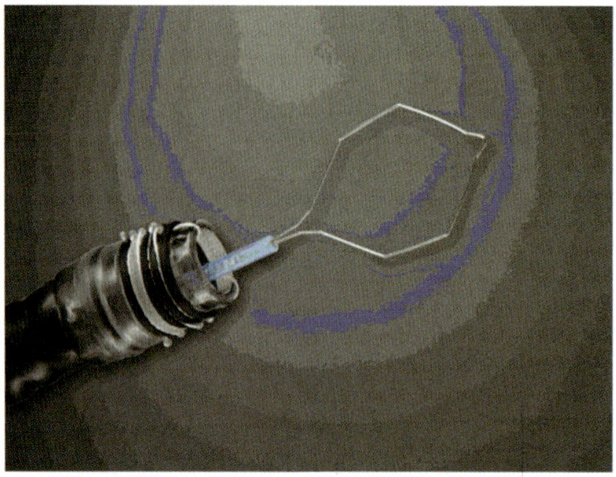

Fig. 5. A variceal ligation device with an electrocautery snare fitted onto an endoscope (Duette, Cook, Medical, Winston-Salem, NC) (Courtesy of Cook Medical).

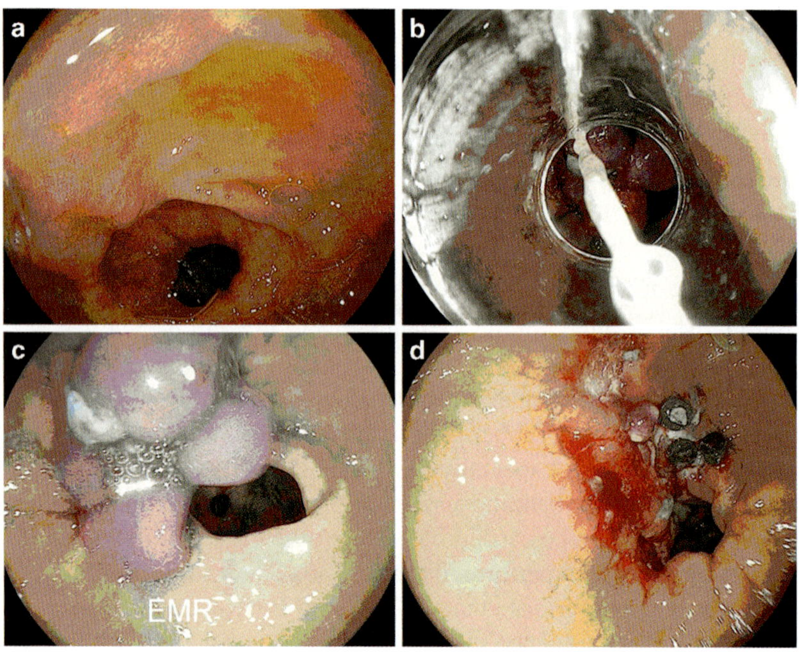

Fig. 6. A 75-year-old man with a gastric ulcer in the antrum. Multiple endoscopic biopsies were negative for malignancy, but positive for dysplasia. He was referred for EMR to obtain larger and deeper biopsies to rule out malignancy. (**a**) A 1-cm gastric ulcer in the antrum with raised and irregular edges. (**b** and **c**) after the area was marked with electrocautery, the abnormal area was suctioned into the cap without prior submucosal injection and rubber bands were released capturing the mucosa and superficial submucosa. (**d**) A hexagonal polypectomy snare, passed alongside the strings of the ligation device, was used to resect the created pseudopolyps below the rubber band. The area was resected without complications. Pathological specimens confirmed adenocarcinoma. The patient was then sent for surgical resection.

Retrieval of Resected Lesion

After EMR-C, the resected lesions can be suctioned into the cap and retrieved from the patient. With the other EMR techniques, the resected lesions can be retrieved by specially designed retrieval devices (Fig. 7).

The resected specimen must be carefully examined for accurate pathologic staging to guide further management and treatment recommendations. In the presence of poor prognostic factors (such as poorly differentiated carcinoma, lymphovascular invasion, cancer at the resected margin, or submucosal invasion), surgical resection should be considered because of the high risk of metastasis. If the lesion is partially resected, further evaluation and treatment will be necessary.

Complications

As with any endoscopic procedure, complication rates with EMR are highly operator dependent and diminish with increased experience. Bleeding is the most common complication of EMR, with an average rate of 10% (Binmoeller et al. 1996; Kodama and Kakegawa 1998; Iishi et al. 2000). Most bleeding occurs during the procedure or within the first 12 h and can be treated endoscopically. Perforation is uncommon with reported rates of 0.1–0.5% (Kaneko et al. 1995). Small perforations recognized during the procedure can be managed with placement of endoclips (Yoshikane et al. 1997; Kim et al. 2000). Large perforations require surgical repair. Stricture formation has been reported in 0–30% of patients after circumferential resections of the esophagus, pylorus, or colon (Katada et al. 2003). These strictures usually respond to endoscopic dilatation.

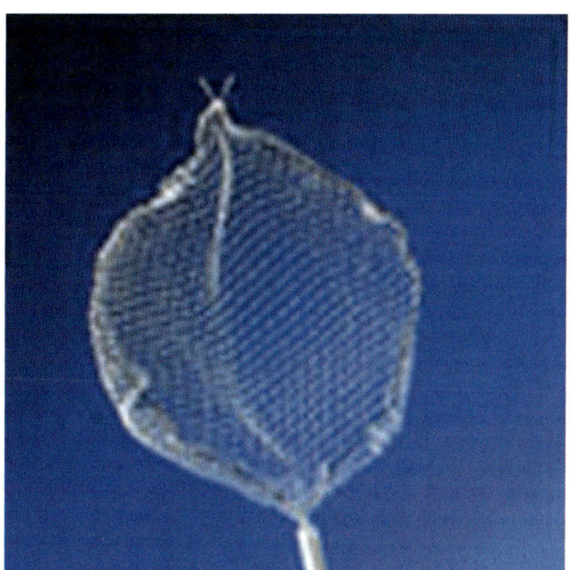

Fig. 7. Roth netTM for retrieval of EMR specimens (Courtesy of US Endoscopy).

Postoperative Care

EMR is generally an outpatient procedure. Hospitalization is not required unless serious complications have occurred. No specific postoperative care is required for EMR of the colorectum.

Following gastric or esophageal EMR, a clear liquid diet is recommended for 24 h. Many patients have pain localized over the resection site, and analgesics are often required for a couple of days. There is increasing evidence that use of a PPI postoperatively for a month may reduce the risk of bleeding and promote ulcer healing after EMR (Watanabe et al. 2006; Uedo et al. 2007).

Patients are offered regular surveillance examinations to exclude local recurrence and to detect synchronous or metachronous lesions.

RESULTS

With proper selection of patients for EMR, the risk of recurrence in lymph node or distant metastasis is very low. Local recurrence is usually due to incomplete resection.

Esophagus

Squamous Cell Carcinoma

Following EMR, superficial squamous cell carcinoma (SCC) has a disease-specific 5-year survival rate of up to 95%, which is not significantly different from 93% after surgical resection (Inoue et al. 2002; Takeshita et al. 1997; Ciocirlan et al. 2007; Shimizu et al. 2002). Nodal metastases were found in 0% of patients who had tumor confined to the lamina propria, in 8% who had tumor invasion into the muscularis mucosa, and in 30% who had invasion into the submucosa (Inoue et al. 2002; Takeshita et al. 1997; Ciocirlan et al. 2007).

Barrett's Esophagus with High-Grade Dysplasia and Early Cancer

Outcome data on BE have been limited. In the largest prospective study published to date evaluating the efficacy of EMR for treatment of high-grade dysplasia (HGD) and early cancer, complete local remission was achieved in 97% of patients with a 5-year survival rate of 84% (Pech et al. 2008). However, during a mean follow-up of 12 months, recurrent or metachronous cancer was found in 21% of patients (Pech et al. 2008). To improve eradication of neoplastic tissue and decrease recurrence, the combined use of EMR with ablative techniques such as argon plasma coagulation (APC) and photodynamic therapy (PDT) has been proposed (May et al. 2002a, b). Risk factors most frequently associated with recurrence were piecemeal resection, long-segment Barrett's esophagus, no ablative therapy of Barrett's esophagus after EMR, time to achieve complete response >10 months, and multifocal neoplasia. Patients with these risk factors may, therefore, require more intensive follow-up. Nevertheless, these results suggest that endoscopic therapy can be highly effective and safe for BE with HGD and early cancer, with an excellent long-term survival rate.

Stomach

The largest experience in endoscopic treatment of early gastric cancer has been in Japan where a high proportion of patients with gastric cancer were diagnosed at an early stage through screening programs. In a review of a total of 1,832 cases from 12 major institutions in Japan, the complete resection rate was 76% (Kojima et al. 1998). In incompletely resected cases, residual cancer was successfully treated with endoscopic retreatment or surgery. Recurrence was observed in only 1.9% of the patients (Kojima et al. 1998). The disease-specific survival rate was 99% with a follow-up period of 4 months to 11 years (Kojima et al. 1998). These results are comparable to those achieved by surgery.

Colorectum

EMR has been successfully used for early-stage colon cancer and large sessile polyps (Tung and Wu 2003; Conio et al. 2004; Arebi et al. 2007; Luigiano et al. 2009; Bories et al. 2006). Sessile polyps are considered to be large when they are greater than 2 cm in size. Their prevalence has been reported to be 0.8–5.2% in patients undergoing colonoscopy (Fukami and Lee 2006). The rate of malignancy in these large lesions has been reported to be 5–15% (Fukami and Lee 2006). Resection of these large lesions can usually be achieved in a piecemeal fashion with injection-assisted polypectomy in over >95% of cases (Fig. 8). Reported recurrence rates following EMR, however, can be as high as 16–40%, which justifies aggressive surveillance strategies after EMR (Tung and Wu 2003; Conio et al. 2004; Arebi et al. 2007). A few studies have suggested that application of APC to the edge and base of the polypectomy site post-EMR may reduce adenomatous recurrence by 50% (Brooker et al. 2002; Zlatanic et al. 1999).

ALTERNATIVE PROCEDURES

Surgical resection has been regarded as the gold standard treatment for GI cancers including those detected at an early stage. However, surgical resection is associated with substantial costs as well as risks. As an example, esophagectomy carries a high morbidity (18–48%) and a significant mortality rate of 3–5% (Kato et al. 1993; Roth and Putnam 1994). Gastrectomy has been reported to have a mortality of 6% (Ichikawa et al. 2004). Complications of gastrectomy, such as anastomotic leakage (3%), wound infection (2.8%), development of pancreatic fistulae (2.2%), and intraabdominal abscesses (1.5%), may shorten the overall postoperative survival (Ichikawa et al. 2004). Furthermore, studies have

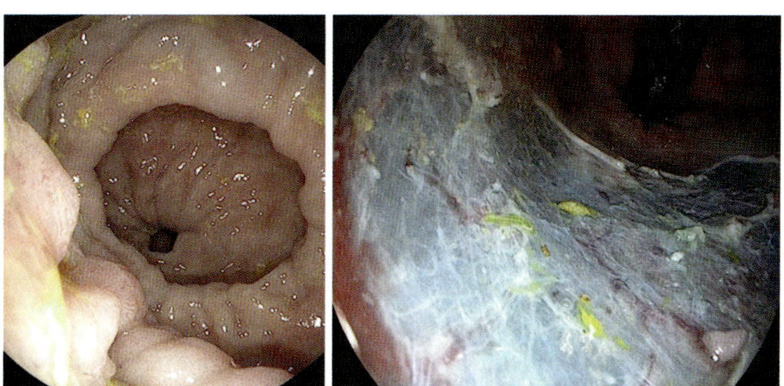

Fig. 8. A large sessile tubulovillous adenoma in the lower rectum resected by injection-assisted EMR. A small amount of methylene blue was added to the injectate to demarcate the resection margins.

shown esophagectomy and gastrectomy to significantly impair overall quality of life (QOL) because of postoperative GI symptoms (Wu et al. 2008; Djarv et al. 2008). For colon cancer and large colorectal polyps, laparoscopy-assisted colectomy has gained acceptance as an alternative to open colectomy in recent years (Nelson et al. 2004). However, the morbidity (11%) and mortality (3.5%) associated with laparoscopy-assisted colectomy are not insignificant (Nassiopoulos et al. 2005).

Endoscopic ablation methods such as photodynamic therapy (PDT), Nd:YAG laser, and argon plasma coagulation (APC) have been used to treat early GI cancers (Karanov 2002; Dumot and Greenwald 2008). Unlike EMR, these techniques do not provide the opportunity for histological assessment of the specimen.

Cost

To date, there have been no published studies on the cost-effectiveness of EMR and surgery for the treatment of early GI cancers. Evidence suggests that EMR is equally effective as surgery in the treatment of early GI cancers. If equally effective, EMR might be a more cost-effective approach, as this strategy does not require expensive equipment, operating room time, general anesthesia, and hospitalization. Furthermore, EMR is less invasive and carries lower morbidity and mortality than surgery.

Although EMR has obvious benefits for patients with early cancers, these techniques are labor-intensive, technically demanding, time consuming, and are not adequately reimbursed at the present time (Kochman et al. 2007). There are no unique Current Procedural Terminology (CPT) or billing codes for EMR in the United States or Canada. Also, the dedicated EMR devices do add to the facility cost of the procedure without added reimbursement.

CONCLUSIONS

EMR has emerged as a safe and effective treatment approach for superficial early cancers of the GI tract. The indications for EMR are ever expanding. This advanced endoscopic technique is minimally invasive and carries a lower morbidity and mortality compared with traditional surgical approaches. Increasing evidence suggests that EMR provides outcomes comparable to surgery for selected indications. To ensure optimal outcomes, appropriate selection of patients for EMR is crucial. Only those with early superficial GI cancers without lymph node involvement or distant metastasis are candidates for EMR. The long-term outcome of EMR will also depend on careful pathological specimen analysis and close endoscopic follow-up. Current challenges facing the wide adoption of EMR in North America include access to training and lack of appropriate reimbursement for this technically demanding and time consuming procedure.

SUMMARY OF KEY POINTS

- EMR is an advanced endoscopic technique with both diagnostic and therapeutic capabilities.
- Current indications for EMR include resection of early superficial GI cancers limited to the mucosa without any lymph node involvement or distant metastasis; removal of premalignant or potentially malignant lesions; obtain deeper and larger biopsies when conventional endoscopic biopsies fail to yield a diagnosis.

- Contraindications for EMR include carcinoma invading into the submucosa of the bowel wall, lymph node, or distant metastasis, non-lifting of the lesion after submucosal injection, and uncorrectable coagulopathy.
- Increasing evidence suggests EMR is a safe and highly effective alternative to surgery for treatment of esophageal dysplasia or cancer, gastric cancer, large flat colorectal polyps, and colorectal cancer.
- Resection techniques can be classified as (1) injection-assisted EMR, (2) cap-assisted EMR (EMR-C), and (3) ligation-assisted EMR (EMR-L).
- Submucosal injection of lesions prior to EMR may reduce the risk of perforation and bleeding. Non-lifting of lesion is predictive of invasive carcinoma.
- Appropriate selection of patients for EMR, careful pathologic specimen analysis, and close endoscopic follow-up are crucial to ensure optimal patient outcomes.

REFERENCES

Tada M, Murata M, Murakami K. Development of the strip-off biopsy. Gastroenterol Endosc. 1984;26:833–9.

Davila RE. Chromoendoscopy. Gastrointest Endosc Clin N Am. 2009;19(2):193–208.

Dubuc J, Legoux JL, Winnock M, et al. Endoscopic screening for esophageal squamous-cell carcinoma in high-risk patients: a prospective study conducted in 62 French endoscopy centers. Endoscopy. 2006;38(7):690–5.

Moschler O, Spahn TW, Middelberg-Bisping C, et al. Chromoendoscopy is a valuable tool for screening of high-risk patients with head and neck cancer for early detection of esophageal cancer. Digestion. 2006;73(2–3):160–6.

Inoue H, Rey JF, Lightdale C. Lugol chromoendoscopy for esophageal squamous cell cancer. Endoscopy. 2001;33(1):75–9.

Kawahara Y, Takenaka R, Okada H, et al. Novel chromoendoscopic method using an acetic acid-indigocarmine mixture for diagnostic accuracy in delineating the margin of early gastric cancers. Dig Endosc. 2009;21(1):14–9.

Ngamruengphong S, Sharma VK, Das A. Diagnostic yield of methylene blue chromoendoscopy for detecting specialized intestinal metaplasia and dysplasia in Barrett's esophagus: a meta-analysis. Gastrointest Endosc. 2009;69(6):1021–8.

Connor MJ, Sharma P. Chromoendoscopy and magnification endoscopy for diagnosing esophageal cancer and dysplasia. Thorac Surg Clin. 2004;14(1):87–94.

Hurlstone DP, Fujii T. Practical uses of chromoendoscopy and magnification at colonoscopy. Gastrointest Endosc Clin N Am. 2005;15(4):687–702.

Tischendorf JJ, Schirin-Sokhan R, Streetz K, et al. Value of magnifying endoscopy in classifying colorectal polyps based on vascular pattern. Endoscopy. 2010;42(1):22–7.

Mannath J, Subramanian V, Hawkey CJ, Ragunath K. Narrow band imaging for characterization of high grade dysplasia and specialized intestinal metaplasia in Barrett's esophagus: a meta-analysis. Endoscopy. 2010;42(5):351–9.

Muto M, Horimatsu T, Ezoe Y, Morita S, Miyamoto S. Improving visualization techniques by narrow band imaging and magnification endoscopy. J Gastroenterol Hepatol. 2009;24(8):1333–46.

Endo M, Yoshino K. Analysis of 1125 cases of early esophageal carcinoma in Japan. Dis Esophagus. 1991;4:71–6.

Tajima Y, Nakanishi Y, Ochiai A, et al. Histopathologic findings predicting lymph node metastasis and prognosis of patients with superficial esophageal carcinoma: analysis of 240 surgically resected tumors. Cancer. 2000;88(6):1285–93.

Kurihara N, Kubota T, Otani Y, et al. Lymph node metastasis of early gastric cancer with submucosal invasion. Br J Surg. 1998;85(6):835–9.

Wilcox GM, Anderson PB, Colacchio TA. Early invasive carcinoma in colonic polyps A review of the literature with emphasis on the assessment of the risk of metastasis. Cancer. 1986;57(1):160–71.

Japanese Gastric Cancer Association. Japanese classification of gastric carcinoma – 2nd English Edition. Gastric Cancer. 1998;1(1):10–24.

Murata Y, Napoleon B, Odegaard S. High-frequency endoscopic ultrasonography in the evaluation of superficial esophageal cancer. Endoscopy. 2003;35(5):429–35.

Saitoh Y, Obara T, Einami K, et al. Efficacy of high-frequency ultrasound probes for the preoperative staging of invasion depth in flat and depressed colorectal tumors. Gastrointest Endosc. 1996;44(1):34–9.

Akahoshi K, Chijiwa Y, Hamada S, et al. Pretreatment staging of endoscopically early gastric cancer with a 15 MHz ultrasound catheter probe. Gastrointest Endosc. 1998;48(5):470–6.

Uno Y, Munakata A. The non-lifting sign of invasive colon cancer. Gastrointest Endosc. 1994;40(4):485–9.

Gotoda T, Yamamoto H, Soetikno RM. Endoscopic submucosal dissection of early gastric cancer. J Gastroenterol. 2006;41(10):929–42.

Binmoeller KF, Bohnacker S, Seifert H, Thonke F, Valdeyar H, Soehendra N. Endoscopic snare excision of "giant" colorectal polyps. Gastrointest Endosc. 1996;43(3):183–8.

Kodama M, Kakegawa T. Treatment of superficial cancer of the esophagus: a summary of responses to a questionnaire on superficial cancer of the esophagus in Japan. Surgery. 1998;123(4):432–9.

Iishi H, Tatsuta M, Iseki K, et al. Endoscopic piecemeal resection with submucosal saline injection of large sessile colorectal polyps. Gastrointest Endosc. 2000;51(6):697–700.

Kaneko E, Hanada H, Kasugai T, Sakita T. The results of a multi-center analysis from 1988–1992 (in Japanese). Gastroenterol Endosc. 1995;37:642–52.

Yoshikane H, Hidano H, Sakakibara A, et al. Endoscopic repair by clipping of iatrogenic colonic perforation. Gastrointest Endosc. 1997;46(5):464–6.

Kim HS, Lee DK, Jeong YS, et al. Successful endoscopic management of a perforated gastric dysplastic lesion after endoscopic mucosal resection. Gastrointest Endosc. 2000;51(5):613–5.

Katada C, Muto M, Manabe T, Boku N, Ohtsu A, Yoshida S. Esophageal stenosis after endoscopic mucosal resection of superficial esophageal lesions. Gastrointest Endosc. 2003;57(2):165–9.

Watanabe Y, Kato N, Maehata T, et al. Safer endoscopic gastric mucosal resection: preoperative proton pump inhibitor administration. J Gastroenterol Hepatol. 2006;21(11):1675–80.

Uedo N, Takeuchi Y, Yamada T, et al. Effect of a proton pump inhibitor or an H2-receptor antagonist on prevention of bleeding from ulcer after endoscopic submucosal dissection of early gastric cancer: a prospective randomized controlled trial. Am J Gastroenterol. 2007;102(8):1610–6.

Inoue H, Fukami N, Yoshida T, Kudo SE. Endoscopic mucosal resection for esophageal and gastric cancers. J Gastroenterol Hepatol. 2002;17(4):382–8.

Takeshita K, Tani M, Inoue H, et al. Endoscopic treatment of early oesophageal or gastric cancer. Gut. 1997;40(1):123–7.

Ciocirlan M, Lapalus MG, Hervieu V, et al. Endoscopic mucosal resection for squamous premalignant and early malignant lesions of the esophagus. Endoscopy. 2007;39(1):24–9.

Shimizu Y, Tsukagoshi H, Fujita M, Hosokawa M, Kato M, Asaka M. Long-term outcome after endoscopic mucosal resection in patients with esophageal squamous cell carcinoma invading the muscularis mucosae or deeper. Gastrointest Endosc. 2002;56(3):387–90.

Pech O, Behrens A, May A, et al. Long-term results and risk factor analysis for recurrence after curative endoscopic therapy in 349 patients with high-grade intraepithelial neoplasia and mucosal adenocarcinoma in Barrett's oesophagus. Gut. 2008;57(9):1200–6.

May A, Gossner L, Pech O, et al. Local endoscopic therapy for intraepithelial high-grade neoplasia and early adenocarcinoma in Barrett's oesophagus: acute-phase and intermediate results of a new treatment approach. Eur J Gastroenterol Hepatol. 2002a;14(10):1085–91.

May A, Gossner L, Pech O, et al. Intraepithelial high-grade neoplasia and early adenocarcinoma in short-segment Barrett's esophagus (SSBE): curative treatment using local endoscopic treatment techniques. Endoscopy. 2002b;34(8):604–10.

Kojima T, Parra-Blanco A, Takahashi H, Fujita R. Outcome of endoscopic mucosal resection for early gastric cancer: review of the Japanese literature. Gastrointest Endosc. 1998;48(5):550–4.

Tung SY, Wu CS. Clinical outcome of endoscopically removed early colorectal cancer. J Gastroenterol Hepatol. 2003;18(10):1175–9.

Conio M, Repici A, Demarquay JF, Blanchi S, Dumas R, Filiberti R. EMR of large sessile colorectal polyps. Gastrointest Endosc. 2004;60(2):234–41.

Arebi N, Swain D, Suzuki N, Fraser C, Price A, Saunders BP. Endoscopic mucosal resection of 161 cases of large sessile or flat colorectal polyps. Scand J Gastroenterol. 2007;42(7):859–66.

Luigiano C, Consolo P, Scaffidi MG, et al. Endoscopic mucosal resection for large and giant sessile and flat colorectal polyps: a single-center experience with long-term follow-up. Endoscopy. 2009;41(10):829–35.

Bories E, Pesenti C, Monges G, et al. Endoscopic mucosal resection for advanced sessile adenoma and early-stage colorectal carcinoma. Endoscopy. 2006;38(3):231–5.

Fukami N, Lee JH. Endoscopic treatment of large sessile and flat colorectal lesions. Curr Opin Gastroenterol. 2006;22(1):54–9.

Brooker JC, Saunders BP, Shah SG, Thapar CJ, Suzuki N, Williams CB. Treatment with argon plasma coagulation reduces recurrence after piecemeal resection of large sessile colonic polyps: a randomized trial and recommendations. Gastrointest Endosc. 2002;55(3):371–5.

Zlatanic J, Waye JD, Kim PS, Baiocco PJ, Gleim GW. Large sessile colonic adenomas: use of argon plasma coagulator to supplement piecemeal snare polypectomy. Gastrointest Endosc. 1999;49(6):731–5.

Kato H, Tachimori Y, Mizobuchi S, Igaki H, Ochiai A. Cervical, mediastinal, and abdominal lymph node dissection (three-field dissection) for superficial carcinoma of the thoracic esophagus. Cancer. 1993;72(10):2879–82.

Roth JA, Putnam Jr JB. Surgery for cancer of the esophagus. Semin Oncol. 1994;21(4):453–61.

Ichikawa D, Kurioka H, Yamaguchi T, et al. Postoperative complications following gastrectomy for gastric cancer during the last decade. Hepatogastroenterology. 2004;51(56):613–7.

Wu CW, Chiou JM, Ko FS, et al. Quality of life after curative gastrectomy for gastric cancer in a randomised controlled trial. Br J Cancer. 2008;98(1):54–9.

Djarv T, Lagergren J, Blazeby JM, Lagergren P. Long-term health-related quality of life following surgery for oesophageal cancer. Br J Surg. 2008;95(9):1121–6.

Nelson H, Sargent DJ, COST Study Group. A comparison of laparoscopically assisted and open colectomy for colon cancer. N Engl J Med. 2004;350(20):2050–2059.

Nassiopoulos K, Pavlidis TE, Menenakos E, Chanson C, Zografos G, Petropoulos P. Laparoscopic colectomy in the management of large, sessile, transformed colorectal polyps. JSLS. 2005;9(1):58–62.

Karanov SI. Long-term results after photodynamic therapy (PDT) of T1N0M0 gastrointestinal (GI) tumors. Hepatogastroenterology. 2002;49(48):1579–81.

Dumot JA, Greenwald BD. Argon plasma coagulation, bipolar cautery, and cryotherapy: ABC's of ablative techniques. Endoscopy. 2008;40(12):1026–32.

Kochman ML, Antillon M, Brill JV, Marcello PW, Margolin D. Alphabet soup: EMR, WEMR, ESD, SAP, ESR. What is it and what is it worth to you? Gastrointest Endosc. 2007;66(1):208.

8 Enteral Nutrition: From Formulations to Delivery

Mark H. DeLegge

CONTENTS

Keywords: Enteral, Nutrition, Formulations, Delivery, Protein, Fiber

In hospitalized and chronically ill patients, malnutrition is associated with impaired immune function, increased infections, increased lengths of hospital stay, and a reduction in overall body function (Isabel and Correia 2003). Malnutrition is present in up to 40% of intensive care unit (ICU) patients and is associated with increased morbidity and mortality (Giner et al. 1996). With these facts, nutritional intervention often plays an important role in the overall therapy of at-risk patient populations.

The approaches to nutritional intervention are seen in Table 1. Often, oral nutrition therapy or pharmacologic appetite stimulation are not options because of a patient's inability or unwillingness to adequately consume nutrition or medications by mouth. In these instances, the use of parenteral nutrition (intravenous nutrition – PN) or enteral tube feeding (EN) becomes necessary. There have been numerous evaluations comparing the use of EN versus PN as a nutrition intervention. The use of EN requires placement of a feeding tube. The use of PN requires placement of a central venous catheter. A recent meta-analysis examining the use of EN versus PN in patients with acute pancreatitis noted a reduction in infectious complication and hospital length of stay with the use of EN (Marik and Zaloga 2004).

Enteral nutrition or feeding through the gut helps set the tone for systemic immunity through stimulation of Th-2 pathways of CD_4 helper lymphocyte proliferation (a process which opposes proliferation of Th-1 proinflammatory cellular pathways) (Kudsk 2002; Spiekermann and Walker 2001; Coffman et al. 1988). Maintaining gut integrity and preventing

From: *Clinical Gastroenterology: Diagnostic and Therapeutic Procedures in Gastroenterology*,
Edited by: G. Y. Wu, S. Sridhar, DOI 10.1007/978-1-59745-044-7_8,

Table 1
Nutritional interventions

Dietary education, oral supplements
Pharmacologic appetite stimulation
Enteral nutrition tube feeding
Parenteral nutrition intravenous feedings

increased permeability helps attenuate oxidative stress and, in some cases, actually reduces disease severity such as seen in acute pancreatitis (Windsor et al. 1998). The effect of these physiologic changes is a dramatic favorable impact on patient outcomes.

The positive published clinical outcomes associated with EN cannot be attributed to a deleterious effect of PN alone. Improved outcomes are seen with use of enteral feeding compared with standard therapy in which no nutritional support is provided (Lewis et al. 2001). In a large meta-analysis, Lewis et al. showed that early EN provided postoperatively (day 1) reduced infections, length of hospital stay, and anastomotic dehiscence compared with awaiting for the presence of bowel sounds before feeding (usually day 4 or 5) (Lewis et al. 2001).

In order to provide EN, enteral access must be obtained. This can be accomplished by an endoscopist, a radiologist, or a surgeon. For a detailed explanation of enteral access, please see the chapter on Percutaneous Enterostomy Tubes from Humana Press, *An Internist's Illustrated Guide to Gastrointestinal Surgery*, by Gaspar Nazareno and George Y. Wu.

Once a decision to use EN has been determined, the clinician must choose the appropriate EN formula, determine a method of EN delivery, and be vigilant to diagnose and treat complications associated with the use of EN.

ENTERAL FEEDING FORMULAS

Enteral formulations are nutritionally complete when given in the recommended amount. They can be used as a sole source of nutrition. Enteral supplements are generally nutritionally incomplete when used as the sole source of nutrition. Enteral formulations contain macronutrients in various forms and concentrations, along with vitamins and minerals. Specialty nutrients, such as arginine, glutamine, and alternative lipid sources, may be added to design "disease specific" formulations. Enteral formulations may or may not contain fiber. Water is present in various concentrations allowing the formulas to be delivered in a "dilute" or a "concentrated" form. With these variations in the content of enteral formulations, a classification system has been designed (Table 2).

Standard Formulas

These formulas contain macronutrient and micronutrient concentrations appropriate for the "standard" population. They generally contain long-chain triglycerides and whole proteins. They do not contain gluten or lactose. They may or may not contain fiber. They are generally available in a 1, 1.5, and 2 cal/cm^3 formulation. The more concentrated formulations can be used for patients who are fluid restricted (e.g., renal disease).

Table 2
Categorization of enteral formulas

Oral supplements
- Generally 1 or 1.5 kcal/cm^3
- Flavor variety
- Carnation Instant Breakfast, Boost (Nestle), Ensure (Ross)

Enteral formulations
- *Standard*
  - 1 kcal/mL
  - Standard protein (35–45 g/L)
  - Examples – Osmolite, Isocal, Nutren, Isosource
- *High protein*
  - 1.5 kcal/mL
  - Higher protein content (45–65 g/L)
  - Examples – Osmolite HN (Ross) Promote (Nestle)
- *High caloric density*
  - 2 kcal/mL
  - Reduced free water content
  - Examples – 2 cal (Ross), Nutren 2.0 (Nestle)
  - Often used for patients with renal disease
- *Fiber containing*
  - Examples – Jevity (Ross), Nutren with Fiber (Nestle)
- *Elemental*
  - Protein as individual amino acids, nearly fat-free
  - High osmolarity
  - Examples – Vivonex TEN (Nestle) Vital HN (Ross)
- *Semielemental or peptide-based*
  - Protein as small chain peptides,
  - Fat mostly as MCT oil
  - Examples – Peptamen (Nestle)

Specialty formulas
- *Pulmonary*
  - Higher fat:carbohydrate ratio
  - Examples – Pulmocare (Ross)
- *Hepatic*
  - Higher branch chain:to aromatic amino acids
  - Examples – Nutrihep (Nestle)
- *Renal*
  - Higher essential AA to ↑ nitrogen cycling, better electrolyte profile
  - Nepro – (Nestle)
- *Diabetic*
  - Lower nonprotein calorie t:nitrogen ratio,
  - Alternate carbohydrate sources
  - Examples – Glucerna (Ross)

(continued)

Table 2
(continued)

Immune modulating
Arginine to ↑ immunity, Omega-3 fish oil to ↓inflammation
Examples – Impact (Nestle), Pivot (Ross)
Ross Laboratories – Columbus, OH
Nestle Nutrition, Glendale, CA

Fiber Containing Formulas

In general, these are fiber supplemented standard formulations. Fiber can be classified by its solubility in water. Soluble fibers, such as pectin, are fermented by colonic bacteria potential resulting in improved fluid and electrolyte absorption in the colon. Insoluble fiber, such as soy fiber, increases fecal weight and may have an effect on intestinal transit time. The use of fiber containing formulas to control diarrhea in the tube-fed patient has resulted in conflicting results (Frankenfeld and Beyer 1989; Shankardass et al. 1990).

High Protein Formulas

These formulas provide 20% or more of total formula macronutrients as protein. This is denoted on the formulation as HN (high nitrogen). These formulas are often used in very catabolic patients such as seen in trauma or sepsis.

Peptide-Based Formulas

Protein content in this formulation is in peptide form of (2–50) amino acids in length. They are usually low fat or contain a high percentage of medium chain triglycerides. These formulas have been formulated for patients with mucosal nutrient malabsorption. It is postulated that the low fat, predigested formulations are more easily absorbed. There has been a paucity of research in this arena supporting the effectiveness of peptide-based formulas.

Elemental Formulas

The protein content of these formulas exists as single peptides, dipeptides, or tripeptides. Generally, they are very low in fat content. These formulas are recommended for patients with "malabsorptive disorders" because of their predigested state. The osmolarity of this formulation is high based on the small particle size of the nutrients. There has been a paucity of research on the utility of these formulations for malabsorptive disorders.

Disease Specific

Disease-specific enteral formulations have been designed to meet the presumptive special nutritional requirements of individual disease states. Many of the available clinical studies evaluating the usefulness of these formulations are from a number of years ago.

Renal-specific formulas: These are generally lower in free water, lower in protein content, calorie dense, and have a reduction in levels of potassium, magnesium, and phosphorous. There are no clinical trials comparing renal-specific products against standardized enteral formulations in the patient with renal disease.

Hepatic disease: These formulations contain higher levels of branched-chain amino acids (BCAA) believed to be associated with a reduction in hepatic encephalopathy. In general, clinical trials have not demonstrated a benefit in the patient with liver failure in terms of improved nitrogen balance nor decreased episodes of encephalopathy using a BCAA enteral formula when compared with standard-based enteral formulations (Cerra et al. 1985; Michel et al. 1985).

Diabetes: These formulas generally contain a lower amount of total carbohydrate and a higher content of fat when compared with standard formulations. Carbohydrate sources usually consist of fructose, cornstarch, fiber, and/or oligosaccharides. There are few randomized, controlled trials evaluating the use of diabetic formulas in the hospitalized diabetic patients. To date, these trials have not shown an effect on patient outcomes, such as intensive care unit days, ventilator days, or mortality (Masejo et al. 2003).

Chronic obstructive pulmonary disease: Early formulations attempted to reduce the carbon dioxide retention associated with high amounts of carbohydrates in enteral formulas by replacing some carbohydrate calories with fat calories resulting in a high-fat enteral formula. Overall, there was no reported evidence report that these specialty disease formulas improved outcomes in this patient population.

Acute respiratory distress syndrome (ARDS): A specialized enteral formula containing modified lipids, including borage and fish oil, as well as increased amount of antioxidants has been tested in the ARDS population. The formula is designed to reduce the associated inflammatory response that develops in at-risk, critically ill patients. Although still controversial, there have been reports of improvement in lung function using this enteral formula (Singer et al. 2006).

Immune enhancing: The innate benefits of early EN may be further enhanced by the addition of immune modulatory agents (Montejo et al. 2003). Adding arginine and nucleotides to an enteral formula, both of which are direct immune stimulants, may enhance proliferation of Th-2 lymphocyte cell populations. Substitution of omega-3 fatty acids from fish oil for the more routinely used omega-6 fatty acids help modify the leukotrienes, thromboxanes, and prostaglandins produced by immune active cells and help generate an anti-inflammatory effect. Agents such as glutamine, vitamin C, and selenium act as antioxidants, reducing the overall level of oxidative stress. A recent meta-analyses by Montejo of 26 studies in which immune active formulas were compared with standard enteral formulas demonstrated that infections were reduced by 46–74%, organ failure was reduced by 79%, and length of stay in the ICU and hospital was reduced between 1.6 and 3.4 days using immune-enhanced formulas (compared with standard formulas) (Montejo et al. 2003) (Table 3).

There is some concern with the use of arginine containing immune formulations in those patients who are critically ill who have ongoing sepsis. This concern is related to the possibility that arginine would stimulate inducible nitric oxide synthetase, leading to production of nitric oxide and worsening hypotension. In a study by Bower et al., mortality was 2–2½ times greater in patients receiving the immune-enhanced formula compared with controls receiving standard formula (Bower et al. 1995). In contrast, in a study by Galban et al., in

Table 3
Immune-enhancing enteral formulations

Product	*Type of formula*	*Arginine per 1,000 cal*	*Omega-3 fish oil/canola oilper L*	*Borage oil*	*Manufacturer*
Impact 1.5	Immune-enhancing	12.5 g	2.6 g combined		Novartis Medical Nutrition (St. Louis Park, MN)
Crucial	Immune-enhancing	10 g	4.3 g combined		Nestle Nutrition (Glendale, CA)
Pivot 1.5	Immune-enhancing	8.6 g	3.9 g combined	2.86 g/ 1,000 cal	Ross Division, Abbott Labs (Columbus, OH)
Optimental	Immune-enhancing	≈5 g	Unspecified amount		Ross Division, Abbott Labs (Columbus, OH)
Perative	Immune-enhancing	≈6 g	Unspecified amount		Ross Division, Abbott Labs
Oxepa	Antiinflamatory	1.4 g	Unspecified amount		Ross Division, Abbott Labs (Columbus, OH)
PeptamenAF	Antiinflamatory	0.0 g	9.3 g fish oil		Nestle Nutrition (Glendale, CA)

which 100% of the patients were septic, using high arginine formula improved mortality compared with controls receiving a standard formula (Galban et al. 2000). In animal models with sepsis, supplementation with arginine in most studies improved survival (Zaloga et al. 2004).

ENTERAL FORMULA DELIVERY METHODS

The actual delivery of EN through a feeding tube may be accomplished by a variety of methods. Patients may be fed by bolus, intermittent, or continuous methods. Bolus feeding generally allows the delivery of a relatively large volume of tube feeding over a short period of time (usually, 5–15 min). In general, the bolus delivery system requires the use of a funnel or the barrel of a large syringe (100 cm^3) attached to the end of the feeding tube (Fig. 1). Tube feeding is slowly poured through the feeding tube into the gastrointestinal tract. In general, bolus feedings are often used in patients who are awake and active.

Intermittent tube-feeding delivery may be useful for patients who cannot tolerate bolus feedings, but do not require the precise delivery of enteral feeding by continuous method. In general, a large volume (200–500 cm^3) of tube feeding is delivered over a specified time, for example, over 1 h. This may be delivered by gravity method (a bag of tube-feeding hung on a bedside pole) or by a pump. Continuous feedings are usually delivered over 12–24 h by a mechanical pump. It allows the precise delivery of tube feeding over a period

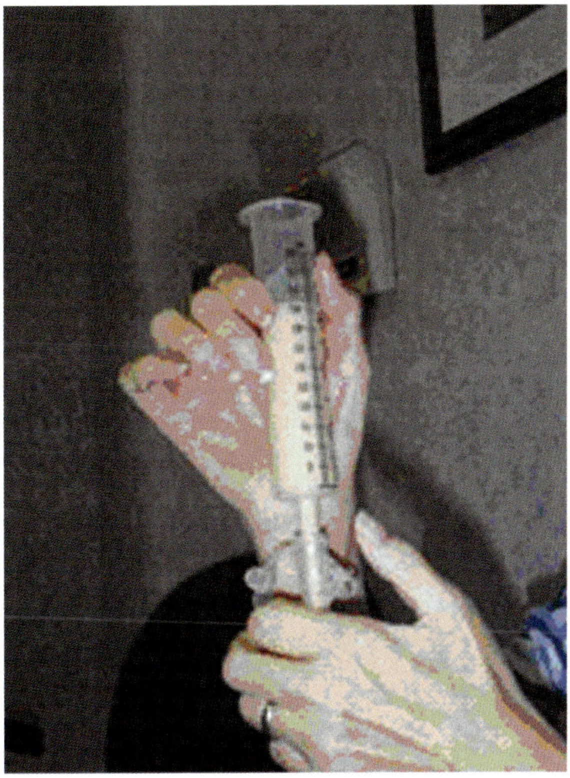

Fig. 1. A photograph of a typical setup for bolus gastrostomy tube feeding.

of time (cm^3/h) (Fig. 2). Patients fed into the small intestine (jejunal feeding) are usually fed by the continuous method.

The use of intermittent or continuous feedings versus bolus feeding to improve patient tolerance of EN by reducing associated symptoms of bloating, abdominal pain, nausea, vomiting, and diarrhea is a common practice. However, there is little clinical data supporting this practice. Recently, Serpa et al. randomized 28 critically ill patients to either bolus or continuous EN (Serpa et al. 2003). There was only one documented case of aspiration. There were some reported associated gastrointestinal complications such as vomiting, diarrhea and abdominal distention, although there was no difference between the two groups.

MONITORING TUBE FEEDING

Gastrointestinal Tolerance

Once feeding has been initiated, monitoring for tolerance is important. In general, evidence that the gut has function is important to the initiation of EN. Evidence that the stomach is functioning is indicated by a nasogastric output <1,200 mL/day (in light of the fact that over 3,000 mL/day can be produced through salivary and gastric secretion). Small bowel contractility may be evaluated by abdominal distention, presence of bowel sounds, and air–fluid levels on an abdominal radiograph. Contractility in the colon may be indicated by passage of flatus and stool. In reality, none of these markers by themselves is

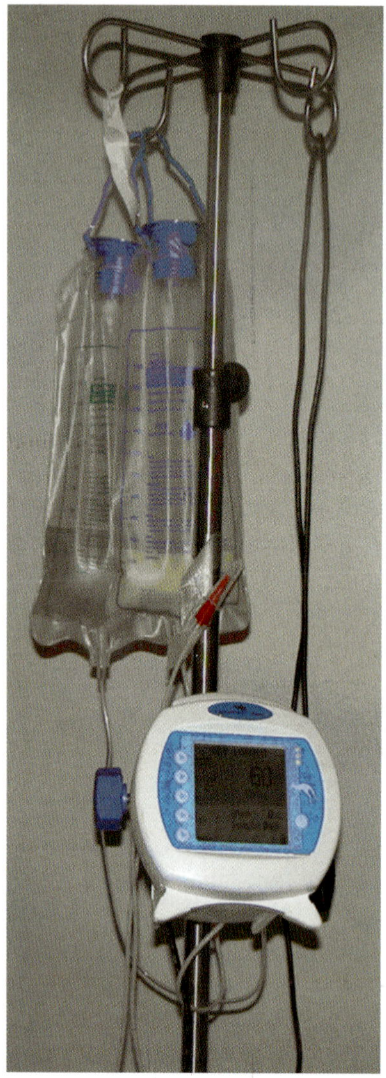

Fig. 2. A photograph of a typical setup for pump-driven gastrostomy tube feeding.

completely reliable in predicting gut function. It is often a combination of these markers that can help to identify a patient with presumed poor gut function.

Nausea and Vomiting

Patients who are awake are able to express symptoms of nausea. Visceral afferent nerves from the gastrointestinal tract (vagus or sympathetic nerves) inform the brainstem of gastrointestinal distention or mucosal irritation. These receptors are most prominent in the proximal small bowel, especially the duodenum. There are also afferent nerves from outside the luminal gut, such as in the bile duct and peritoneum. Vomiting is demonstrated by the active regurgitation of food substances out of the oral cavity either in the awake or in the comatose patients. Nausea and vomiting have a number of etiologies including gastrointestinal

Table 4
Common causes of acute nausea and vomiting in enteral nutrition patients

Bacterial or viral gastroenteritis
Medications
Fever
Severe gastroparesis
Ileus
Gastroesophageal reflux disease
Peptic ulcer disease
Cholecystitis
Pancreatitis
Peritonitis
Gastric outlet obstruction
Small bowel or colon obstruction
Gut volvulus

pathology such as peptic ulcer disease, gastric outlet obstruction, small bowel obstruction, colon obstruction, and ileus (Table 4). In additional medications, fever or active tissue inflammation from any disease process may also lead to symptoms of nausea and/or vomiting. Vomiting may not be an indicator of tube-feeding intolerance, but may be a symptom of the patient's primary disease state.

Gastric Residual Volume

In the gastric-fed patient, it is believed that monitoring of gastric residual volumes will allow the clinician to predict who will experience vomiting or regurgitation of tube feeding. This practice is based on the theory that increased gastric residuals leads to increased intragastric pressures resulting in regurgitation and vomiting (Lin and Van Critters 1997). This theory would hold true for a "fixed" volume container. However, the stomach is a distensible container that has the ability to hold liters of fluid. This use of GRV measurements to determine tube-feeding tolerance does not take into account the 1,500 cm^3 of saliva and 2,000 cm^3 of gastric secretions produced each day. Fluctuations of 10–20% in the production of these secretions would be expected to significantly impact the validity of GRV as a marker of tube-feeding tolerance. Clinically, it is further hypothesized that preventing regurgitation and vomiting in the tube-fed patient population will reduce the incidence of aspiration pneumonia.

The threshold level of GRV tolerated by clinicians is a point of great debate. It is certainly of no clinical significance at volumes <200 cm^3 (Mullan et al. 1992). More recently, McClave et al. evaluated 40 ventilated intensive care unit (ICU) patients who were receiving gastric enteral feedings containing fluorometric beads (McClave et al. 2005). More than 1,000 oral and tracheal aspirates were collected and analyzed for the presence of fluorometric beads (defined as aspiration). The mean frequency of aspiration was 22.1% with a mean GRV for aspiration of 30.6 mL. There was no difference in aspiration events when GRV were increased to 400 cm^3. There was no difference in aspiration events if patients were fed through an NG tube or a PEG tube.

More importantly, aspiration events, especially in the critically ill population, can be reduced by maintaining a patient's head of the bed elevated during tube feeding and providing good oral hygiene to reduce the presence of pharyngeal bacteria and oral–tracheal aspiration (McClave et al. 2002).

Diarrhea

Alterations in fecal output are common in patients receiving EN. This includes both diarrhea and constipation, although diarrhea is more common. There have been numerous methods employed to clinically document the characteristics of diarrhea including stool frequency, stool consistency, and stool weight. Because of this, the clinical definition of diarrhea associated with EN varies tremendously from institution to institution.

The etiologies of diarrhea are numerous. Most diarrheas can be categorized into a secretory or a malabsorptive etiology. In general, diarrhea with tube feeding is believed to be most often secondary to either an infectious cause (e.g., *Clostridium difficile* enterocolitis), concurrent medication use (e.g., sorbitol containing elixirs), or malabsorption. Malabsorptive etiologies of diarrhea generally require significant disease of the small intestine or specific nutrient malabsorption.

A common etiology of diarrhea associated with EN is best explained by three published experiments. Breath test studies have shown that breath hydrogen is increased markedly in post-surgical patients just prior to an episode of diarrhea. This is most likely a result of malabsorbed small intestinal carbohydrates spilling over into the colon causing an osmotic diarrhea (Hammer et al. 1989). Microorganisms in the colon ferment malabsorbed enteral diet carbohydrates to short-chain fatty acids (SCFA). These SCFA stimulate colon mucosal cell hypertrophy, thereby increasing colon water and electrolyte absorption (Bowling et al. 1994). It is believed that the use of antibiotics in tube-fed patients decreases colonic microorganisms, thereby reducing the production of SCFA, resulting in a net colon wasting of sodium and water (Jorgensen et al. 2001).

In clinical practice, an increase in a patient's stool output may be documented as "diarrhea." When using the term diarrhea, it suggests that a threshold for the clinician has been reached and that the patient requires some evaluation or medical intervention. The overall incidence of TF-related diarrhea in the literature has been reported from 2% to 95% (Debnam and Grimble 2001). In these reports, there were over 33 different definitions of diarrhea (Lebak et al. 2003). This includes an increase in stool frequency, stool consistency, stool weight (>300 g/day), and multiple combinations of the above. This lack of definition, clarity, and clinical relevance makes clinical studies of tube-feeding-related diarrhea difficult to perform and difficult to interpret. The use of verbal and pictorial descriptions of diarrhea is only slightly more reliable than a subject's verbal description alone (Lebak et al. 2003). Recently, Whelan et al. developed a standardized scoring system of stool frequency, stool consistency, and stool weight using a standardized chart for data tabulation.

This chart provided significant intraobserver reproducibility for describing clinical diarrhea (Whelan et al. 2004). This consistency in diarrhea reporting will help to adequately determine the true incidence of TF-related diarrhea and will also assist in determining which interventions are effective for controlling TF-related diarrhea.

Most diarrheas associated with tube-fed patients are treatable and should not result in withholding of EN. This would include diarrheas related to *Clostridium difficile* enterocolitis, the use of diarrhea causing medications, bacterial overgrowth, and pancreatic insufficiency. Using anticholinergic agents, such as loperamide, is appropriate to decrease bowel transit time and improve the chances of nutrient and water absorption. Some physicians will empirically treat patients with metranidazole or a quinolone antibiotic in hopes that altering the patient's gut flora will improve the patient's diarrhea. Pancreatic enzymes may be helpful in the patient with pancreatic insufficiency and steatorrhea. Enteral nutrition should be held for clinically significant diarrhea that worsens with TF and improves with withholding of TF. Clinically significant diarrhea includes those that result in volume depletion, weight loss, decubitus ulcer formation, or worsening abdominal pain.

Current algorithms for the treatment of diarrhea in the tube-fed patient include changing the tube feeding to a more readily absorbed tube-feeding product, such as an elemental or semi-elemental tube-feeding formula. Although there are reports of success with the change to a more readily absorbed tube-feeding product, prospective clinical trials have shown no benefit. A prospective analysis of 40 patients with multiple comorbid disease processes at a subacute medical center used a Malbsorption Index, which was applied to individual patients to predict which class of enteral formulas should be initiated to avoid GI intolerance, specifically the development of diarrhea (DeLegge et al. 2000) (Fig. 1). The scoring system took into account multiple clinical parameters including the patient's medical condition, serum albumin level, and nutritional status. The use of this scoring system was effective for matching patients and a class of tube feeding to avoid tube-feeding-related diarrhea.

More recently, the use of probiotics for the treatment of diarrhea in the tube-fed patient has been evaluated. A recent meta-analysis of six trials demonstrated a significant reduction in the risk of developing antibiotic-associated diarrhea in patients treated with probiotics at the initiation of their antibiotic treatment (Jenkins et al. 2005). Recent clinical trial analysis also suggests that probiotics may be useful for the prevention and treatment of *Clostridium difficile* associated diarrhea (Dendukuri et al. 2005).

Bloating and Distention

Abdominal bloating and distention is a common physical finding in patients who are in the hospital. Although frequently used as a rationale to hold or discontinue tube feedings, the pathophysiology and clinical significance of these symptoms remains poorly defined.

Three factors are believed to be important in the pathophysiology of bloating. This includes the subjective sensation of bloating, the objective presence of abdominal distention, and the volume of intraabdominal contents (Lasser et al. 1975). Patients with a heightened sensation for intestinal distention, usually by gas, most likely have an abnormality of the sensory loop of the enteric (gut) nervous system. Excess bowel gas production may be a more significant problem for patients who are hospitalized, have an altered bowel flora, and are predisposed to nutrient maldigestion, especially carbohydrates. Applications of hydrogen breath tests have shown that maldigestion of small quantities of carbohydrates can lead to chronic complaints of gas, abdominal pain, and flatulence (Ravich et al. 1982). Several studies measuring abdominal girth changes, either with a tape measure or CT scan, have shown that the subjective sensation of abdominal distention is often associated with some objective abdominal distention (Harder et al. 2003). Gas transit studies have shown that patients with bloating have some impaired handling of intestinal contents. Elaborate studies of gut gas transit demonstrate that gas retention is usually due to impaired propulsion of gut contents in the most proximal portions of the small bowel. Studies using xenon-labeled gas indicate that the small bowel is responsible for impaired gas transit, not the colon, as is often believed (Slavioli et al. 2005).

Determination of Adequate Gut Function

The symptoms of abdominal bloating and the finding of abdominal distention are believed to be indicators of a poorly functioning bowel. However, these symptoms are not, by themselves, proven indicators for withholding or terminating the use of EN. Often, these symptoms and signs are combined with other radiographic and/or bedside findings in the decision-making process to withhold tube feedings because of poor intestinal motility. Mechanisms of an adynamic ileus are poorly understood. They are a combination of neurogenic, myogenic, and humoral mechanisms. Any of these mechanisms may reduce or abolish motor activity. In general, small bowel motility function returns more rapidly than does colonic motor function following an episode of adynamic ileus (Smith et al. 1977).

The presence of bowel sounds is often used as a determinant of the adequacy of intestinal motility. Unfortunately, most clinicians do not spend the time on the auscultation component of the abdominal exam to reliably characterize bowel sounds. In addition, there is tremendous intraobserver variability in the interpretation of the presence and type of bowel sounds, both in normal volunteers and in patients with significant pathologic disease (Gade et al. 1998). The use of bowel sounds, by itself, to determine the function of the gut is unreliable.

Radiographic interpretation of the abdomen is frequently used to confirm the diagnosis of ileus or intestinal obstruction. The plain abdominal radiograph demonstrates the amount and the distribution of solids, gas, and fluid in the GI tract. In the normal patient, there is almost no gas in the small intestine and only scattered air bubbles and feces in the colon. It is often the degree of intestinal distention that a radiologist will use to identify GI pathology and help to identify an ileus or a GI obstruction (Grassi et al. 2004). However, many hospitalized patients have abnormal abdominal radiographs with increased air, fluid, and feces in the small bowel and colon as a result of inactivity and their overall "disease state." The gold standard for delineating an ileus from a bowel obstruction is a contrast radiographic study such as a small bowel follow through, barium enema, or a computerized tomography of the abdomen. Patients with intestinal obstruction should not receive EN. However, patients with a diagnosis of ileus by abdominal radiograph will often not have difficulty tolerating EN. Thus, the use of an abdominal radiograph alone to determine the adequacy of intestinal function can be misleading. The patient with a triad of an ileus on abdominal radiograph, abdominal distention on physical examination, and lack of bowel sounds is usually the patient who will not tolerate EN.

SUMMARY OF KEY POINTS

- Enteral nutrition is the nutrition intervention of choice in patients with a functioning gastrointestinal tract.
- Obtaining enteral access is the first step required for initiating EN therapy.
- The clinician ordering EN should also be familiar with the varied enteral formulations available, methods of tube-feeding delivery, and the knowledge of the potential complications and associated treatments of EN-related complications

REFERENCES

Isabel TD, Correia M. The impact of malnutrition on morbidity, mortality, length of hospital stay and costs evaluated through a multivariate model analysis. Clin Nutr. 2003;22:235–42.

Giner M, Laviano A, Mequid MM, et al. In 1995, a correlation between malnutrition and poor outcomes in critically ill patients still exist. Nutrition. 1996;12:23–9.

Marik P, Zaloga GP. Meta-analysis of parenteral nutrition versus enteral nutrition in patients with acute pancreatitis. BMJ. 2004;328:1407–12.

Kudsk KA. Current aspects of mucosal immunology and its influence by nutrition. Am J Surg. 2002; 183:390–8.

Spiekermann GM, Walker WA. Oral tolerance and its role in clinical disease. J Pediatr Gastroent Nutr. 2001; 32:237–55.

Coffman RL, Seymour BW, Lebman DA, et al. The role of helper T cell products in mouse B cell differentiation and isotype regulation. Immuno Rev. 1988;102:5–28.

Windsor AC, Kanwar S, Li AG, Barnes E, et al. Compared with parenteral nutrition, enteral feeding attenuates the acute phase response and improves disease severity in acute pancreatitis. Gut. 1998;42:431–5.

Lewis SJ, Egger M, Sylvester PA, Thomas S. Early enteral feeding versus "nil by mouth" after gastrointestinal surgery: systematic review and meta-analysis of controlled trials. BMJ. 2001;6:773–6.

Frankenfeld DC, Beyer PL. Soy-polysaccharide fiber: effect on diarrhea in tube-fed, head-injured patients. Am J Clin Nutr. 1989;50:533–8.

Shankardass K, Chuchman S, Chelwick K, et al. Bowel function of long-term tube-fed patients containing formulas with and without dietary fiber. J Parent Ent Nutr. 1990;14:508–12.

Cerra FB, Cheung NK, Fischer JF. Disease specific amino acid infusion in hepatic encephalopathy: a prospective, randomized double-blinded controlled trial. J Parenteral Enteral Nutr. 1985;9:288–95.

Michel H, Bories P, Aubin JP, et al. Treatment of acute hepatic encephalopathy in cirrhotics with branched-chain amino acids enriched versus a conventional amino acid mixture. Liver. 1985;5:282–9.

Masejo A, Acosta JA, Ortega C, et al. Comparison of a high-protein, disease-specific enteral formula in hypeglycemic critically ill patients. Clin Nutr. 2003;22:295–305.

Singer P, Theilla M, Fisher H, et al. Benefit of an enteral diet enriched with eicosapentaenoic acid and gamma-linolenic acid in ventilated patients with acute lung injury. Crit Care Med. 2006;34:1033–8.

Montejo JC, Zarazaga A, Lopez-Martinez J, et al. Immunonutrition in the intensive care unit. A systematic review and consensus statement. Clin Nutr. 2003;22:221–33.

Bower RH, Cerra FB, Bershadsky B, et al. Early enteral administration of a formula (Impact) supplemented with arginine, nucleotides, and fish oil in intensive care unit patients: results of a multicenter, prospective, randomized, clinical trial. Crit Care Med. 1995;23:436–49.

Galban C, Montejo JC, Mesejo A, et al. An immune-enhancing enteral diet reduces mortality rate and episodes of bactermia in septic intensive care unit patients. Crit Care Med. 2000;28:643–8.

Zaloga GP, Siddiqui R, Terry C, et al. Arginine: mediator or modulator of sepsis? Nutr Clin Pract. 2004;19:201–15.

Serpa LF, Kimura M, Faintuch J, et al. Effects of continuous versus bolus infusion of enteral nutrition in critical patients. Rev Hosp Clin Fam Med. 2003;58:9–14.

Lin HC, Van Critters GW. Stopping of enteral feeding for arbitrary gastric residual volumes may not be physiologically sound. Results of a computer stimulation model. JPEN. 1997;21:286–8.

Mullan H, Roubenoff RA, Roubenoff R. Risk of pulmonary aspiration among patients receiving enteral nutrition support. JPEN. 1992;16:160–4.

McClave SA, Lukan JK, Stefater JA, et al. Poor validity of residual volumes as a marker for risk of aspiration in critically ill patients. Crit Care Med. 2005;33:324–30.

McClave SA, DeMeo MT, DeLegge MH, et al. North American summit on aspiration in the critically ill patient: consensus statement. JPEN. 2002;26(suppl):S80–5.

Hammer HF, Santa Ana CA, Schiller LR, et al. Studies of osmotic diarrhea induced in normal subjects by the ingestion of polyethylene glycol and lactulose. J Clin Invest. 1989;84:1056–62.

Bowling TE, Ramundo AH, Grimble GK, et al. Colonic secretory effect in response to enteral feedings in humans. Gut. 1994;36:1734–41.

Jorgensen JR, Fitch MD, Mortensen PB, et al. In vivo absorption of medium-chain fatty acids by the rat colon exceed that of short-chain fatty acids. Gastroenterology. 2001;120:452–61.

Debnam ES, Grimble GK. Methods for assessing intestinal absorptive function in relation to enteral nutrition. Curr Opin Clin Nutr Met Care. 2001;4:355–67.

Lebak KJ, Bliss DZ, Savik K, et al. What's new on defining diarrhea in tube-feeding studies. Clin Nurs Res. 2003;12:174–204.

Whelan K, Judd PA, Taylor MA. Assessment of fecal output in patients receiving enteral tube feedings: validation of a novel chart. Eur J Clin Nutr. 2004;58:1030–7.

DeLegge M, Rhodes B, Hennessey K, et al. The Malabsorption Index(A). ASPEN Conference, Chicago, 2000.

Jenkins B, Holsten S, Bengmark S, et al. Probiotics: a practical review of their role in specific clinical scenarios. Nutr Clin Pract. 2005;20:262–70.

Dendukuri N, Costa V, McGregor M, et al. Probiotic therapy for the prevention and treatment of Clostridium difficle-associated diarrhea: a systemic review. CMAJ. 2005;173:167–70.

Lasser RB, Bond JH, Levitt MD. The role of intestinal gas in functional abdominal pain. New Engl J Med. 1975;293:524–6.

Ravich WJ, Bayless TM, Thomas M. Fructose: increased intestinal absorption in humans. Gastroenterology. 1982;84:26–32.

Harder H, Serra J, Azpiroz F, et al. Intestinal gas distribution determines abdominal symptoms. Gut. 2003;52:1708–13.

Slavioli B, Serra J, Azpiroz F, et al. Origin of gas retention in patients with bloating. Gastroenterology. 2005; 128:574–9.

Smith J, Kelly KA, Weinschilbaum RM. Pathophysiology of postoperative ileus. Arch Surg. 1977;112:203–8.

Gade J, Kruse P, Anderson OP, et al. Physician's abdominal examination A multi-rater agreement. Scand J Gastrol. 1998;33:773–7.

Grassi R, DiMinzio R, Pinto A. Serial plain abdominal films findings in the assessment of acute abdomen: spastic ileus, hypotonic ileus, mechanical ileus and paralytic ileus. Radiol Med. 2004;108:56–70.

9 Capsule Endoscopy

Sherman M. Chamberlain, Akit Patel, and Subbaramiah Sridhar

Contents

INTRODUCTION

Wireless video capsule endoscopy (VCE) is a significant advancement in gastrointestinal (GI) imaging for the evaluation of small bowel mucosa. VCE is a noninvasive endoscopic tool comprised of an ingestible 11×26 mm capsule. It is a self-contained camera and antenna that transmits images to a sensor array/data recorder worn by a patient. The recorded images captured by the data recorder are downloaded to a computer work station, allowing a physician to visualize the recorded data. The VCE was first adjunctively approved by the Food and Drug Administration (FDA) in 2001 for the evaluation of obscure gastrointestinal bleeding (OGIB), presumptively from the small bowel, after failure of other small bowel studies imaging modalities (such as small bowel follow-through or enteroclysis) to identify the source (Appleyard et al. *2001*). In 2003, the FDA approved VCE as a first-line diagnostic for examining the small bowel after nondiagnostic standard upper and lower endoscopies.

From: *Clinical Gastroenterology: Diagnostic and Therapeutic Procedures in Gastroenterology*,
Edited by: G. Y. Wu, S. Sridhar, DOI 10.1007/978-1-59745-044-7_9,

VCE technology made by Given Imaging (Yoqneam, Israel) has further expanded beyond small bowel imaging (*Pillcam SB*) to include esophageal imaging by a double-headed camera capsule (*Pillcam ESO*) (Figs. 1–4). There is also a larger, not yet FDA-approved, 11 × 31 mm double-headed camera capsule (*Pillcam Colon*) that provides colon imaging. Recently, Olympus (Center Valley, PA) has released another FDA-approved 11 × 26 mm small bowel camera capsule called *EndoCapsule*.

The limitation of all VCE modalities is that there is no control over capsule movement (Box 1). Because insufflation is not possible, lesions may be hidden behind folds, and

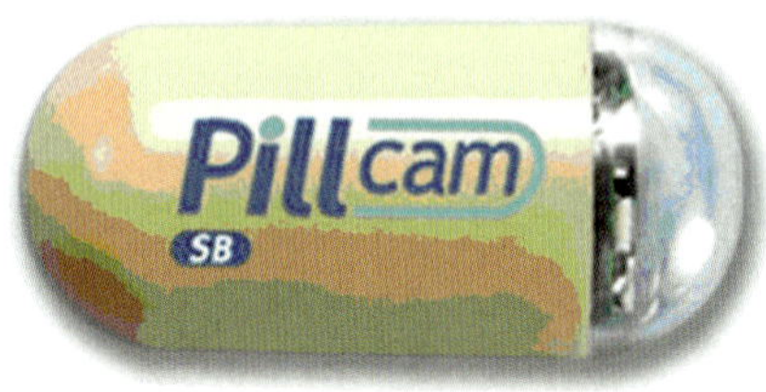

Fig. 1. Pillcam SB.

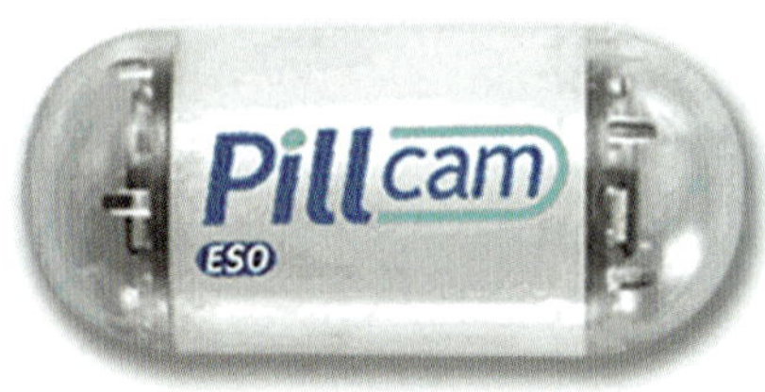

Fig. 2. Pillcam ESO.

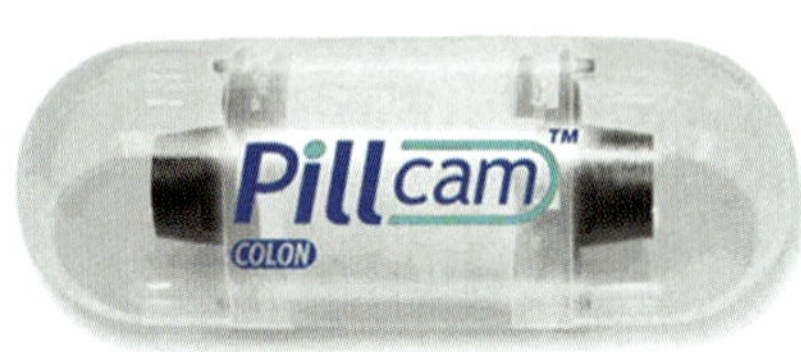

Fig. 3. Pillcam colon.

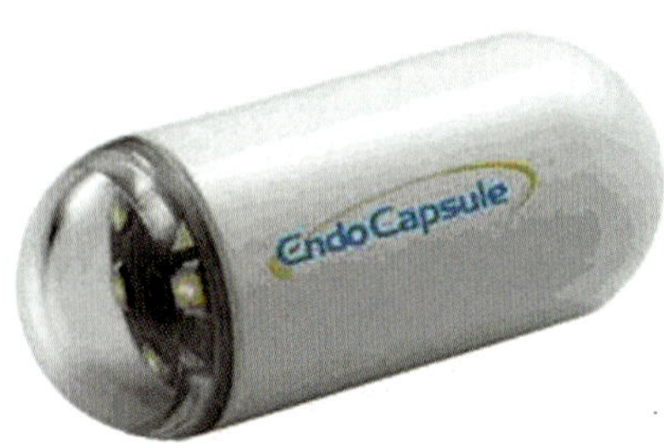

Fig. 4. Endocapsule.

Box 1
Limitations of all VCE

- No control over capsule movement
- Lack of insufflation allows lesions to remain hidden
- Debris and bubbles obscure visualization
- Only a diagnostic technique, endoscopy still required for biopsy and therapeutics

debris and bubbles may obscure mucosal visualization. VCE is only an initial diagnostic technique, with clinically suspicious findings requiring invasive endoscopic techniques for biopsy or application of therapeutics.

Obscure GI Bleeding

VCE was originally designed to evaluate OGIB, the source of which was presumptively from the small bowel, Box 2 (Appleyard et al. *2001*). Current indications have expanded to the evaluation of Crohn's disease and celiac disease. Small bowel bleeding sources may

Box 2
Small bowel VCE indications

- Obscure GI bleed
- Small bowel tumor
- Crohn's Disease
- Celiac Disease

represent 3–5% of all gastrointestinal bleeding (American Gastroenterological Association medical position statement of occult and obscure gastrointestinal bleeding. Gastroenterol *2000*). A substantial number, 33–50%, of patients who do not receive appropriate therapy may bleed again from their small bowel sources. Previously, the average lag time to diagnose small bowel OGIB was 36 months, utilizing multiple radiographic and endoscopic procedures at great expense (Lewis and Godfarb *2003*). Pooled analysis of OGIB showed VCE to be 63–87% sensitive versus 28% for invasive enteroscopy and 8–13% sensitive for radiography (Figs. 5–12) (Lewis et al. *2005*). Recently, double-balloon enteroscopy (DBE) (Fujinon, Inc. Wayne, NJ) has become available, which allows an endoscopist to view the full length of the small bowel and enables diagnosis and therapy of small bowel lesions. Yet, OGIB diagnostic yield for VCE have remained superior to DBE on meta-analysis (60% vs 57%) (Chen et al. *2007*). The procedures can be considered complementary to each other, with VCE for diagnosis prior to DBE, which can be used for therapy in OGIB. We propose the following algorithm below for the use of VCE in OGIB, Table 1.

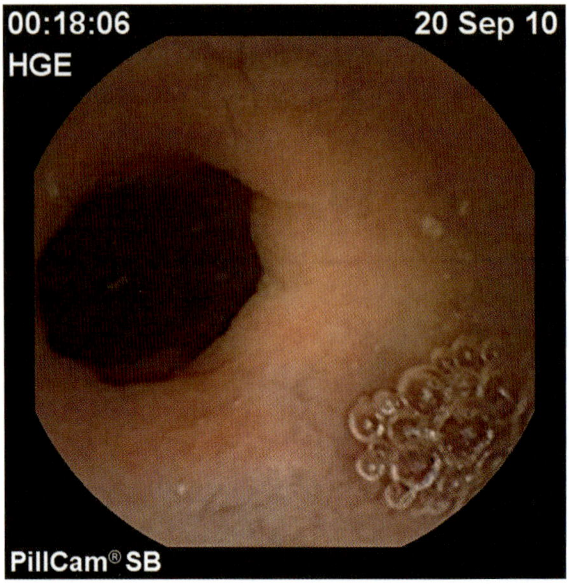

Fig. 5. Normal pylorus.

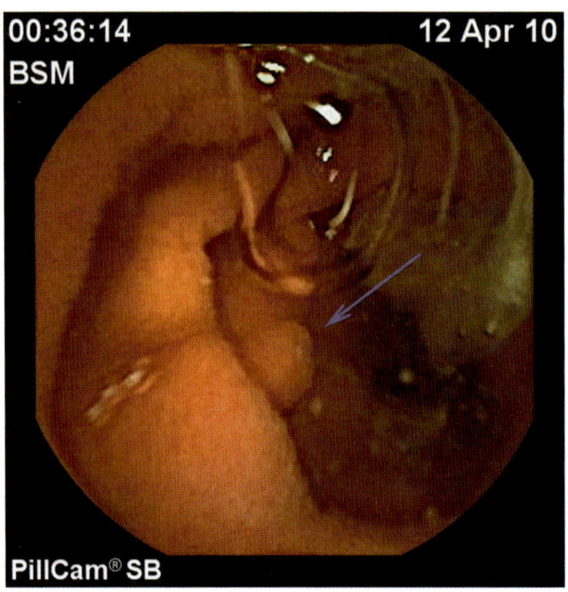

Fig. 6. Normal ampulla of Vater.

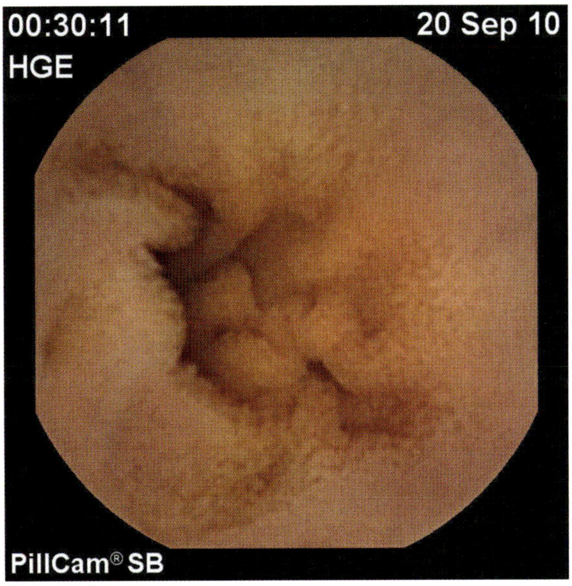

Fig. 7. Normal small bowel villi.

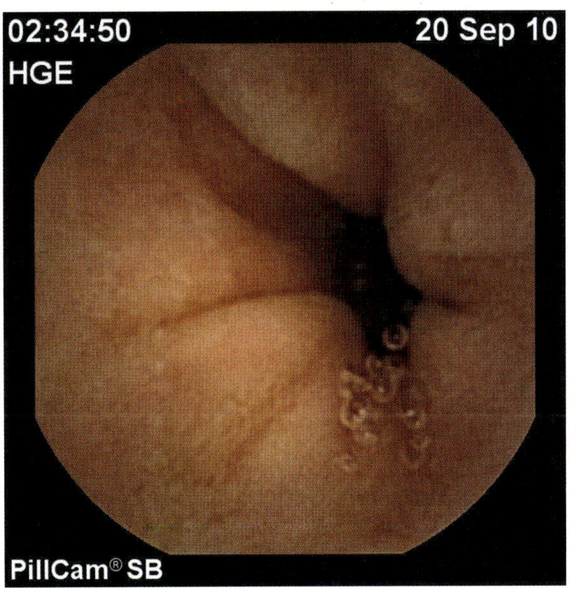

Fig. 8. Normal ileocecal valve.

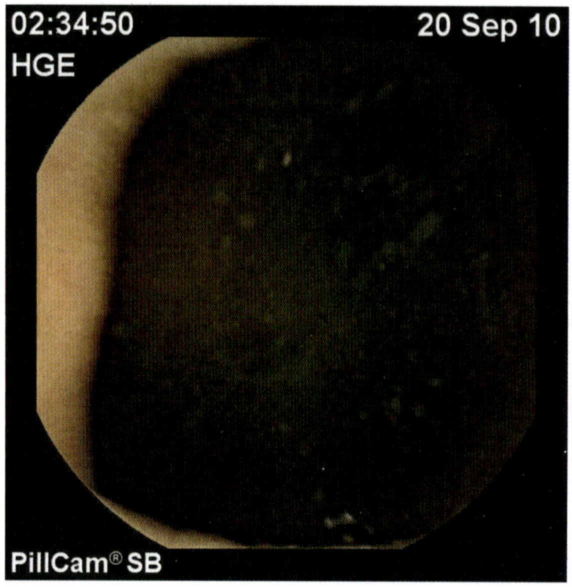

Fig. 9. Normal cecum and ileocecal valve.

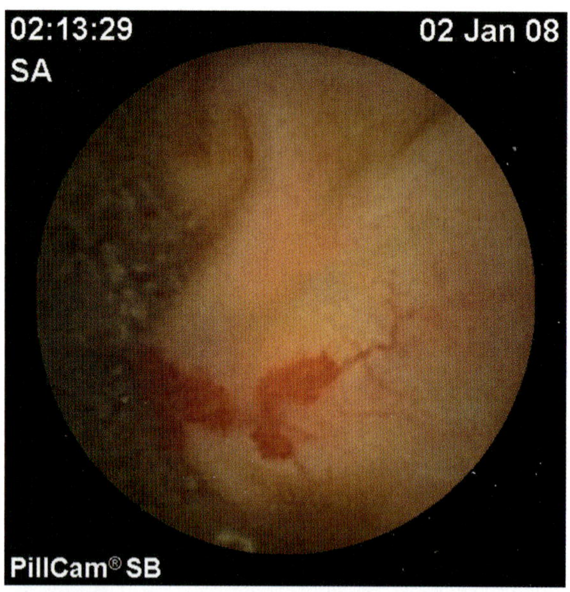

Fig. 10. Small bowel telangiectasia.

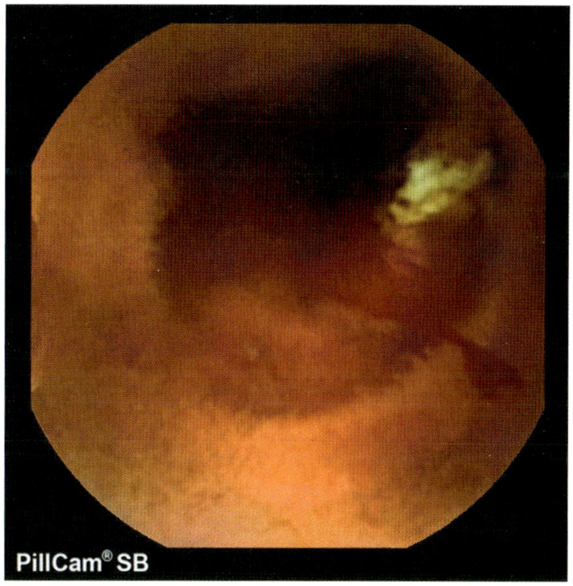

Fig. 11. Active bleeding in an obscure GI bleeder.

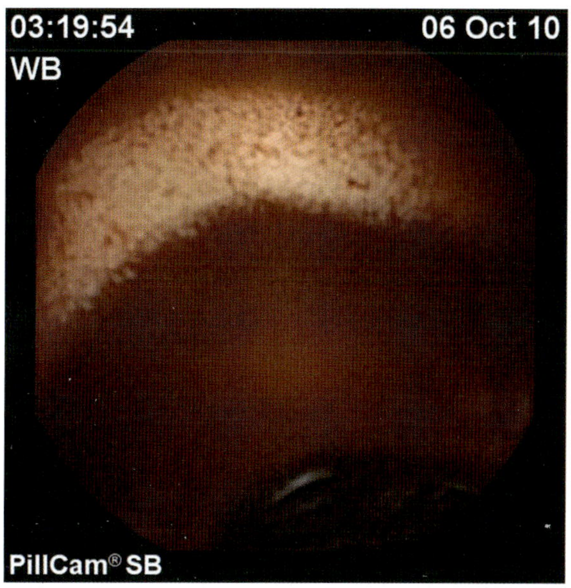

Fig. 12. Jejunum with active bleeding.

Table 1
VCE in OGIB

Limitations of All VCE:

- No control over capsule movement
- Lack of insufflation allows lesions to remain hidden
- Debris and bubbles obscure visualization
- Only a diagnostic technique, endoscopy still required for biopsy and therapeutics

Small Bowel Tumors

Small bowel tumors account for 1–3% of all gastrointestinal neoplasms. The frequency of tumor detection is higher with VCE than with other radiographic modalities (Cobrin et al. *2006*). Patients younger than age 50 with OGIB have an increased risk of small bowel tumors as a bleeding source, whereas those older than 50 are significantly more likely to have angioectasias (Fig. 13a and b) as their small bowel bleeding source (Cobrin et al. *2006*). A multicenter European study involving 5,129 patients, of whom 124 had small bowel tumors, found that the most common small bowel tumor VCE diagnoses were gastrointestinal stromal tumors (32%) (Fig. 14), adenocarcinomas (20%) and carcinoids (Fig. 15) (15%), and metastatic tumors (10%), with 75% of these being melanoma (Rondonotti et al. *2008*). Of the tumors (Figs. 16 and 17), 80.6% were diagnosed solely by

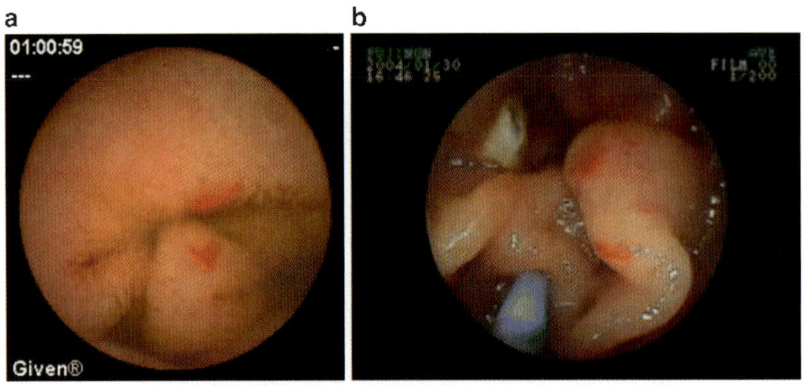

Fig. 13. (**a**) VCE image of an angioectasia. (**b**) DBE with ablation therapy of angioectasias (Chen et al. *2007*).

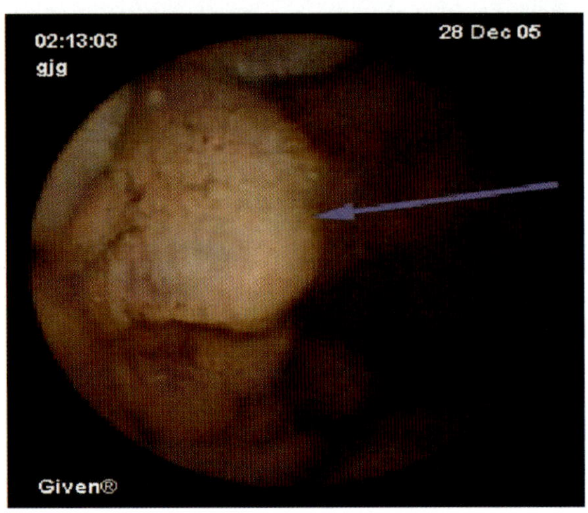

Fig. 14. Small bowel stromal tumor.

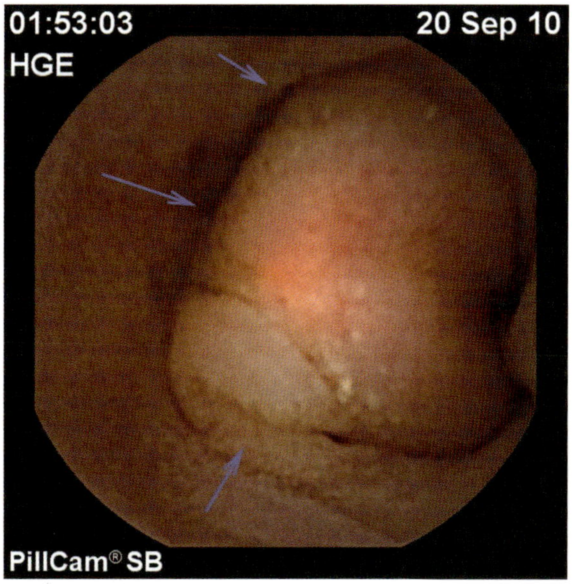

Fig. 15. Ileal carcinoid tumor.

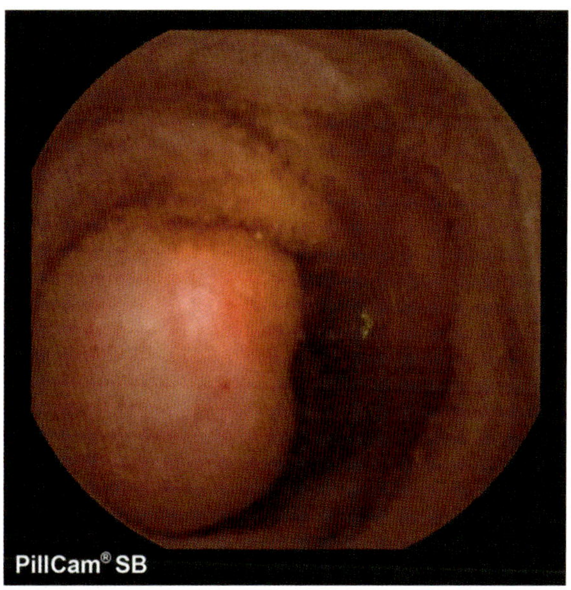

Fig. 16. Submucosal jejunal mass.

VCE, other modalities failing to make the diagnosis of small bowel tumors. Capsule retention occurred in one of these patients. Additional benign tumors found by VCE include hamartomas, cystic lymphangiomas, amyloidosis, and lipomas (Rondonotti et al. *2008*). While VCE is currently the most sensitive method of diagnosing small bowel tumors, the VCE findings of small bowel tumors remain quite non-specific.

Crohn's Disease

VCE is currently the most accurate diagnostic modality in detecting the presence and extent of small bowel Crohn's disease (Figs. 18 and 19). Meta-analyses found VCE to be significantly more accurate than both small bowel radiography (63% vs 23%) and colonoscopy with ileoscopy (61% vs 46%) in the diagnosis of nonstricturing small bowel Crohn's disease (Buchman et al. *2004*; Triester et al. *2006*). Common VCE findings of Crohn's

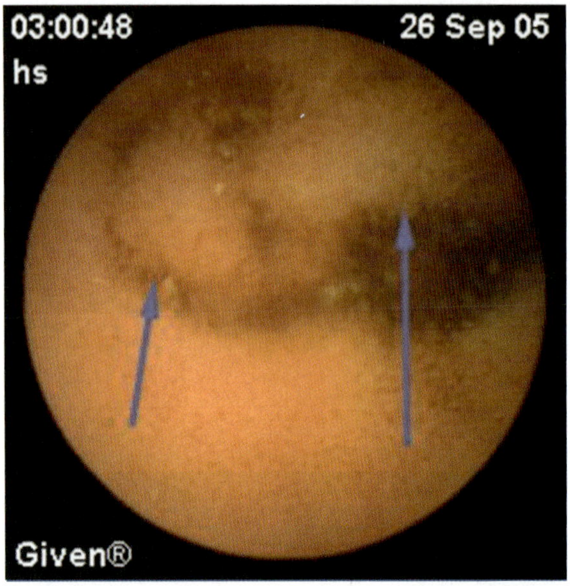

Fig. 17. Small bowel polypoid mass.

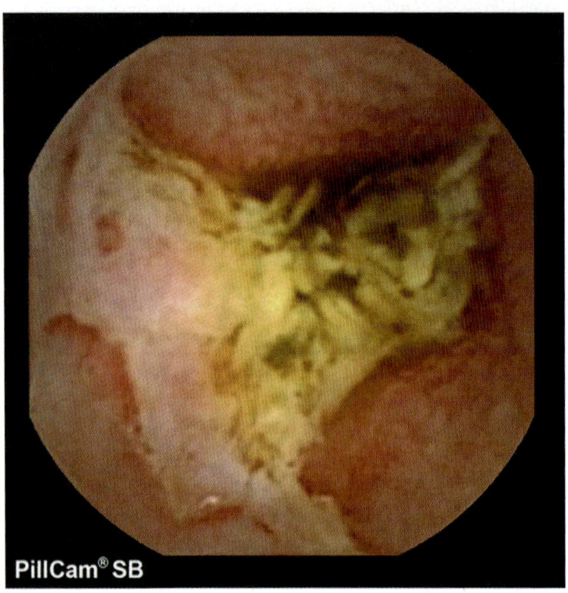

Fig. 18. Crohn's ulcers with inflammatory exudates.

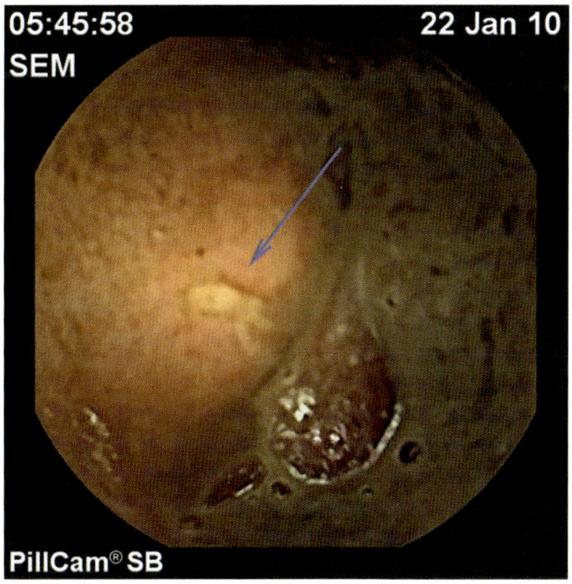

Fig. 19. Jejunal Crohn's ulcer.

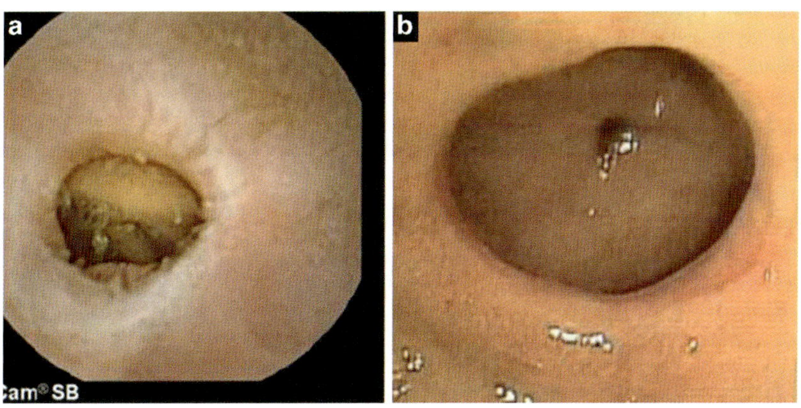

Fig. 20. NSAID-induced ulceration.

disease include mucosal breaks, focal villus denudation, erosions and frank ulceration, and stricture formation (Kornbluth et al. *2005*). A standardized VCE scoring index remains to be validated (Lewis et al. *2004*). VCE study findings are not specific and, thus, not sufficient for the diagnosis of Crohn's disease. Abnormal findings such as mucosal breaks and minor lesions may be seen in up to 13% of normal patients (Goldstein et al. *2005*). Crohn's disease must be diagnosed based on clinical, histological, radiological, and biochemical patient findings. Other small bowel pathologic processes that appear similar to Crohn's on VCE include celiac disease, infectious, immunodeficiency-related, allergic, and NSAID and other enteropathies. NSAID-enteropathy may cause diaphragms, webs, and strictures that are particularly indistinguishable from Crohn's disease on VCE (Fig. 20).

Celiac Disease

There is growing evidence that VCE is a sensitive small bowel imaging modality in the evaluation of mucosal changes associated with celiac disease such as villus atrophy, "scalloping," layered or stacked folds, and a mosaic appearance of the mucosa (Figs. 21 and 22). VCE may also be a preferred modality for evaluating extent of small bowel involvement,

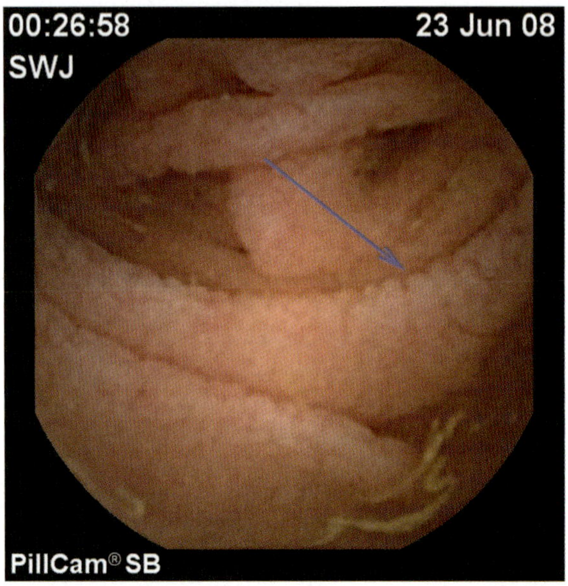

Fig. 21. Celiac disease with scalloped mucosa.

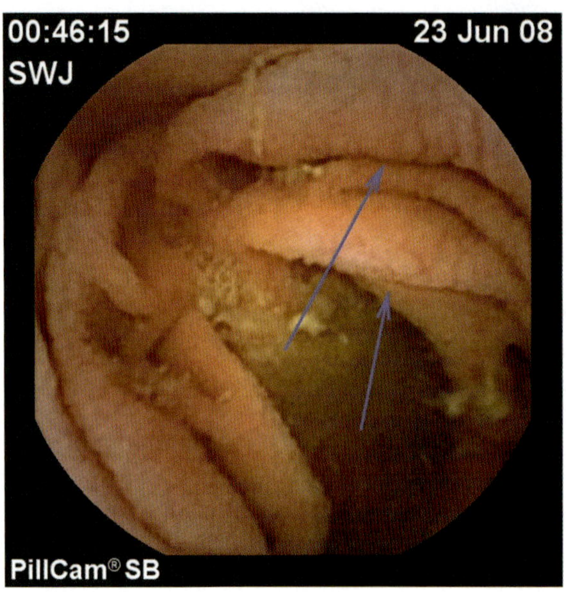

Fig. 22. Celiac with atrophy of villi.

and complications such as chronic ulcerative jejunoileitis, small bowel lymphoma, and adenocarcinoma (Murray et al. *2004*). VCE is also effectively employed in patients suspected of celiac disease, with positive serology and negative upper endoscopy and small bowel biopsies. However, Petroniene found good interobserver agreement for celiac disease findings only among expert VCE readers (Petroniene et al. *2005*). Common VCE findings of patients with complicated or refractory celiac disease include: ulcerations, ulcerated nodular mucosa, small bowel cancer and polyps, strictures, and submucosal masses (Culliford et al. *2005*). Specificity of VCE images for celiac disease remains poor as other ulcerative small bowel diseases such as Crohn's disease, Behçet's disease, and ulcerated small bowel tumors, all appear similar on VCE. The exact role of VCE for the evaluation and management of celiac disease remains to be established.

Contraindications

Relative contraindications for VCE include patients with known small bowel strictures, prior major abdominal surgeries with obstructive symptoms, which would significantly raise the likelihood of strictures, dysphagia, gastroparesis (not allowing the capsule to traverse the small bowel without the battery life expiring), implantable pacemaker, age less than 10 years, and pregnancy (Box 3) (Mishkin et al. *2006*).

Box 3
Small bowel VCE contraindications

- Known or suspected GI obstruction, strictures, or fistulas
- Abdominal surgeries
- Dysphagia/swallowing disorders
- Gastroparesis
- Cardiac pacemaker or other implanted electromedical devices
- <10 years of age
- Pregnancy

EQUIPMENT

The VCE capsule captures two images per second during 8 h of battery life. The VCE capsule consists of a short focal lens, white LED lights, an image manager (Given *Pillcam SB*). It contains complementary metal oxide semiconductor technology and Olympus *EndoCapsule*, which utilizes charge coupled-device technology, a battery, an antenna, and transmitter. The VCE capsule provides an eight-times magnified, wide-angle view of bowel mucosa (156° for newest *Pillcam SB2*, and 145° for *EndoCapsule*.) The small bowel capsule system contains three main components: the VCE capsule, a data recorder that records the 8 h of data via radiofrequency signals (RF) received from the VCE capsule, and a computer work station where the health care provider will read and interpret the VCE images (Figs. 23–27).

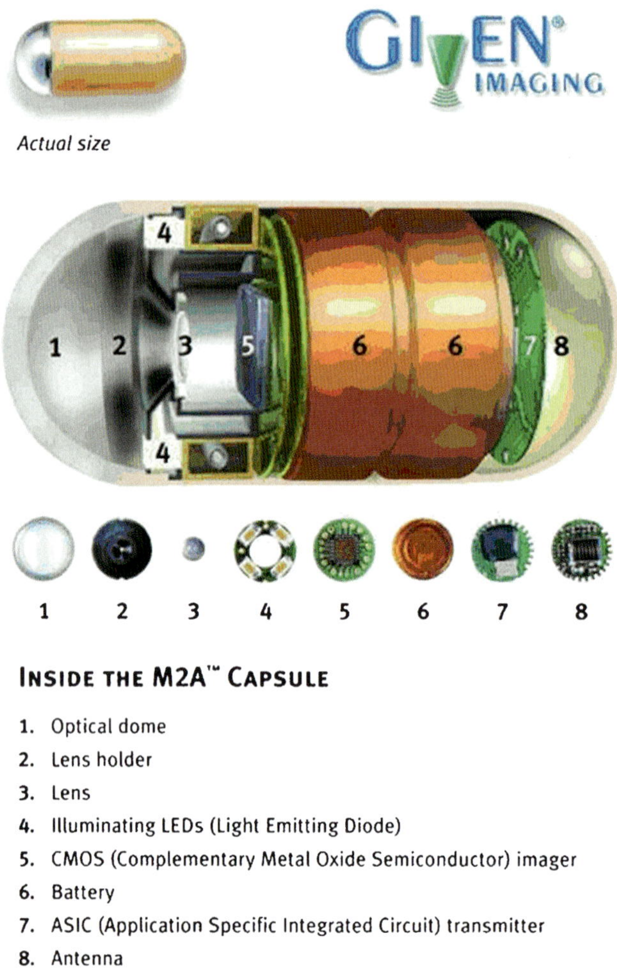

Fig. 23. Given M2A/Pillcam Capsule.

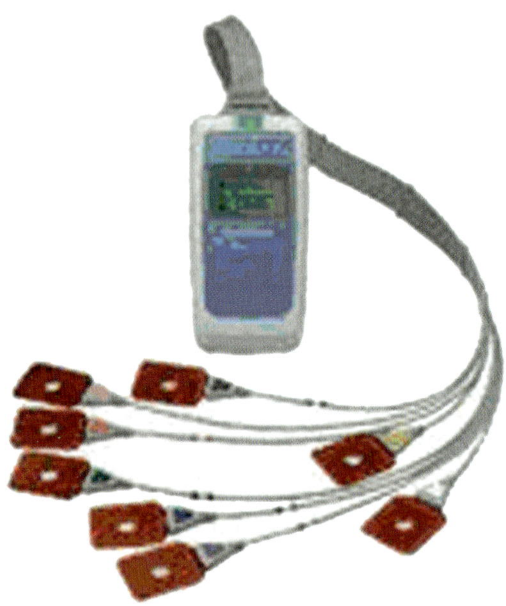

Fig. 24. EndoCapsule data recorder.

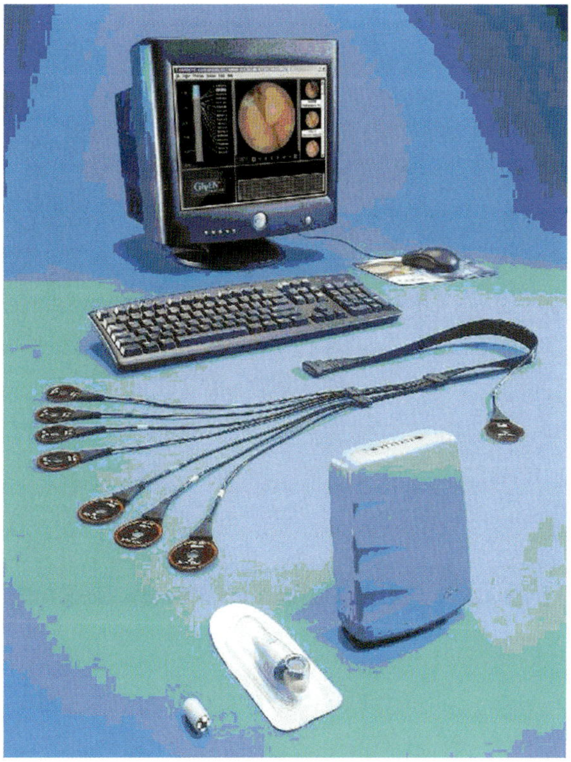

Fig. 25. VCE Equipment: Capsule, sensory array, leads, recorder, and computer workstation.

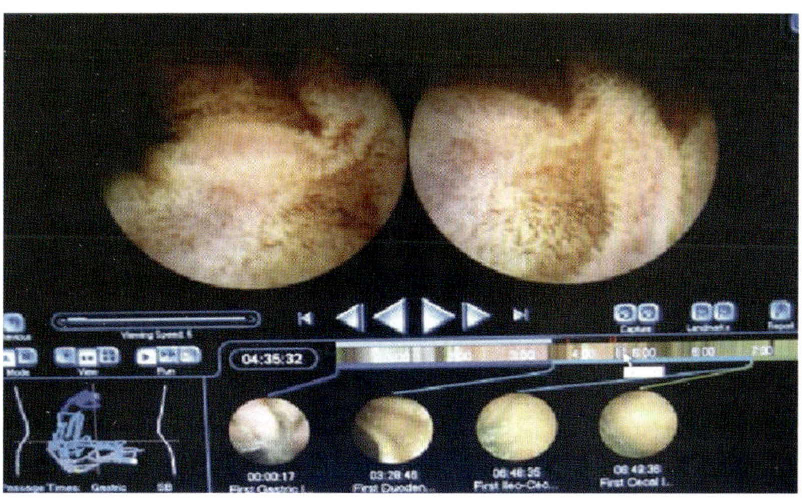

Fig. 26. Given Imaging software interface for VCE.

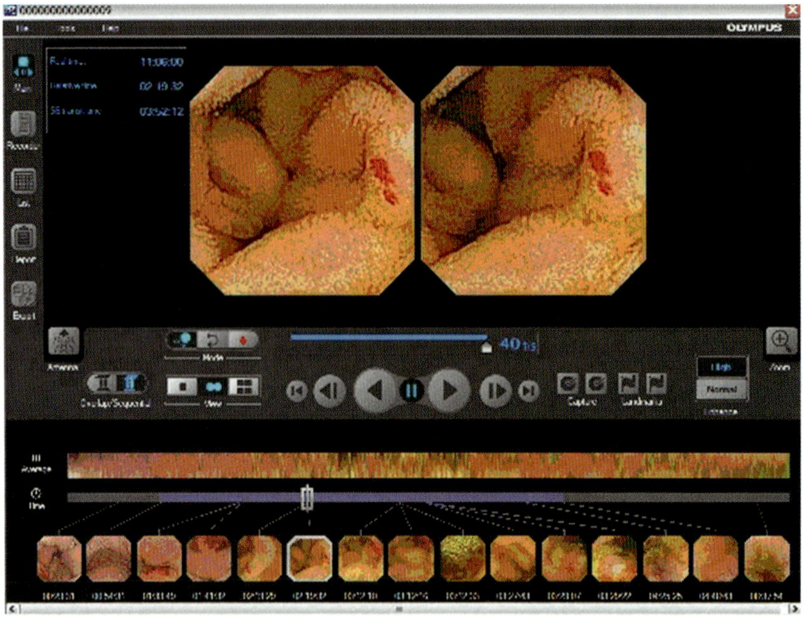

Fig. 27. EndoCapsule computer software for VCE.

TECHNIQUE

All patients should be educated regarding the potential complications, and an informed written consent should be obtained. Gut-cleansing regimens and prokinetic agents prior to VCE capsule ingestion can be used to improve visualization and transit times (Box 4). However, their use remains controversial and should be tailored to each individual case. In our institution, we instruct our patients to take a clear fluid diet and one bottle of magnesium citrate or 2 L of polyethylene glycol the day before the procedure

Box 4
Small bowel VCE technique

- Patient fasts 8 h or administer pre-procedure gut-cleansing agents, prokinetic agents, or simethicone
- Fit patient with sensor array, leads, and recorder
- Activate VCE capsule by removing from package and confirm sensor array/recorder placement by running capsule over attached leads
- Ingest capsule with 30–60 cc of water
- Patient remains NPO for 2 h after capsule ingestion then advances to clear liquids for additional 2 h
- Patient returns to clinic after 8 h
- Sensor array, leads, and recorder removed from patient and images downloaded onto computer workstation receiver
- Capsule passes with bowel movement within 24 h

(Niv and Niv *2004*). We generally avoid sodium phosphate cleansing as it may cause mucosal changes of inflammation (Niv et al. *2005*). Some institutions administer 80 mg of simethicone by mouth prior to VCE examination (Ge et al. *2006*). This may minimize missed lesions, thus, enhancing mucosal viewing. Prior to VCE ingestion, patients are fitted with a sensor array with leads attached to their abdomen at appropriate locations, and a recorder worn on a belt throughout the 8 h VCE study time. The VCE capsule is removed from its magnet containing packaging to activate the capsule. Appropriate sensor array/recorder placement is confirmed by running the capsule over all the attached sensor array leads, which illuminates the recorder via RF. The capsule is swallowed with 30–60 cc of water. After the VCE capsule is ingested, the patient leaves the endoscopy unit and remains with nothing by mouth for 2 h, followed by clear liquids for the next 2 h.

The patient returns to the endoscopy unit after 8 h by which time the VCE battery has expired. The sensor array and recorder are removed from the patient, the recorder placed in the computer work-station receiver, and the VCE images are then downloaded into the computer workstation.

READING

After the VCE video is downloaded, the video is read and interpreted using the available software features. The video can be read in single, dual (2 × 1), and quad (2 × 2) formats at speeds of 5–40 images per second that are adjusted to accommodate viewer comfort. Currently, there is no minimal amount of reading time proven to minimize missed lesions. Small bowel VCEs are read in the quad format at the rate of 18–24 frames per second, resulting in an average of 20–45 min to accurately read each VCE study. Given Imaging software also includes a suspected blood indicator that automatically flags images of suspected bleeding. However, this has been shown to be of little utility due to a high number of false-positive results (Buscaglia et al. *2008*). Given Imaging provides its viewing platform with an atlas feature that allow the viewer to match selected images with a set standard VE image atlas to facilitate image interpretation. Another helpful software feature is the video time bar, which allows the provider to move quickly throughout the images on the VCE video. The time bar also contains a color bar that averages the image color through each section of video, to facilitate rapid location of anatomic transitions in the gastrointestinal tract.

OUTCOMES

Common VCE findings (Fig. 28) include angioectasias and telangiectasias, Crohn's disease, celiac disease, small bowel neoplasms (5% of GI tract tumors), ulcers (Fig. 29), small bowel diverticula (Fig. 30) (e.g., Meckel's diverticula), infections (e.g., CMV, histoplasmosis, and GI tuberculosis) (Fig. 31), and small bowel Dieulafoy's lesions (Fig. 32) (Carey et al. *2007*).

The timing and nature of OGIB is important for VCE yields, with overt OGIB at the time of VCE having a significantly increased yield over remote overt OGIB or occult OGIB (60% vs 46%) (Saperas et al. *2007*). However, VCE studies may have false-negative

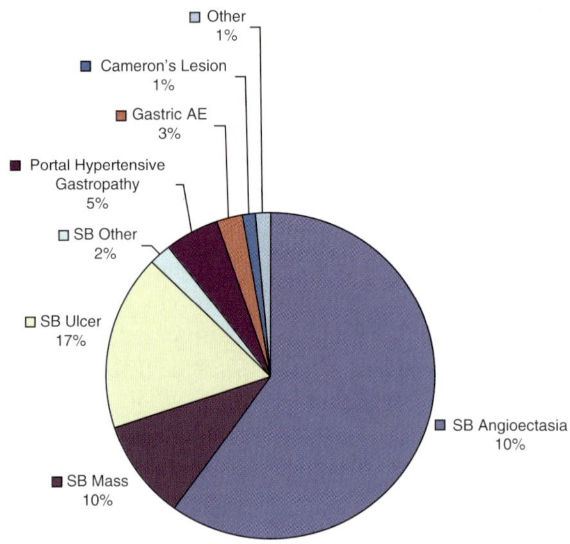

Fig. 28. Common VCE Findings (*AE* angioectasia, *SB* small bowel) (Carey et al. *2007*).

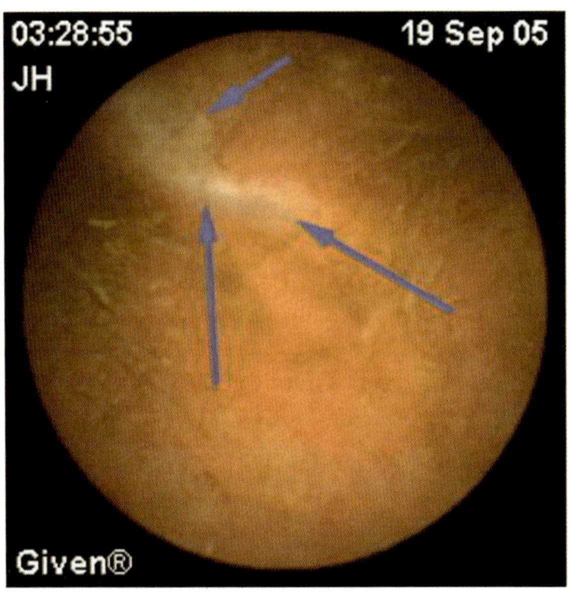

Fig. 29. Small bowel ulcer.

results due to the presence of only a single-headed camera and lack of insufflation of small bowel. Patients who have a negative VCE with continuing bleeding may have significant findings with a repeat VCE, with a reported 75% yield on repeat examination. (Jones et al. *2005*)

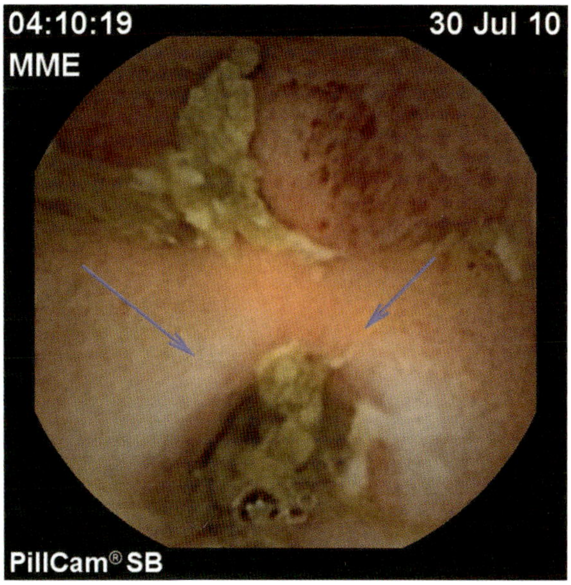

Fig. 30. Small bowel diverticula.

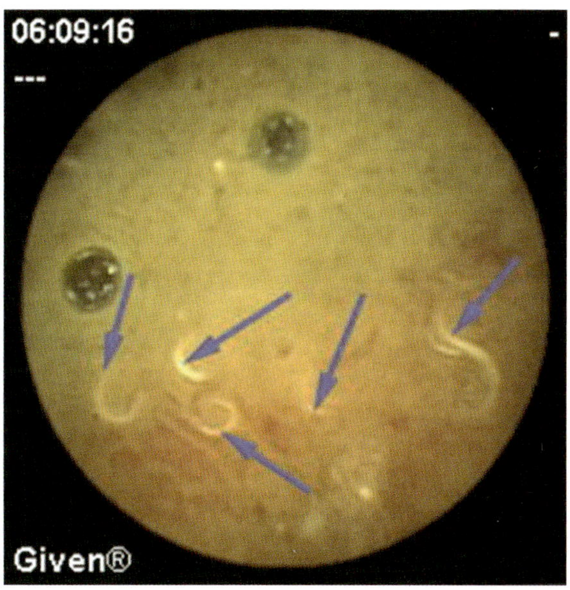

Fig. 31. Nematodes.

PROBLEMS

Capsule retention is the most feared complication of using VCE in Crohn's patients (Box 5, Fig. 33). Chiefetz found a 1.6% capsule retention rate in patients with suspected Crohn's disease and a 13% capsule retention rate in those with known Crohn's disease (Chiefetz et al. *2006*). Retained capsules have been removed surgically or with double bal-

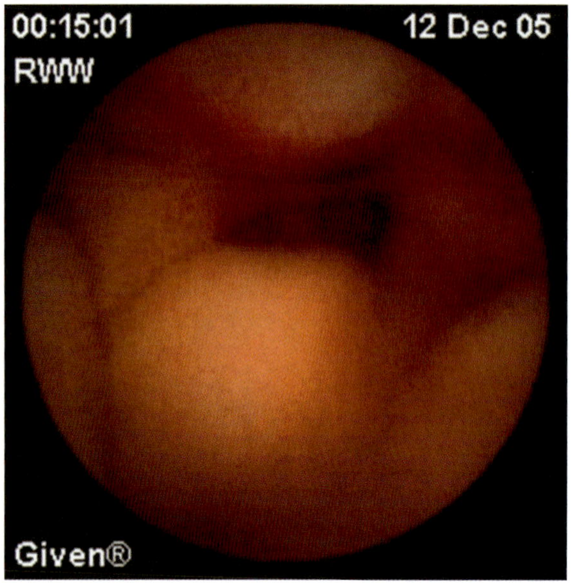

Fig. 32. Jejunal Dieulafoy's lesion with active bleeding.

Box 5
Small bowel VCE problems

- Capsule retention
- Incomplete VCE examination
- Pacemaker interference

loon enteroscopy. Most patients will remain asymptomatic after capsule retention, with the diagnosis made only when the provider fails to see the capsule enter the cecum on VCE images. Diagnosis of capsule retention must be confirmed radiographically as most patients will fail to see the capsule in their stool even with its normal passage.

Up to 25% of patients will have incomplete VCE examinations of the small bowel (Oosterveen et al. *2006*). Incomplete exams may be due to delayed gastric emptying, primary small bowel motility issues, or lack of patient mobility. For the above reasons, VCE should ideally be avoided in hospitalized patients. The examinations are best performed in mobile outpatients to increase the likelihood of complete small bowel examinations (Oosterveen et al. *2006*). Options for the practitioner when faced with an incomplete small bowel VCE study include: repeating the study with a promotility agent, endoscopically placing the VCE capsule into the small bowel (described below), or using an alternative radiographic technique (e.g., CT enterography).

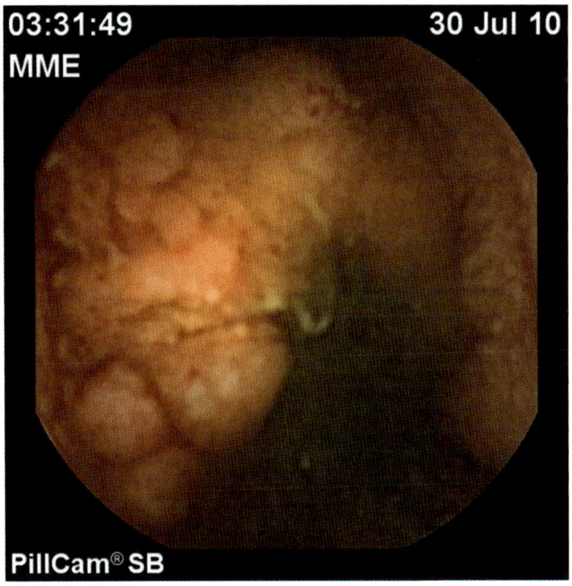

Fig. 33. Retained small bowel capsule.

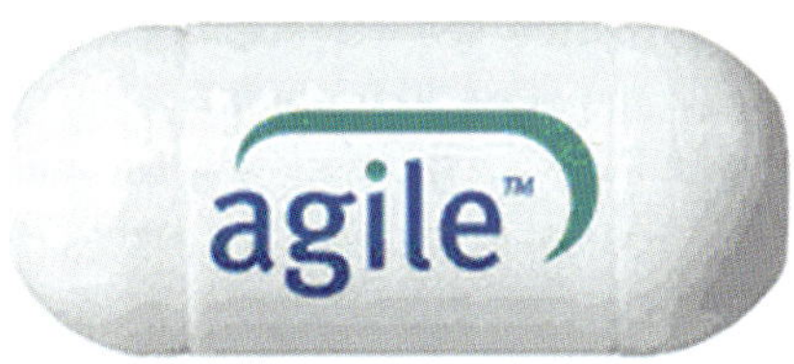

Fig. 34. Self-dissolvable agile patency capsule.

The RF emitted from the VCE capsule has the potential to interfere with cardiac pacemakers function, and pacemakers themselves also have the potential to inactivate VCE capsules (Dirks et al. *2008*). Several studies of more than 50 patients found no pacemaker interference from VCE RF, and only one case of temporary VCE capsule inactivation by a pacemaker (Dirks et al. *2008*). Thus, use of VCE in pacemaker patients is likely safe and remains only a relative contraindication, and could be considered in those patients for whom it is deemed medically necessary.

OVERCOMING THE PROBLEMS

The Agile Patency Capsule (Given Imaging, Inc.) was recently FDA approved for patients with known or suspected small bowel obstructing lesions to assess the ability of the VCE capsule to traverse the small bowel prior to performing an actual VCE (Spada et al. *2005*). The Agile Patency Capsule is 11×26 mm, like a standard VCE capsule, but is composed of lactose with barium, a radiofrequency identification (RFID) tag, and 2-sided timer plugs with exposed windows (Fig. 34). It remains intact for a minimum of

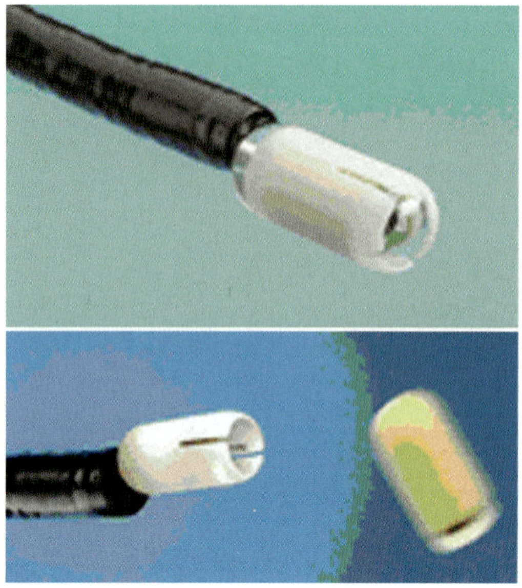

Fig. 35. AdvanCE capsule delivery system.

30 h and then disintegrates. The system comes with an RFID patency scanner that can detect the RFID tag. If the patient witnesses excretion of the intact patency capsule or the scanner does not detect the RFID tag after 30 h, then it is safe to proceed with VCE. If the patient has a pacemaker, the signal of which could be interfered with by the RFID scanner, then a plain X-ray or fluoroscopy could be used to detect the Agile Patency Capsule. A multicentered trial using the Agile Patency Capsule in patients with known small bowel obstruction prior to VCE found no cases of VCE capsule retention after appropriate passage of the patency capsule prior to the VCE studies (Herrerias et al. *2008*).

The AdvanCE capsule delivery system (US Endoscopy, Mentor, Ohio) was released in 2005 for the endoscopic delivery of VCE capsules into the small bowel of patients with known dysphagia, gastroparesis, or abnormal upper-GI anatomy, which could inhibit normal VCE capsule passage (Holden et al. *2007*). The AdvanCE delivery system (Fig. 35) consists of a plastic sleeve that holds a VCE capsule and screws onto a firing device that is threaded through the biopsy channel of a standard diagnostic upper endoscope. Prior to using the AdvanCE system, the patient is appropriately fitted with the VCE sensor array and recording device. The patient is then sedated and the VCE capsule activated and fitted into the AdvanCE capsule sleeve, which has been loaded onto the upper endoscope (Fig. 36). The upper endoscope with the VCE capsule-loaded AdvanCE delivery system is blindly inserted into the patient's posterior oropharynx and pushed beyond the upper esophageal sphincter into the esophagus and stomach. The AdvanCE VCE-loaded delivery catheter is then visually advanced through the pylorus into the duodenum and manually fired by an endoscopy assistant, thus delivering the free VCE capsule into the duodenum. The emptied AdvanCE fitted upper endoscope is then removed from the patient, and a normal VCE study is performed. A recent study of 16 consecutive patients with dysphagia, gastroparesis, and abnormal upper-GI anatomy found successful VCE capsule delivery in all patients with the use of the AdvanCE system (Holden et al. *2007*).

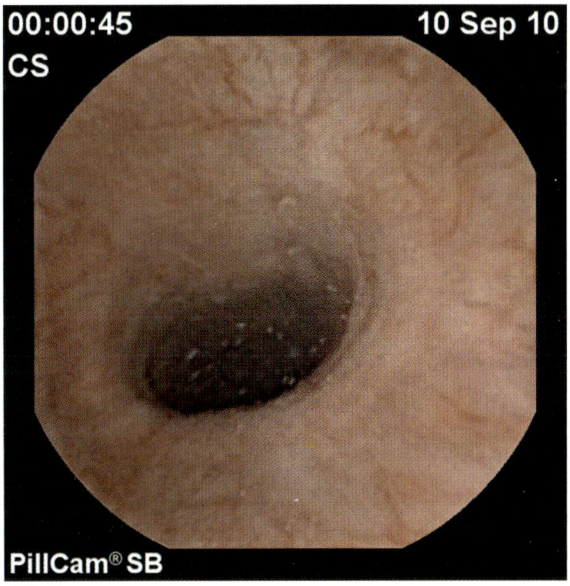

Fig. 36. Normal esophagus.

ESOPHAGEAL VCE

Introduction

Esophageal VCE (ECE) first became clinically relevant after a 2003 pilot study established that standard small bowel VCE attached to a 100 cm string could accurately evaluate esophageal pathology (Neu et al. *2003*). ECE initially was performed utilizing an 11 × 26 mm dual-headed capsule camera that took four images per second with a total of 20 min of battery life. Several years ago, it was replaced by *Pillcam ESO*, which could capture 14 images per second (seven frames per second on each camera) with ECE images taken in a 140° field of view over 20 min of battery life. *Pillcam ESO* utilizes the same transmission frequency as *Pillcam SB* VCE. Thus, the same VCE equipment is used. More recently, a new-generation *Pillcam ESO2* has been released, which takes18 images per second with a wider 169° field of view and over a longer (30 min) battery life. The optics and illumination of *Pillcam ESO2* have also significantly improved over the original *Pillcam ESO* (Gralnek et al. *2008*).

Indications

Esophageal VCE in commonly indicated as an alternative to standard endoscopy for the evaluation of reflux esophagitis, Barrett's esophagus, and may be useful for the evaluation of esophageal varices in cirrhotic patients (Box 6).

Box 6
Esophageal VCE indications

- Reflux esophagitis
- Barrett's esophagus

Gastroesophageal Reflux and Barrett's Esophagus

ECE is primarily used as a non-invasive method for the evaluation of gastroesophageal reflux (GERD) and the feared complication of Barrett's esophagus (BE) (Figs. 37–45). To date, studies have addressed the diagnostic accuracy of ECE for reflux esophagitis and BE compared to standard upper endoscopy. One study with 109 patients used four frame per second (FPS) technology, two studies with 196 patients used 14 FPS technology, and one

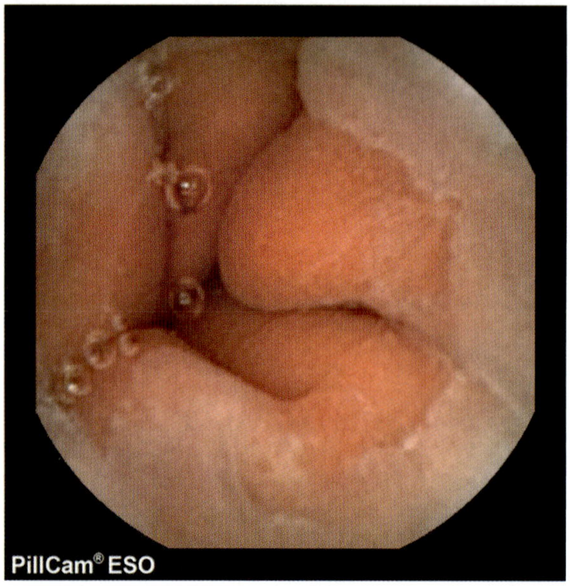

Fig. 37. Normal Z-line.

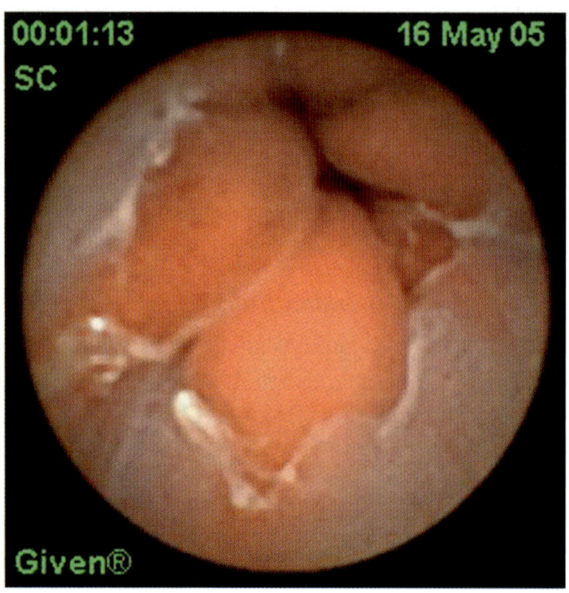

Fig. 38. Distal esophagitis.

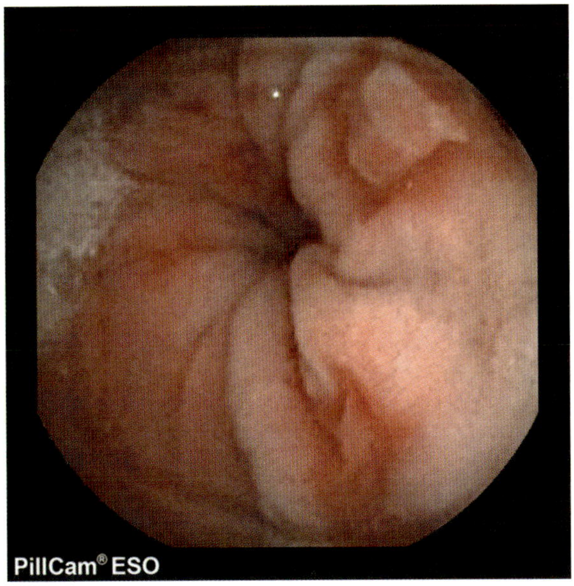

Fig. 39. Esophageal ulcer at GE junction.

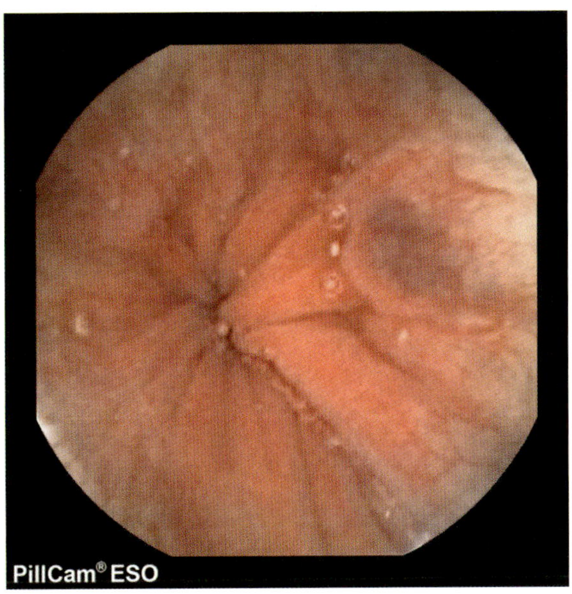

Fig. 40. Esophageal varices.

used both (25 patients each) (Wilkins et al. *2008*). For the studies using 14 FPS technology, the sensitivity was 77%. Because of the heterogeneity of the studies, the specificity ranged from 75% to 100%. Capsule retention requiring endoscopic removal was surprisingly high at a rate of 0.5%. No studies have clearly assessed ECE cost effectiveness in the evaluation and management of GERD and BE (Hur *2007*).

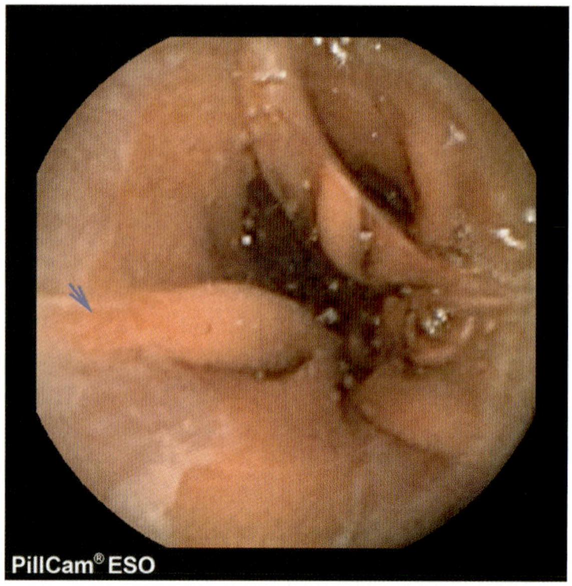

Fig. 41. Barrett's esophagus.

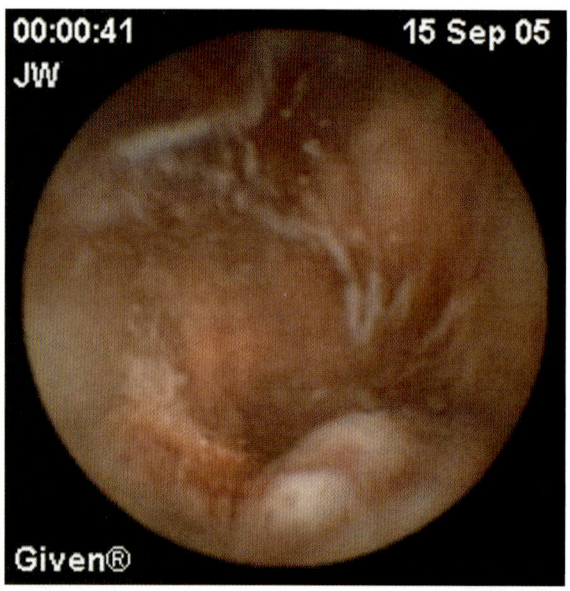

Fig. 42. Esophageal tumor.

ECE may be uniquely suited as a non-invasive tool for the diagnosis of esophageal varices (EV) and other portal hypertensive upper GI findings in difficult to sedate patients with liver disease or in those with comorbidities that preclude standard upper endoscopy. It has been estimated that up to 90% of patients with cirrhosis will develop EV, with 50% of patients with Childs A or B cirrhosis having medium or large varices found at index screening endoscopy (Kovalak et al. *2007*). When medium and large varices are detected

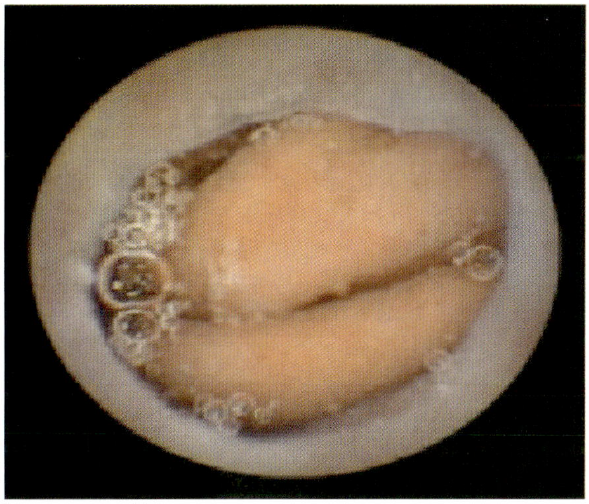

Fig. 43. Schatzki's ring.

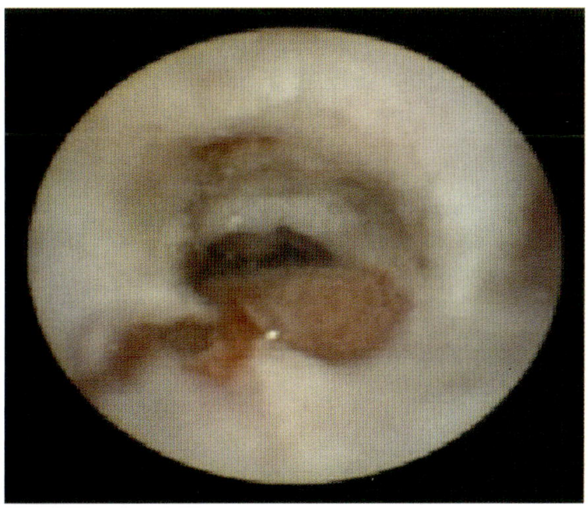

Fig. 44. Erosive esophagitis with stricture.

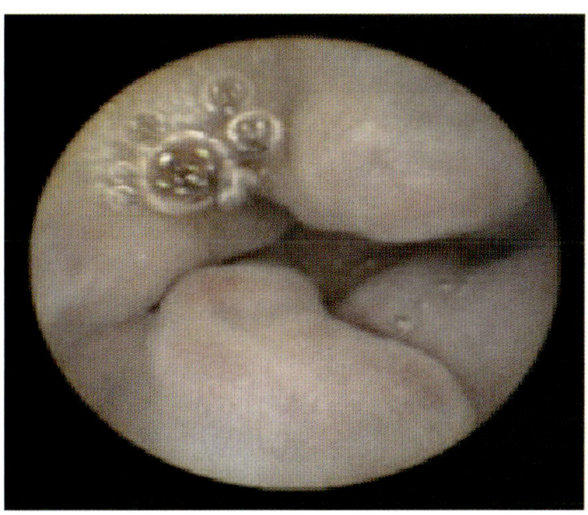

Fig. 45. Large esophageal varices.

in cirrhotic patients, pharmacologic and/or endoscopic therapy is required. Thus, universal endoscopic screening for EV for cirrhotic patients is endorsed by both American and European GI societies. ECE sensitivity, for the detection of medium and large EV, was found to be 84% (compared to EGD), and there was reasonable interobserver variability (κ=0.73), in the largest study to date (de Franchis et al. *2008*). Other smaller studies had higher sensitivities (94% and 100%). However, one had no clear grading system, and the other was a small study. Because of the heterogeneities of the studies, a summary of estimated sensitivity was not possible in our meta-analysis on ECE for EV detection, but specificity was found to be 88%. We found ECE to have an acceptable utility and safety for ruling out EV in cirrhotic patients, but further studies will be required before ECE can be judged as an effective grading tool for EV. (Raina et al. *2008*) No studies have clearly assessed ECE cost effectiveness for EV screening.

Contraindications

The contraindications are suspicion of esophageal stricture and the other contraindications outlined in the section of VCE (Box 7).

Box 7
Esophageal VCE contraindications

- Esophageal strictures
- Small bowel strictures
- Abdominal surgeries
- Dysphagia
- Gastroparesis
- Implanted pacemaker
- <10 years of age
- Pregnancy

TECHNIQUE

ECE should be performed with the patient fasting for a minimum of 4 h. The sensor array is applied to the patient and the recorder connected. The patient undergoes an ingestion protocol that requires ECE capsule ingestion with the patient in the supine position. The patient remains in the supine position for 2 min, followed by gradually inclination of the head by 30° every 2 min until the sitting position is reached, and maintained for the next 20 min. The provider administering the examination may allow the use of 100 cc of water with simethicone to clear saliva and bubbles. Recently, investigators have proposed to modify the ingestion protocol to enhance viewing of the esophagogastric junction (Gralnek et al. *2006*). The patient swallows 100 cc of water while standing followed by the ingestion of the ECE capsule in the supine right lateral decubitus position. While remaining in this position, the patient then drinks 15 cc sips of water every 30 s for 7 min. The patient then sits upright for 20 min (Box 8).

Box 8
Esophageal VCE technique

- Patient fasts 4 h
- Fit patient with sensory array, leads, and recorder
- Ingest capsule while supine and remain supine for 2 min
- Gradually raise patient 30° every 2 min until in sitting position and remain in sitting position for additional 20 min
- Ingest 100 cc of water with simethicone

COLON VCE

Pillcam Colon is currently the only colon VCE and is an 11 × 31 mm dual-headed camera capsule capturing four frames per second (two frames per second on each camera) with 10 h of battery life. Optimized optics and enhanced light control are thought to provide better mucosal coverage and depth of view compared to SB VCE. Details of the procedure technique are not available at the time of writing this chapter due to its current experimental status in the USA. There have been a few studies to date evaluating the use of colon VCE (Figs. 46 and 47). In the largest study, Eliakim compared colon VCE with conventional optical colonoscopy (OC) in 91 patients, and clinically significant findings (one polyps 6 mm or larger or greater than three polyps of any size) were noted in 70% of patients with colon VCE and 80% of patients using OC (Eliakim et al. *2006*). However, 15 patients (33%) had false-positive findings on colon VCE (Eliakim et al. *2006*). The large number of false-positive findings remains a concern, as this occurred similarly in another prospective study. (Schoofs et al. *2006*) Colon VCE could have the potential for use in patients who have contraindications for OC, for patients with incomplete colonoscopy and for monitoring of patients with colonic involvement of inflammatory bowel disease. Cost effectiveness of colon VCE remains unknown as its procedural costs, and its impact on colon cancer screening rates remain to be determined (Boxes 10, 11, 12).

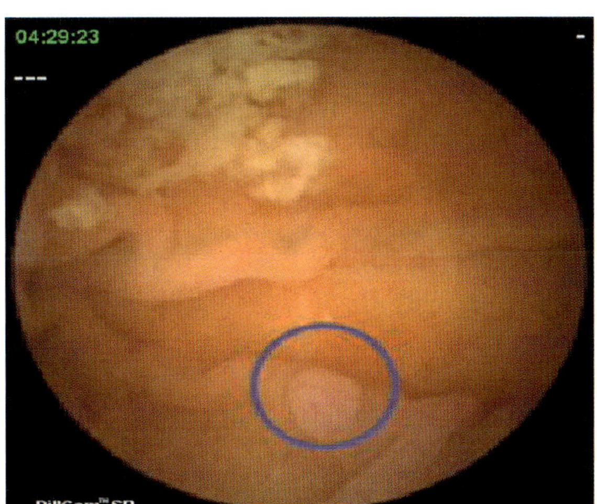

Fig. 46. Polyp in colon.

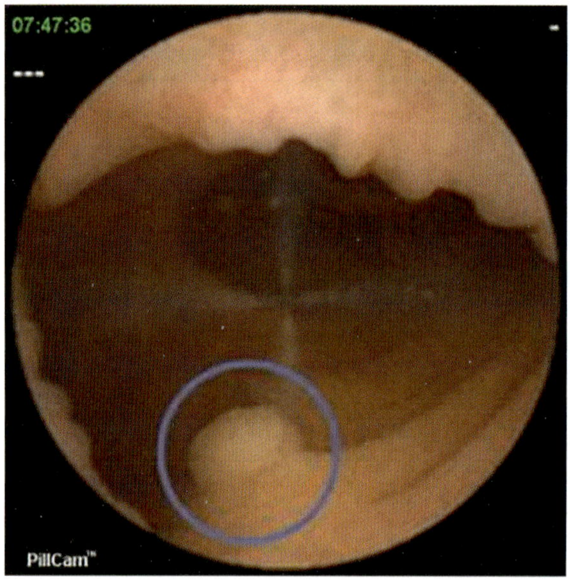

Fig. 47. Polyp in colon.

Box 9
Review

- Wireless video capsule endoscopy (VCE) is a very significant advancement in GI imaging that provides a non-invasive method for the evaluation of the esophagus, the small bowel, and potentially the colon.
- VCE has become a standard tool for the evaluation and management of small bowel bleeding, small bowel tumor detection, Crohn's disease, and Celiac disease.
- ECE is a procedural option for diagnosis and management of GERD and Barrett's esophagus and possibly for esophageal varices in patients with liver disease.
- Colon VCE could be a promising option for colon polyp screening. However it remains experimental and further studies are required.

Box 10
Indications for VCE

Small Bowel VCE

- Obscure gastrointestinal bleeding
- Evaluation of the site and extent of Crohn's disease
- Evaluation, extent and complications of celiac disease

Esophageal VCE

- Barrett's esophagus detection
- Possibly for esophageal variceal screening

Colon VCE

- Possibly for colon polyp screening

Box 11
Relative contraindications and solutions

- Small bowel strictures-consider Agile patency capsule prior to VCE
- Dysphagia - consider AdvanCE capsule delivery by endoscopy
- Gastroparesis - consider AdvanCE capsule delivery by endoscopy
- Pacemakers - theoretical risk, need to consider on an individual patient basis

Box 12
VCE procedure checklist

- Inform patient of indications for VCE, risk of retention, and study limitations
- Consider prepping patient with a small bowel purge and possibly simethicone prior to VCE
- Confirm sensor array placement and capsule detection by leads prior to VCE ingestion
- After small bowel VCE ingestion, patient waits a full 8 h prior to dropping off the recorder
- Read study carefully, limiting disruptions and interruptions

SUMMARY OF KEY POINTS

- VCE has emerged from its introduction in 2001 to become a standard endoscopic tool for the evaluation and management of small bowel bleeding, small bowel tumor detection, and other small bowel mucosal disorders.
- ECE may be a procedural option for the diagnosis and management of GERD and BE; however, its cost effectiveness remains to be determined.
- ECE may prove to be an option for the diagnosis of EV in cirrhotic patients; however, further studies will be required to evaluate its usefulness.
- Colon VCE could be a promising option for colon polyp screening. However, it remains experimental at the time; therefore, its role in the evaluation of colon pathology remains to be determined.

REFERENCES

American Gastroenterological Association medical position statement: evaluation and management of occult and obscure gastrointestinal bleeding. Gastroenterol. 2000;118:197–201.

Appleyard M, Glukhovsky A, Swain P. Wireless-capsule diagnostic endoscopy for recurrent small bowel bleeding. N Engl J Med. 2001;344:232–3.

Buchman A, Miller F, Wallin A, et al. Video-capsule endoscopy versus barium contrast studies for the diagnosis of Crohn's recurrence involving the small intestine. Am J Gastroenterol. 2004;99:2171–77.

Buscaglia J, Giday S, Kantsevoy S, et al. Performance characteristics of the suspected blood indicator feature in capsule endoscopy according to indication for study. Clin Gastroenterol Hepatol. 2008;6:298–301.

Carey E, Leighton J, Heigh R, et al. A single-center experience of 260 consecutive patients undergoing capsule endoscopy for obscure gastrointestinal bleeding. Am J Gastroenterol. 2007;102:89–95.

Chen X, Ran ZH, Tong JL. A meta-analysis of the yield of capsule endoscopy compared to double-balloon enteroscopy in patients with small bowel diseases. World J Gastroenterol. 2007;13:4372–8.

Chiefetz A, Kornbluth A, Legnani P, et al. The risk of retention of the capsule endoscope in patients with known or suspected Crohn's disease. Am J Gastroenterol. 2006;101:2218–22.

Cobrin G, Pittman R, Lewis B. Increased diagnostic yield of small bowel tumors with capsule endoscopy. Cancer. 2006;107:22–7.

Culliford A, Daly J, Diamond B, et al. The value of wireless capsule endoscopy in patients with complicated celiac disease. Gastrointest Endosc. 2005;62:55–61.

de Franchis R, Eisen G, Laine L, et al. Esophageal capsule endoscopy for screening and surveillance of esophageal varices in patients with portal hypertension. Hepatology. 2008;47:1595–603.

Dirks M, Costea F, Seidman E. Successful videocapsule endoscopy in patients with an abdominal cardiac pacemaker. Endoscopy. 2008;40:73–5.

Eliakim R, Fireman Z, Gralnek I, et al. Evaluation of the PillCam Colon capsule in the detection of colonic pathology: results of the first multicenter, prospective, comparative study. Endoscopy. 2006;38:963–70.

Ge Z, Gao Y, Hu Y, et al. The role of simethicone in small bowel preparation for capsule endoscopy. Endoscopy. 2006;38:836–40.

Goldstein J, Eisen G, Lewis B, et al. Video capsule endoscopy to prospectively assess small bowel injury with celecoxib, naproxen plus omeprazole and placebo. Clin Gastroenterol Hepatol. 2005;3:133–41.

Gralnek I, Rabinovitz R, Afik D, et al. A simplified ingestion procedure for esophageal capsule endoscopy: initial; evaluation in healthy volunteers. Endoscopy. 2006;38:913–18.

Gralnek I, Adler S, Yassin K, et al. Detecting esophageal disease with second-generation capsule endoscopy: initial evaluation of the PillCam ESO2. Endoscopy. 2008;40:275–79.

Herrerias J, Leighton J, Costmanga G, et al. Agile patency system eliminates risk of capsule retention in patients with known intestinal strictures who undergo capsule endoscopy. Gastrointest Endosc. 2008;67:902–09.

Holden J, Dureja P, Pfau P, et al. Endoscopic placement of the small-bowel video capsule by using a capsule endoscope delivery device. Gastrointest Endosc. 2007;65:842–47.

Hur C. Esophageal capsule endoscopy for Barrett's esophagus screening: a hard pill to swallow. Clin Gastroenterol Hepatol. 2007;5:312–18.

Jones B, Fleischer D, Sharma V, et al. Yield of repeat wireless video capsule endoscopy in patients with obscure gastrointestinal bleeding. Am J Gastroenterol. 2005;100:1058–64.

Kornbluth A, Colombel J, Leighton J, et al. ICCE: concensus for inflammatory bowel disease. Endoscopy. 2005;37:1051–54.

Kovalak M, Lake J, Mattek N, et al. Endoscopic screening for varices in cirrhotic patients data from a national endoscopic database. Gastrointest Endosc. 2007;65:82–8.

Lewis B, Godfarb N. The advent of capsule endoscopy- a not so futuristic approach to obscure gastrointestinal bleeding. Aliment Pharmacol Ther. 2003;17:1085–96.

Lewis B, Legnani P, Gralnek I, et al. The Crohn's disease capsule endoscopic scoring index: a new disease activity scale. Gastroenterology. 2004;126:A 124.

Lewis B, Eisen G, Friedman S. A pooled analysis of capsule endoscopy trials. Endoscopy. 2005;37:960–5.

Mishkin D, Chutlani R, Croffie J, et al. Technology Assessment Committee, American Society of Gastrointestinal Endoscopy. ASGE Technology Status Evaluation Report: wireless capsule endoscopy. Gastrointest Endosc. 2006;63:539–45.

Murray J, Brogan D, Van Dyke C, et al. Mapping the extent of untreated celiac disease with capsule endoscopy. Gastrointest Endosc. 2004;59:AB101.

Neu B, Wettschureck E, Rosch T. Is esophageal capsule endoscopy feasible? Results of a pilot study. Endoscopy. 2003;35:957–61.

Niv Y, Niv G. Capsule endoscopy: role of bowel preparation in successful visualization. Scan J Gastroenterol. 2004;39:1005–09.

Niv Y, Niv V, Wiser K, et al. Capsule endoscopy a comparison of two strategies of bowel preparation. Aliment Pharmacol Ther. 2005;22:957–62.

Oosterveen S, Rahimi R, Losurdo J, et al. Inpatient capsule endoscopy leads to frequent incomplete small bowel examinations. Gastrointest Endosc. 2006;63:AB149.

Petroniene R, Dubcenco E, Baker J, et al. Given capsule endoscopy in celiac disease: evaluation of diagnostic accuracy and interobserver agreement. Am J Gastroenterol. 2005;100:685–94.

Raina D, Wilkins T, Chamberlain S, et al. The accuracy and safety of esophageal capsule endoscopy for the detection of esophageal varices: a meta-analysis. Gastroenterology. 2008;134:A343.

Rondonotti E, Pennazio M, Toth E, et al. Small bowel neoplasms in patients undergoing video capsule endoscopy: a multicenter European study. Endoscopy. 2008;40:488–95.

Saperas E, Dot J, Videla S, et al. Capsule endoscopy versus computer tomographic or standard angiography for diagnosis of obscure gastrointestinal bleeding. Am J Gastroenterol. 2007;102:731–37.

Schoofs S, Devière J, Van Gossom A. PillCam colon capsule endoscopy compared with colonoscopy for colorectal tumor diagnosis: a prospective pilot study. Endoscopy. 2006;38:971–77.

Spada C, Spera G, Riccioni M, et al. A novel diagnostic tool for detecting functional patency of the small bowel: the Given patency capsule. Endoscopy. 2005;37:793–800.

Triester S, Leighton J, Leontiadis G, et al. A meta-analysis of the yield of capsule endoscopy compared to other diagnostic modalities in patients with non-stricturing small bowel Crohn's disease. Am J Gastroenterol. 2006;1010:954–64.

Wilkins T, Raina D, Chamberlain S, et al. The safety and accuracy of esophageal capsule endoscopy for the diagnosis of Barrett's esophagus: a systematic review and meta-analysis. Gastroenterology. 2008;103:S2.

10 Double Balloon Enteroscopy

Prithvi Sreenivasan and Seth A. Gross

CONTENTS

Keywords: Double Ballon, Enteroscopy, DBE, Enteroscope

INTRODUCTION

Endoscopic examination of the small bowel, until recently, has been elusive because of the bowel's relative inaccessibility. Standard endoscopic examinations evaluate only short segments of the proximal and distal small bowel. Until recently, intraoperative enteroscopy was considered the gold standard, providing the highest diagnostic and therapeutic yield in patients with bleeding from the small bowel. This was, however, associated with a substantial risk for complications and mortality (Desa et al. 1991). The double-balloon enteroscope (DBE) is a instrument that was first described by Yamamoto in 2001 (Yamamoto et al. 2001), and its system was first developed by the Fujinon Corporation in 2003 (Yamamoto et al. 2003). It has a high success rate of intubation into the deep small intestine (Kaffes et al. 2006; Yamamoto et al. 2004) and allows endoscopic evaluation of the small bowel with interventional capabilities. Its use has subsequently grown worldwide. The first

From: *Clinical Gastroenterology: Diagnostic and Therapeutic Procedures in Gastroenterology*,
Edited by: G. Y. Wu, S. Sridhar, DOI 10.1007/978-1-59745-044-7_10,

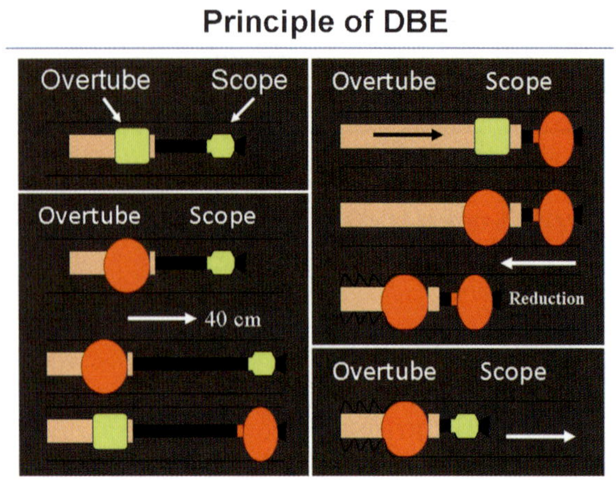

Fig. 1. "The sequence of overtube and scope advancement during DBE".

international workshop on DBE was held in Japan in August 2006 (Sugano and Marcon 2007). This chapter aims to describe the DBE procedure and its progress in recent years.

PRINCIPLE OF DBE

The most important principle for insertion of the enteroscope is to effectively transmit the force from the shaft of the scope to its tip. When the enteroscope bends to form a loop, the force applied to the shaft is not transmitted to the tip, and, as a result, the tip does not advance. The challenge of deep insertion is not the bending and the formation of loops itself, but the stretching of the intestine causing the loop. Inserting the enteroscope stretches the intestine, and, hence, the force on the enteroscope shaft is not transmitted to the tip of the enteroscope. The DBE overcomes this issue because the scope is inserted through an overtube. The inflated balloon at the tip of the overtube offers the potential to anchor the intestine in place from inside and prevents the tip of the overtube from slipping. With alternate inflation and deflation of the balloons of the enteroscope and the overtube and the relative movement of the scope with respect to the overtube, the small intestine is pleated over the overtube (Fig. 1). This decreases looping, shortens the intestine, and helps to maximize insertion (Yamamoto and Kita 2006).

DEVICE DESCRIPTION

A double-balloon enteroscope system consists of a high-resolution video endoscope with a balloon on the distal end, an overtube equipped with a balloon, and a pump for inflating and deflating the balloons (Fig. 2). There are two versions of the enteroscope currently available, one for general use (Fujinon EN-450P5/20; p type; Fujinon Inc., Saitama City, Japan) and the other for therapeutic intervention (Fujinon EN-450 T5; t-type). The working length of the enteroscope is 200 cm, and the overtube length is 145 cm. The difference between the two types of enteroscopes is the difference in their diameters. The enteroscope for general use is thinner with an external diameter of 8.5 mm, and a working channel of 2.2 mm in diameter. This enteroscope used in combination with an overtube has

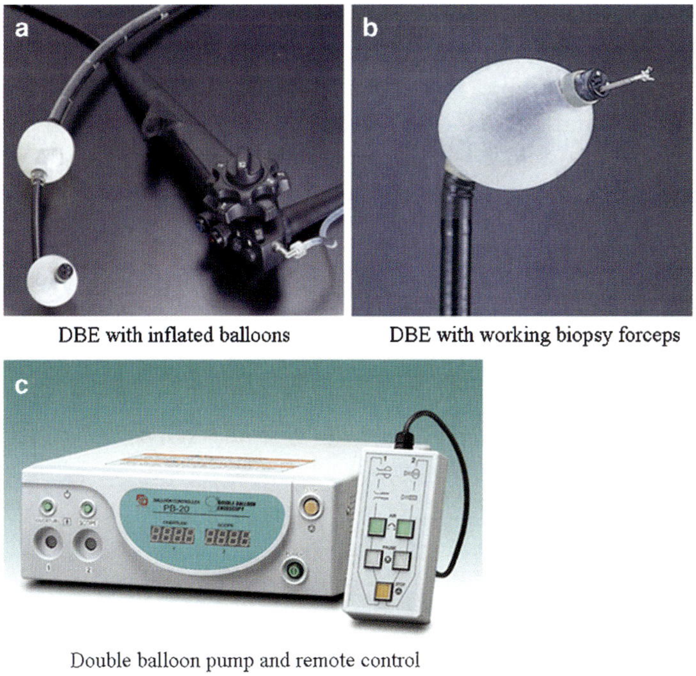

Fig. 2. DBE Equipment. (**a**) DBE with both scope and overtube balloons inflated; (**b**) the tip of the DBE with balloons inflated and opened biopsy forceps; (**c**) DBE balloon pump processor with remote control.

Table 1
Enteroscope characteristics

Scope	*EN450P5*	*EN450T5*
Working length (cm)	200	200
Total length (cm)	230	230
External diameter (mm)	8.5	9.5
Working channel (mm)	2.2	2.8
Field of view (degrees)	120	140
Overtube	Diagnostic	Therapeutic
External diameter (mm)	12.2	13.2
Inner diameter (mm)	10	10.8
Distal end diameter (mm)	8.7	9.8
Total length (cm)	145	145

an external diameter of 12.2 mm and an inner diameter of 10 mm. The therapeutic enteroscope has an external diameter of 9.5 mm, with a working channel diameter of 2.8 mm. This enteroscope is used in combination with an overtube with an external diameter of 13.2 mm and an inner diameter of 11 mm. The DBE has a built-in air route provided for inflating the distal end balloon (Table 1). The inner and outer surfaces of the tube have a hydrophilic coating. Both balloons are soft and made from latex, with a thickness of about 0.1 mm. Inflating and deflating operations for the balloon can be controlled with one-touch controls using a dedicated pump. The minimum balloon pressure that is required to grip the small bowel safely and cause minimal discomfort to the patient is 45 mmHg. The tip of the DBE has bending capability (up and down, left and right), allowing for targeted biopsies and therapeutic intervention.

PREPROCEDURE PREPARATION

Anterograde (oral) Approach: The procedure is similar to routine upper endoscopy. The patient is placed in a left lateral decubitus position with regular monitoring of electrocardiogram and oxygen saturation. No bowel prep is required

Retrograde (rectal) Approach: The procedure is the same as with colonoscopy but bowel preparation is required

Sedation

The duration of intubation using a DBE is long; therefore, it is common to use conscious sedation or general anesthesia. In a multicenter US study, there was no difference in the time taken, outcomes, and rate of complications between centers that used either of the above (Mehdizadeh et al. 2006a). In a German study, general anesthesia was not used in any of the 248 patients (May et al. 2005a). In the USA, many of the endoscopists prefer propofol-based sedation as the main modality to sedate their patients, but general anesthesia for DBE is typically not required.

PROCEDURE

After lubrication of its inner surface, the overtube is back-loaded onto the DBE prior to intubation. During an oral approach also known as the anterograde DBE the endoscopist advances the scope with both balloons deflated to the level of the duodenum. Upon reaching these points, the overtube balloon is inflated to grip the intestinal wall, and the enteroscope is advanced as far as possible. As previously mentioned, this prevents the small intestine from forming redundant loops. The double-balloon enteroscope advances by holding the intestine alternately by the balloon on the enteroscope and the balloon on the overtube. When the tip of the enteroscope is inserted as far as possible, the balloon on the enteroscope tip is inflated, the balloon on the overtube is deflated, and the overtube is advanced along the enteroscope. When the distal end of the overtube reaches the end of the enteroscope, the balloon on the overtube is inflated to fix a second point to the intestine. After this "push" procedure has been completed, the "pull" procedure begins, during which both the enteroscope and the overtube are pulled back under endoscopic and, if necessary fluoroscopic guidance, with both balloons inflated. This causes shortening of the intestine, of a total length of 6–7 m on the overtube, and also simplifies the shape of the intestine distally, thus preventing looping. The sequence is repeated each time with effective pleating of the intestine (Fig. 3). Even in the distal small intestine, precise control of the enteroscope tip is possible as it is controlled from the stabilized point by the overtube balloon, which could be located close to the tip of the enteroscope. The above

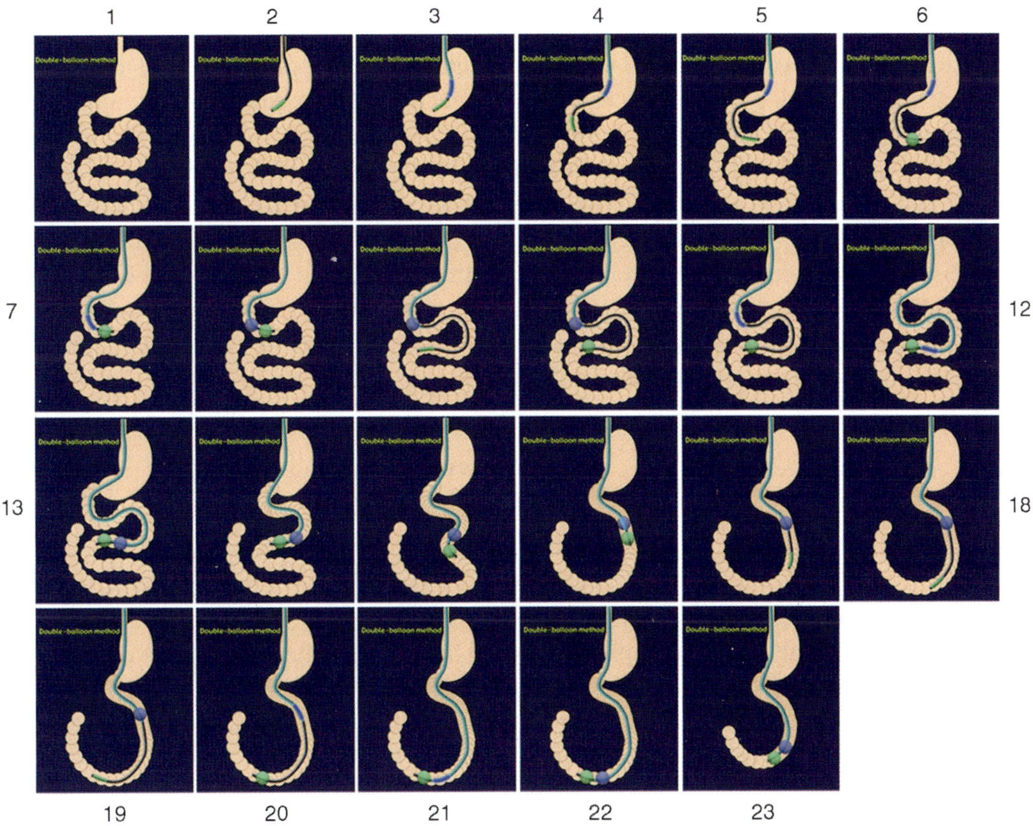

Fig. 3. Anterograde (oral) DBE approachThe DBE is advanced into the small bowel using a push and pull reduction technique accomplished by alternating inflation of the balloons on the scope and overtube.

described technique can also be done via the anal approach also known as Retrograde DBE. For this approach the push and pull technique is used starting in the colon as the enteroscope is advanced to the small intestine.

Total enteroscopy via a unilateral approach, from either side, usually takes too long and is not practical for routine examination. In reports by Yamamoto et al. (2004) and May et al. (2005a), total enteroscopy using one route alone (from mouth to cecum) was possible in only a very small number of patients. Endoscopic insertions via the oral or anal route on an average can reach about half to two thirds of the small intestine (Yamamoto et al. 2004). Thus, bilateral approaches are often used to examine the entire small intestine. However, total enteroscopy is only necessary in less than half of the patients, as indicated by the high diagnostic yield of approximately 80% with partial enteroscopy. Anterograde and retrograde approaches are done on separate days if the target is not reached by the initial approach.

The absence of landmarks in the small bowel can limit precision. To ensure a complete examination is achieved, it is generally well established that tattooing the distal-most portion reached. Tattoos are also used to localize a lesion if future interventions are required, such as surgical resection.

Route of Insertion

DBE can be inserted either from the mouth (anterograde approach) or anus (retrograde approach). Prior imaging studies can be used to direct the initial route of enteroscopy to help provide the highest clinical impact. DBE via retrograde approach has been described to be more technically challenging and examines a shorter length of the small intestine because of difficulty in accessing the small bowel beyond the ileocecal valve or a surgical anastomosis. The rate of terminal ileal intubation has been found to be considerably decreased in patients with adhesions, which is thought to be the main cause for insertion difficulty in these cases. For optimal enteroscope advancement and bowel shortening by the DBE, the bowel needs to be mobile within the abdominal cavity. Fixation of loops of bowel decreases bowel mobility, making scope passage difficult (Mehdizadeh et al. 2007).

Indications

Diagnosis

Obscure GI bleeding

Abnormal findings on capsule endoscopy/small bowel follow-through/CT enterography

Known or suspected small bowel stricture

Evaluation of small bowel tumors (e.g., surveillance of malignancy (adenocarcinoma and lymphoma) in patients with celiac disease, carcinoid)

Tissue sampling/microbiology sampling for disease diagnosis (e.g., Whipple's disease sparing duodenum, diagnosis of *Mycobacterium avium intracellulare* (MAI), AIDS)

Chronic diarrhea

Crohn's disease

Therapeutic

Hemostasis

Retained foreign bodies

Stenting for stricture management

Polypectomy/Resection of small bowel mass to prevent obstruction, bleeding, malignancy (e.g., Peutz–Jeghers syndrome)

Salvage Therapy

Abdominal complaints in gastric bypass patients

PEG placement in gastric bypass anatomy

ERCP in Roux-en-Y situations

Previous failed colonoscopy

The DBE has also been used to demonstrate a variety of small intestinal disorders, including small bowel lesions (aphthae, erosions, ulcers, and strictures) related to Crohn's disease (Oshitani et al. 2006), NSAID-related small bowel injury and diaphragms (Hayashi et al. 2005; Yen et al. 2006; Nosho et al. 2005; Kamata et al. 2006), gastrointestinal stromal tumors (Iwamoto et al. 2005; Kunihiro et al. 2006), carcinoid tumors (Yamaguchi et al. 2005), ileal lymphoma (Yoshida et al. 2004), jejunal diverticulosis (Kamal and Gerson 2006), eosinophilic jejunitis (Chen et al. 2006), an inflammatory polyp causing intussusception (Miyata et al. 2004), an anticoagulant ileus (Shinozaki et al. 2004), Meckel's diverticulum (Gasbarrini et al. 2005; Manner et al. 2006; Park and Sohn 2006), Gorham's disease (Ji et al. 2005), and small intestinal involvement in familial adenomatous polyposis (Matsumoto et al. 2008).

DBE can be used therapeutically. It has been used for sampling or biopsying small bowel mucosa, small bowel polypectomy, placement of stents or dilation of strictures of the small bowel, endoscopic mucosal resection, to achieve hemostasis for bleeding lesions and to retrieve retained video capsules from the small bowel (Fig. 4) (Yamamoto et al. 2004; Sunada et al. 2004, 2005; Ohmiya et al. 2005; Yen et al. 2007; Nishimura et al. 2004; Kita et al. 2005; Lee et al. 2005; May et al. 2005b).

In patients in whom standard colonoscopy has been unsuccessful, it has been used to examine the colon via a retrograde approach (Gay and Delvaux 2007; Moreels and Pelckmans 2008). One report described use of DBE to facilitate endoscopic submucosal dissection of a superficial colon tumor located between the terminal ileum and cecum that could not be achieved with conventional colonoscopy. The tumor was resected successfully en bloc without complications (Kita and Yamamoto 2007).

The DBE has provided access and permitted therapy in patients with surgically modified digestive anatomy and intubation of the bypassed stomach that would have normally precluded standard endoscopic approaches. Examples of therapy include endoscopic retrograde cholangiography, biopsy, lithotripsy, dilatation of biliary stenosis, stent placement, and PEG placement in the excluded stomach of patients with gastric bypass (Kita and Yamamoto 2007;

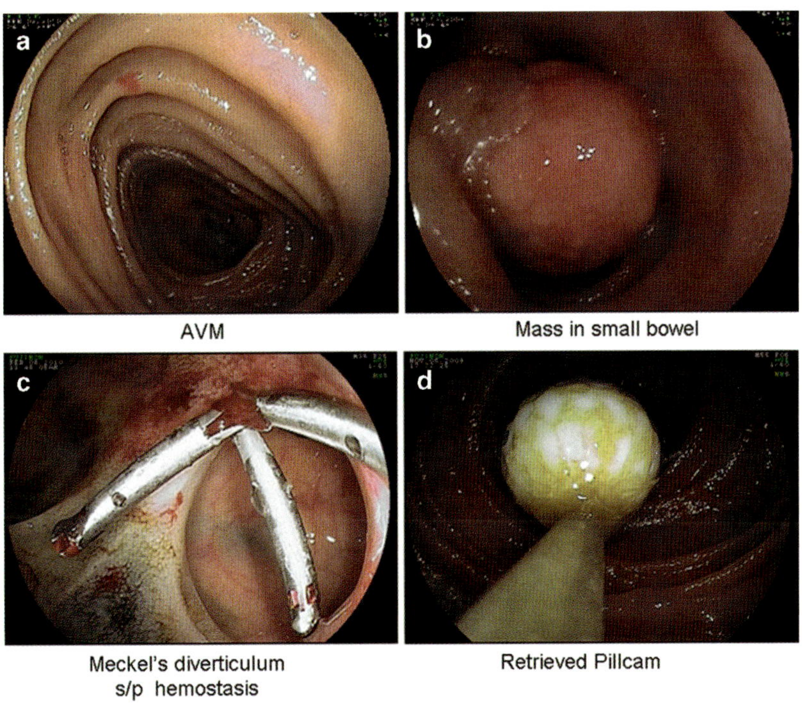

Fig. 4. Examples of clinical findings using a DBE. (**a**) Arteriovenous malformation (*AVM*); (**b**) small bowel mass; (**c**) Meckel's diverticulum with active bleeding treated with clips for hemostasis; (**d**) a pillcam lodged in a small bowel stricture retrieved using a Roth net.

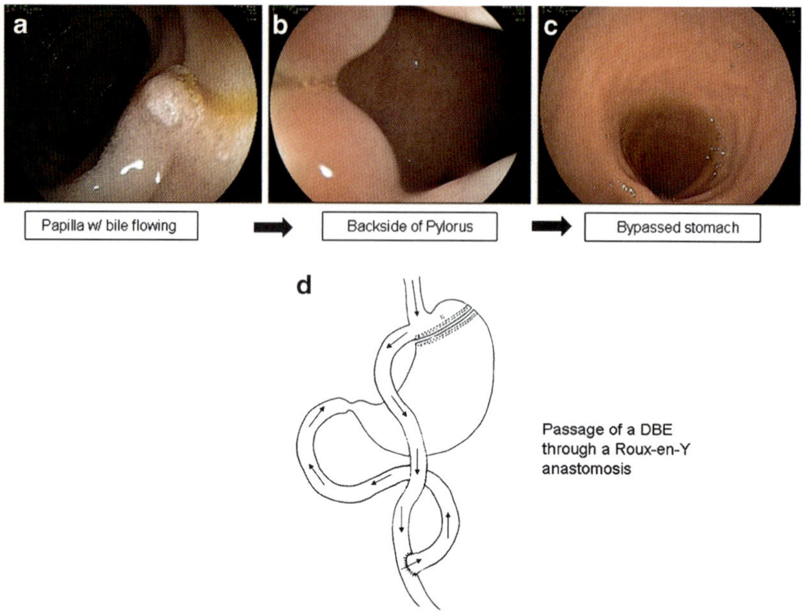

Fig. 5. Passage of a DBE through a gastric bypass Roux-en-Y anastomosis. (**a**) Papilla with bile flow; (**b**) backside of pylorus; (**c**) view of bypassed stomach; (**d**) passage of a DBE through a Roux-en-Y gastric bypass.

Haber 2007; Maaser et al. 2008; Sakai et al. 2005). Endoscopic mucosal resection in the afferent limb of a Roux-en-Y anatomy has also been reported (Kuno et al. 2004) (Fig. 5).

It has allowed for insertion of new devices such as the endoscopic ultrasound miniprobes and miniprobe with confocal microscopy (Delvaux and Gay 2009).

Contraindications

Bleeding tendency
Suspected or predisposition to perforation of the GI tract
Esophageal varices (if antegrade intubation is planned)
Latex allergy
Generalized debilitation

In contrast to a regular endoscope, the traction generated during pushing and pulling of the balloon-anchored endoscope is quite significant. This may predispose to perforation in a preexisting weakened intestinal wall (e.g. recent surgical site, severely ulcerated small intestine, after active chemotherapy for small bowel tumors, with preexisting connective tissue disorders such as Ehlers-Danlos syndrome that renders the small bowel wall very fragile, extensive colonic diverticulosis, eosinophilic esophagitis) or can cause mucosal hemorrhage in patients with underlying coagulopathy. This procedure should not be performed in people with suspected perforation or high-grade intestinal obstruction. Because DBE is often a lengthy procedure, it has been felt that patients with significant anesthetic risks may not be suitable for the procedure (Yamamoto et al. 2004; Simon and Lo 2007; Kuga et al. 2009; Tanaka et al. 2007).

A rare and a potential complication that has been previously described is a latex allergy. The balloons attached to the ends of the DBE and the overtubes are made of latex. This may pose health hazards to patients or health care workers with latex allergy. Latex allergy has become an increasingly prevalent medical problem must be recognized when evaluating a patient for the use of a DBE.

Disadvantages

Examination time is long
Two person procedure
Need for radiological backup

DBE is a time-consuming and a labor-intensive procedure. It may take several hours to visualize the small bowel and patients may be required to be admitted to the hospital. The reported examination time ranges from 70 to 123 min (Yamamoto et al. 2004; Mehdizadeh et al. 2006a; May et al. 2005a; Heine et al. 2006; Di Caro et al. 2005; Gross and Stark 2008; Ell et al. 2005; Akahoshi et al. 2006). The procedure duration has been reported to be longer at US-based centers compared to centers in Europe or Japan. These variations have been attributed to differences in techniques or patient characteristics, with Americans felt to be taller and heavier and, hence, to have larger abdominal cavities with more space when compared to the Japanese. It also requires a high level of staffing and often requires two assistants, one to help perform the procedure (push and pull technique), and the other to provide patient care and help the endoscopist. Fluoroscopic guidance is sometimes required to help guide the scope and to determine enteroscope configuration. Average fluoroscopy time could be anywhere between 2.1 and 5 min, with longer times reported by the American trials compared to the European trials (May et al. 2005a; Gross and Stark 2008; Ell et al. 2005) (Fig. 6).

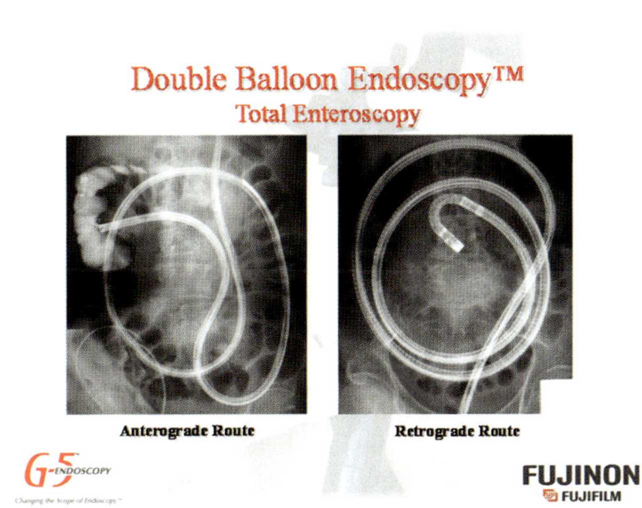

Fig. 6. Fluoroscopic images of DBE after anterograde and retrograde insertions.

Complications

Pancreatitis
Perforation
Aspiration
Bleeding
Abdominal pain from air insufflations and distention

Overall, insertion of the DBE has been considered to be a safe endoscopic procedure with a complication rate of approximately 1%. There have also been cases of acute pancreatitis and perforation associated with the technique. In one of the largest studies specifically designed to evaluate the complication rate of DBE, 85 adverse events were recorded (4 %) out of a total of 2,362 procedures. The complication rate was higher for therapeutic versus diagnostic procedures (4.3% versus 0.8%). No fatal complications were reported. There were seven cases of pancreatitis (overall incidence of 0.3%), six after diagnostic (0.3%) and one after therapeutic (0.2%) DBE (Mensink et al. 2007). A second survey study from Germany reported 48 complications (1.2%). Acute pancreatitis occurred in nine patients (0.34%) with one mortality, and perforation occurred in eight cases, all of them requiring surgery. There was also one procedure-related death. Six perforations occurred after polypectomy, making the perforation rate after polypectomy during DBE, 3.4%. In six cases, major bleeding was reported, four after polypectomy and two after biopsy. All patients required endoscopic treatment and recovered. The authors do suggest that, for diagnostic DBE, pancreatitis has to be taken into consideration in the written informed consent (Moschler et al. 2008). Additionally, there have been reports of esophageal perforation as a result of entrapment of the mucosa between the endoscope and the overtube during the process of sliding the overtube over the enteroscope during its insertion (Dinning and Jaffe 1997). Therefore, if the outer tube does not advance smoothly, one should not use undue force to push it deeper into the small intestine.

Air retention resulting in patient discomfort has been well described in people undergoing lengthy endoscopic procedures. There have been reports to suggest the use of carbon dioxide (CO_2) as an insufflation gas, can mitigate pain due to its capacity to be more rapidly absorbed from the intestine compared to air (Hirai et al. 2007).

Alternative Procedures

Wireless Video Capsule Endoscopy

The wireless video capsule endoscopy (CE) is an innovative technique designed to examine the small bowel and is well established in the USA and Europe. It is a passive imaging technology, has the advantage of being non-invasive, easy to use, and is most widely used in evaluating causes of obscure GI bleeding (Iddan et al. 2000; Gong et al. 2000). The main disadvantage is that it does not permit tissue sampling or therapeutic intervention and is strictly a screening or diagnostic tool. The images are sometimes not sharp enough for judging the precise nature of the lesions, and the capsule does not reach the cecum within recording time in about 20–30% of cases (Westerhof et al. 2009). In a meta-analysis comparing the DBE to capsule endoscopy, the authors concluded that there was a comparable diagnostic yield in pertinent small bowel findings, including causes of obscure gastrointestinal bleeding (Pasha et al. 2008). The yield was also similar when comparing specific types of findings such as vascular malformations, inflammatory lesions, and polyps/tumors (Hadithi et al. 2006; Nakamura et al. 2006; Matsumoto et al. 2005a; Mehdizadeh et al. 2006b). It is now well accepted that capsule endoscopy is preferred as an initial diagnostic test because of its noninvasiveness, patient tolerance, and the ability to view the entire small bowel. DBE is reserved for treatment or to obtain a histopathological diagnosis after detection of bleeding site by CE, cases in which there is a suspicion for a small bowel lesion despite a negative capsule endoscopy, and in patients with active bleeding from the small bowel. Thus, while CE can be regarded as a first-line investigation for small bowel disorders, the DBE is complementary. DBE may, however, be the modality of choice for management if small bowel stricture is suspected. Wireless capsule endoscopy in such patients is associated with a risk of capsule retention.

Enteroscopy

Single Balloon Enteroscopy

Single Balloon Enteroscope is a novel balloon endoscopy system in which only a single balloon is attached to the tip of the over tube (Tsujikawa et al. 2008). In a prospective randomized multicenter study to compare the double balloon and single balloon techniques, complete enteroscopy with the single balloon technique was significantly lower 22% (11/50 cases) with oral and anal routes combined as opposed to 66% (33/50 cases) using a double balloon enteroscope ($p<0.0001$). There were no severe complications with either procedure. Additionally, the rate of therapeutic consequences (relevant findings that confirmed the suspected diagnosis and negative complete enteroscopies influencing further therapy) was significantly higher with the DBE technique (72%) compared to the single balloon technique (48%). The authors concluded that the DBE must, therefore, be still considered as the non-surgical gold standard procedure for small bowel evaluation (May et al. 2010).

Spiral Enteroscopy

The Spiral enteroscopy system consists of a novel spiral shaped overtube device that has been approved for small bowel evaluation. By using a rotating method to advance, similar to the motion of a corkscrew, it converts rotational force into linear force and allows one to pleat the small bowel and advance into the distal small bowel. In a prospective study, the procedure was successfully performed in 96% of the patients with mean time to maximum insertion being 21 min and total procedure time being 34 min. The average estimated depth of insertion beyond the ligament of Treitz was 262 cm. It was well tolerated, and there were no complications. Conclusions were that it was a safe and effective procedure with a comparable depth of insertion compared to a DBE, and the total procedure time was less than that of a DBE (Buscaglia et al. 2009). It has also been used to perform ERCP in post-gastric surgery patients including Roux-en-Y patients and retrograde endoscopies (Esmail et al. 2009; Cantero et al. 2009; Akerman et al. 2009). The diagnostic yield has been comparable with the DBE based on existing studies (Schembre and Ross 2009). The DBE and Spiral enteroscopy are competing technologies. Large prospective studies and long-term data are required to further evaluate and compare these techniques.

Push-Enteroscopy

The push-enteroscope with its diagnostic and therapeutic capabilities became the standard endoscopic method for examination of the proximal small bowel in the 1980s. This is performed with an enteroscope of extended length (200–250 cm), with or without an overtube. The shortcoming of this procedure is its limited insertion depth of approximately 60–100 cm past the ligament of Treitz (Taylor et al. 2001; May et al. 2006). In obscure bleeding, its diagnostic yield ranged from 3% to 70%, with AVMs being diagnosed most commonly in 7–60% of the examinations (Pennazio et al. 1995; Schmit et al. 1996; Descamps et al. 1999). For suspected small-bowel bleeding, DBE was found to be superior to push-enteroscopy for endoscopic examination of the small bowel, both with regard to the length of small bowel visualized, and the overall diagnostic yield. DBE identified additional lesions in distal parts of the small bowel in push-enteroscopy-positive patients in 78% of cases (May et al. 2006; Matsumoto et al. 2005b). Push-enteroscopy may, however, be suitable for detecting suspected proximal small bowel tumors, suspected celiac sprue, polyposis syndromes, malabsorption, and AVMs. Push-enteroscopy with a colonoscope may have an added advantage over DBE, single balloon enteroscope, and spiral enteroscope for dilation of strictures and placement of expandable metal stents. Overall, push-enteroscopy is a reasonable option if DBE, single balloon enteroscopy, or spiral enteroscopy is not available, one that gives moderate yield and involves minimal risk.

Intraoperative Enteroscopy

Intraoperative enteroscopy is an invasive technique with insertion of an enteroscope orally or rectally or through an enterotomy site during surgery and involves a surgeon and an endoscopist. The surgeon manually advances the endoscope by telescoping the bowel over the tip. It enables investigation of the entire small intestine and treatment of pathological findings by endoscopic or surgical means at the same time. The diagnostic rate of intraoperative enteroscopy for mucosal disease has been reported to range from 70% to 100%, depending on the inclusion criteria (Lewis et al. 1991; Ress et al. 1992; Lopez et al. 1996; Desa et al. 1991; Lau et al. 1989; Flickinger et al. 1989; Bhattacharya et al. 1999; Benz et al. 1999). Although the success rate of reaching the ileum approaches 90%, the use of intraoperative enteroscopy does not appear to be associated with lower rates of recurrent GI bleeding, and it is not only invasive and cumbersome but also carries a significant morbidity. Hence, it is recommended only when all other techniques have failed. Some complications described with this procedure are ileus, congestive heart failure, azotemia, intraabdominal abscess, chest infections, postoperative bowel ischemia, and bowel obstruction (Douard et al. 2000; Ress et al. 1992).

Small Bowel Series

In comparing diagnostic yields between DBE and small-bowel series in patients with suspected small bowel bleeding, DBE detected a possible bleeding source in a higher proportion of patients than did small-bowel series (70% vs 44%). Because significant complications associated with DBE did not occur, they suggested that DBE may be superior to small-bowel series in the evaluation of obscure GI bleeding (Byeon et al. 2006).

Costs

The cost for a DBE is not known at the present time. The CPT code 44799 (unlisted procedure, intestine) is currently recommended by some hospital billing departments. It is anticipated that CPT codes for a DBE will be established shortly (Gerson and Kamal 2008).

SUMMARY OF KEY POINTS

- The DBE provides both diagnostic as well as therapeutic intervention to the entire small bowel.
- It is currently being used as first-line therapy in patients with positive findings on capsule endoscopy or other small bowel imaging that requires tissue sampling or therapy out of reach of a standard endoscope, and to further investigate cases with a high suspicion for a small bowel lesion despite a negative capsule study.
- It is also being used as salvage therapy to reach the excluded stomach in bariatric surgery patients, perform ERCP in patients with Roux-en-Y anatomy or to reach the cecum in failed colonoscopy cases.
- The rate of complications is low with the most severe complications being pancreatitis and perforation.
- The main disadvantages of this procedure include the long procedural time, the need for additional staff, anesthesia, and fluoroscopic support.
- The DBE has revolutionized examination of the small bowel.

REFERENCES

Akahoshi K, Kubokawa M, Matsumoto M, et al. Double-balloon endoscopy in the diagnosis and management of GI tract diseases: methodology, indications, safety and clinical impact. World J Gastroenterol. 2006;12(47):7654–9.

Akerman P, Cantero D, Pangtay J, et al. Retrograde small bowel enteroscopy using the Olympus SIF-140 260 cm enteroscope and the Vista-SB spiral overtube. Gastrointest Endosc. 2009;69:AB201.

AU Oshitani N, Yukawa T, Yamagami H, et al. Evaluation of deep small bowel involvement by double-balloon enteroscopy in Crohn's disease. Am J Gastroenterol. 2006 July;101(7):1484–9.

Benz C, Jakobs R, Arnold JC, et al. Outcome of intraoperative enteroscopy in cases of gastrointestinal bleeding of unknown origin after negative push-type enteroscopy (abstract). Gastroenterology. 1999;16:202.

Bhattacharya K, Lopez MJ, Cooley JS, et al. Intraoperative sonde enteroscopy in the management of transfusion dependent small intestinal bleeding [abstract]. Gastrointest Endosc. 1999;49:593.

Buscaglia JM, Dunbar KB, Okolo 3rd PI, et al. The spiral enteroscopy training initiative: results of a prospective study evaluating the Discovery SB overtube device during small bowel enteroscopy (with video). Endoscopy. 2009 Mar;41(3):194–9.

Byeon JS, Choi KD, Yang SK, et al. Comparison of double balloon enteroscopy and small bowel series in the evaluation of small bowel lesion [abstract]. Gastrointest Endosc. 2006;63:AB172.

Cantero D, Akerman P, Pangtay J. Retrograde spiral enteroscopy using the Fujinon EN-450 T5 and Olympus SIF-180 200 cm enteroscopes with the Discovery SB overtube. Gastrointestinal Endoscopy. 2009;69(5):AB192.

Chen YY, Su WW, Soon MS, et al. Eosinophilic jejunitis presenting with acute abdomen: the usefulness of double-balloon enteroscopy. Gastrointest Endosc. 2006;63:532.

Delvaux M, Gay G. Novel applications of balloon endoscopy. Gastrointest Endosc Clin N Am. 2009 July;19(3):509–18.

Desa LA, Ohri SK, Hutton KA, Lee H, Spencer J. Role of intraoperative enteroscopy in obscure gastrointestinal bleeding of small bowel origin. Br J Surg. 1991;78:192–5.
Descamps C, Schmit A, Van Gossum A. "Missed" upper gastrointestinal tract lesions may explain "occult" bleeding. Endoscopy. 1999;31:452–5.
Di Caro S, May A, Heine DG, et al. The European experience with double- balloon enteroscopy: indications, methodology, safety, and clinical impact. Gastrointest Endosc. 2005 Oct;62(4):545–50.
Dinning JP, Jaffe PE. Delayed presentation of esophageal perforation as a result of overtube placement. J Clin Gastroenterol. 1997;24:250–2.
Douard R, Wind P, Panis Y, et al. Intraoperative Enteroscopy for Diagnosis and Management of Unexplained Gastrointestinal Bleeding. Am J Surg. 2000 Sept;180(3):181–4.
Ell C, May A, Nachbar L, et al. Push-and-pull enteroscopy in the small bowel using the double-balloon technique: results of a prospective European multicenter study. Endoscopy. 2005 July;37(7):613–6.
Esmail S, Odstrcil EA, Mallat D, et al. A single center retrospective review of spiral enteroscopy. Gastrointest Endosc. 2009;69:197.
Flickinger E, Stanforth A, Sinar D, et al. Intraoperative videopanendoscopy for diagnosing sites of chronic intestinal bleeding. Am J Surg. 1989;157:137–44.
Gasbarrini A, Di Caro S, Mutignani M, et al. Double-balloon enteroscopy for diagnosis of a Meckel's diverticulum in a patient with GI bleeding of obscure origin. Gastrointest Endosc. 2005;61:779–81.
Gay G, Delvaux M. Double-balloon colonoscopy after failed conventional colonoscopy: a pilot series with a new instrument. Endoscopy. 2007 Sep;39(9):788–92.
Gerson L, Kamal A. Cost-effectiveness analysis of management strategies for obscure GI bleeding. Gastrointest Endosc. 2008 Nov;68(5):920–36.
Gong F, Swain P, Mills T. Wireless endoscopy. Gastrointest Endosc. 2000;51:725.
Gross SA, Stark ME. Initial experience with double-balloon enteroscopy at a U.S. center. Gastrointest Endosc. 2008 May;67(6):890–7.
Haber GB. Double balloon endoscopy for pancreatic and biliary access in altered anatomy (with videos). Gastrointest Endosc. 2007 Sept;66:S47–50.
Hadithi M, Heine GD, Jacobs MA, van Bodegraven AA, Mulder CJ. A prospective study comparing video capsule endoscopy with double-balloon enteroscopy in patients with obscure gastrointestinal bleeding. Am J Gastroenterol. 2006 Jan;101(1):52–7.
Hayashi Y, Yamamoto H, Kita H, et al. Non-steroidal anti-inflammatory drug-induced small bowel injuries identified by double-balloon endoscopy. World J Gastroenterol. 2005;11:4861–4.
Heine GD, Hadithi M, Groenen MJ, Kuipers EJ, Jacobs MA, Mulder CJ. Double-balloon enteroscopy: indications, diagnostic yield, and complications in a series of 275 patients with suspected small-bowel disease. Endoscopy. 2006 Jan;38(1):42–8.
Hirai F, Matsui T, Yao K, Sou S, Seki T. Efficacy of carbon dioxide insufflation in endoscopic balloon dilation therapy by using double balloon endoscopy. Gastrointest Endosc. 2007 Sep;66(3 Suppl):S26–9.
Iddan G, Meron G, Glukhovsky A, Swain P. Wireless capsule endoscopy. Nature. 2000;405:417.
Iwamoto M, Yamamoto H, Kita H, et al. Double-balloon endoscopy for ileal GI stromal tumor. Gastrointest Endosc. 2005;62(3):440–1.
Ji JS, Choi H, Choi KY, et al. Two cases of GI involvement of Gorham's disease diagnosed by double-balloon enteroscopy: Case report and review of the literature. Gastrointest Endosc. 2005;62(2):312–5.
Kaffes AJ, Koo JH, Meredith C. Double-balloon enteroscopy in the diagnosis and the management of small-bowel diseases: an initial experience in 40 patients. Gastrointest Endosc. 2006 Jan;63(1):81–6.
Kamal A, Gerson LB. Jejunal diverticulosis diagnosed by double-balloon enteroscopy. Gastrointest Endosc. 2006;63:864.
Kamata Y, Iwamoto M, Nara H, et al. A case of rheumatoid arthritis with protein losing enteropathy induced by multiple diaphragmatic strictures of the small intestine: successful treatment by bougieing under double-balloon enteroscopy. Gut. 2006;55(9):1372.
Kita H, Yamamoto H. New indications of double balloon endoscopy. Gastrointest Endosc. 2007 Sept;66:S57–9.
Kita H, Yamamoto H, Nakamura T, Shirakawa K, Terano A, Sugano K. Bleeding polyp in the mid small intestine identified by capsule endoscopy and treated by double-balloon endoscopy. Gastrointest Endosc. 2005 Apr;61(4):628–9.

Kuga R, Furuya Jr CK, Ide E, et al. Eosinophilic esophagitis and double-balloon enteroscopy: a dangerous combination. Endoscopy. 2009;41 Suppl 2:E85.

Kunihiro K, Manabe N, Hata J, et al. Gastrointestinal stromal tumor in jejunum: diagnosis using contrast-enhanced ultrasonography and double-balloon enteroscopy. Dig Dis Sci. 2006 July;51(7):1236–40.

Kuno A, Yamamoto H, Kita H, et al. Double balloon enteroscopy through a Roux-en-Y anastomosis for EMR of an early carcinoma in the afferent duodenal limb. Gastrointest Endosc. 2004 Dec;60(6):1032–4.

Lau W, Wong S, Yuen W, Wong K. Intraoperative enteroscopy for bleeding angiodysplasias of small intestine. Surg Gynecol Obstet. 1989;168:341–4.

Lee BI, Choi H, Choi KY, et al. Retrieval of a retained capsule endoscope by double-balloon enteroscopy. Gastrointest Endosc. 2005;62(3):463–5.

Lewis B, Wenger J, Waye J. Small bowel enteroscopy and intraoperative enteroscopy for obscure gastrointestinal bleeding. Am J Gastroenterol. 1991;86:171–4.

Lopez M, Cooley J, Petros J, et al. Complete intraoperative small-bowel endoscopy in the evaluation of occult gastrointestinal bleeding using the sonde enteroscope. Arch Surg. 1996;131:272–7.

Maaser C, Lenze F, Bokemeyer M, et al. Double balloon enteroscopy: a useful tool for diagnostic and therapeutic procedures in the pancreaticobiliary system. Am J Gastroenterol. 2008 April;103(4):894–900.

Manner H, May A, Nachbar L, Ell C. Push-and-pull enteroscopy using the double-balloon technique (double-balloon enteroscopy) for the diagnosis of Meckel's diverticulum in adult patients with GI bleeding of obscure origin. Am J Gastroenterol. 2006 May;101(5):1152–4.

Matsumoto T, Esaki M, Moriyama T, Nakamura S, Iida M. Comparison of capsule endoscopy and enteroscopy with the double-balloon method in patients with obscure bleeding and polyposis. Endoscopy. 2005a;37(9):827–32.

Matsumoto T, Moriyama T, Esaki M, Nakamura S, Iida M. Performance of antegrade double-balloon enteroscopy: comparison with push enteroscopy. Gastrointest Endosc. 2005b;62(3):392–8.

Matsumoto T, Esaki M, Yanaru-Fujisawa R, et al. Small-intestinal involvement in familial adenomatous polyposis: evaluation by double-balloon endoscopy and intraoperative enteroscopy. Gastrointest Endosc. 2008 Nov;68(5):911–9.

May A, Nachbar L, Ell C. Extraction of entrapped capsules from the small bowel by means of push-and-pull enteroscopy with the double-balloon technique. Endoscopy. 2005a;37:591.

May A, Nachbar L, Ell C. Double-balloon enteroscopy (push-and-pull enteroscopy) of the small bowel: feasibility and diagnostic and therapeutic yield in patients with suspected small bowel disease. Gastrointest Endosc. 2005b;62(1):62–70.

May A, Nachbar L, Schneider M, Ell C. Prospective comparison of push enteroscopy and push-and-pull enteroscopy in patients with suspected small-bowel bleeding. Am J Gastroenterol. 2006 Sept;101(9):2016–24.

May A, Färber M, Aschmoneit I, et al. Prospective multicenter trial comparing push-and-pull enteroscopy with the single- and double-balloon techniques in patients with small-bowel disorders. Am J Gastroenterol. 2010 Mar;105(3):575–81.

Mehdizadeh S, Ross AS, Leighton J, et al. Double balloon enteroscopy (DBE) compared to capsule endoscopy (CE) among patients with obscure gastrointestinal bleeding (OGIB): a multicenter U.S. experience [abstract]. Gastrointest Endosc. 2006a;63:AB91.

Mehdizadeh S, Ross A, Gerson L, et al. What is the learning curve associated with double-balloon enteroscopy? Technical details and early experience in 6 U.S. tertiary care centers. Gastrointest Endosc. 2006b;64(5):740–50.

Mehdizadeh S, Han NJ, Cheng DW, Chen GC, Lo SK. Success rate of retrograde double balloon enteroscopy. Gastrointest Endosc. 2007;65(4):633–39.

Mensink PB, Haringsma J, Kucharzik T, et al. Complications of double balloon enteroscopy: a multicenter survey. Endoscopy. 2007 July;39(7):613–5.

Miyata T, Yamamoto H, Kita H, et al. A case of inflammatory fibroid polyp causing small-bowel intussusception in which retrograde double-balloon enteroscopy was useful for the preoperative diagnosis. Endoscopy. 2004 Apr;36(4):344–7.

Moreels TG, Pelckmans PA. Double-balloon endoscope for failed conventional colonoscopy. Clin Gastroenterol Hepatol. 2008 Feb;6(2):259.

Moschler O, May AD, Muller MK, Ell C. Complications in double-balloon-enteroscopy: Results of the German DBE register. Z Gastroenterol. 2008 Mar;46(3):266–70.

Nakamura M, Niwa Y, Ohmiya N, et al. Preliminary comparison of capsule endoscopy and double-balloon enteroscopy in patients with suspected small-bowel bleeding. Endoscopy. 2006 Jan;38(1):59–66.

Nishimura M, Yamamoto H, Kita H, et al. Gastrointestinal stromal tumor in the jejunum: diagnosis and control of bleeding with electrocoagulation by using double-balloon enteroscopy. J Gastroenterol. 2004 Oct;39(10):1001–4.

Nosho K, Endo T, Yoda Y, et al. Diaphragm disease of small intestine diagnosed by double-balloon enteroscopy. Gastrointest Endosc. 2005;62:187–9.

Ohmiya N, Taguchi A, Shirai K, et al. Endoscopic resection of Peutz-Jeghers polyps throughout the small intestine at double-balloon enteroscopy without laparotomy. Gastrointest Endosc. 2005;61:140.

Park JH, Sohn CI. A case of Meckel's diverticulum diagnosed by double balloon enteroscopy. Korean J Gastroenterol. 2006;47(1):1–4.

Pasha SF, Leighton JA, Das A, et al. Double-balloon enteroscopy and capsule endoscopy have comparable diagnostic yield in small-bowel disease: A meta-analysis. Clin Gastroenterol Hepatol. 2008 June;6(6):671–6.

Pennazio M, Arrigoni A, Risio M, Spandre M, Rossini FP. Clinical evaluation of push-type enteroscopy. Endoscopy. 1995 Feb;27(2):164–70.

Ress A, Benacci J, Sarr M. Efficacy of intraoperative enteroscopy in diagnosis and prevention of recurrent, occult gastrointestinal bleeding. Am J Surg. 1992;163:94–9.

Sakai P, Kuga R, Safatle-Ribeiro AV, et al. Is it feasible to reach the bypassed stomach after Roux-en-Y gastric bypass for morbid obesity? The use of the double-balloon enteroscope. Endoscopy. 2005 June; 37(6):566–9.

Schembre D, Ross A. Yield of antegrade double balloon versus spiral enteroscopy for obscure gastrointestinal bleeding. Gastrointest Endosc 2009;Abstract DDW:69.

Schmit A, Gay F, Adler M, Cremer M, Van Gossum A. Diagnostic efficacy of push-enteroscopy and long-term follow-up of patients with small bowel angiodysplasias. Dig Dis Sci. 1996 Dec;41(12):2348–52.

Shinozaki S, Yamamoto H, Kita H, et al. Direct observation with double-balloon enteroscopy of an intestinal intramural hematoma resulting in anticoagulant ileus. Dig Dis Sci. 2004 June;49(6):902–5.

Simon K, Lo MD. Technical matters in double balloon enteroscopy. Gastrointest Endosc. 2007; 66(3):S17–18.

Sugano K, Marcon N. The First International Workshop On Double Balloon Endoscopy: A Consensus Meeting Report. Gastrointest Endosc. 2007 Sep;66(3 Suppl):S7–11.

Sunada K, Yamamoto H, Kita H, et al. Case Report: Successful treatment with balloon dilatation in combination with double-balloon enteroscopy of a stricture in the small bowel of a patient with Crohn's disease. Dig Endosc. 2004;16:237.

Sunada K, Yamamoto H, Kita H, et al. Clinical outcomes of enteroscopy using the double-balloon method for strictures of the small intestine. World J Gastroenterol. 2005;11:1087–9.

Tanaka S, Mitsui K, Tatsuguchi A, et al. Current status of double balloon endoscopy–indications, insertion route, sedation, complications, technical matters. Gastrointest Endosc. 2007 Sep;66(3 Suppl):S30–3.

Taylor AC, Chen RY, Desmond PV. Use of an overtube for enteroscopy: does it increase depth of insertion? A prospective study of enteroscopy with and without an overtube. Endoscopy. 2001;33:227–30.

Tsujikawa T, Saitoh Y, Andoh A, et al. Novel single-balloon enteroscopy for diagnosis and treatment of the small intestine: preliminary experiences. Endoscopy. 2008 Jan;40(1):11–5.

Westerhof J, Weersma RK, Koornstra JJ. Risk factors for incomplete small-bowel capsule endoscopy. Gastrointest Endosc. 2009;69:74.

Yamaguchi T, Manabe N, Tanaka S, et al. Multiple carcinoid tumors of the ileum preoperatively diagnosed by enteroscopy with the double-balloon technique. Gastrointest Endosc. 2005;62(2):315–8.

Yamamoto H, Kita H. Double-balloon endoscopy: from concept to reality. Gastrointest Endosc Clin N Am. 2006 Apr;16(2):347–61.

Yamamoto H, Sekine Y, Sato Y, et al. Total enteroscopy with a nonsurgical steerable double-balloon method. Gastrointest Endosc. 2001;53(2):216–20.

Yamamoto H, Yano T, Kita H, Sunada K, Ido K, Sugano Kl. New system of double-balloon enteroscopy for diagnosis and treatment of small intestinal disorders. Gastroenterology. 2003;125:1556.

Yamamoto H, Kita H, Sunada K, et al. Clinical outcomes of double-balloon endoscopy for the diagnosis and treatment of small-intestinal diseases. Clin Gastroenterol Hepatol. 2004;2(11):1010–6.

Yen HH, Chen YY, Soon MS. Nonsteroidal anti-inflammatory drug-associated ileal ulcers: an evaluation by double-balloon enteroscopy. Gastrointest Endosc. 2006;63:328.
Yen HH, Chen YY, Soon MS, Lin YM. An unusual cause of obscure gastrointestinal bleeding. Gut. 2007 Jan;56(1):12.
Yoshida N, Wakabayashi N, Nomura K, et al. Ileal mucosa-associated lymphoid tissue lymphoma showing several ulcer scars detected using double-balloon endoscopy. Endoscopy. 2004 Nov;36(11):1022–4.

11 Sphincterotomy and Stents in Benign and Malignant Disorders and Biliary ERCP

John Baillie and Nathan J. Shores

CONTENTS

Keywords: Sphincterotomy, Stents, Benign, Malignant, Cystgastrostomy

INTRODUCTION

Advances in cross-sectional imaging, including magnetic resonance cholangiopancreatography (MRCP) and endoscopic ultrasound (EUS), have rendered endoscopic retrograde cholangiopancreatography (ERCP) a primarily therapeutic modality. Biliary sphincterotomy and stent placement are frequently part of the management of large bile duct stones, the relief of obstructive jaundice associated with benign and malignant strictures, the treatment of iatrogenic biliary leaks, etc. An individual's training largely dictates their ERCP technique.

SPHINCTEROTOMY

Endoscopic sphincterotomy has many benefits, but carries significant risk; manipulating the sphincter of Oddi (SO) should never be undertaken lightly. Incising the duodenal papilla is the primary therapy for papillary stenosis, sphincter of Oddi dysfunction (SOD), choledocholithiasis, and AIDS cholangiopathy (Farman et al. 1994). Extending the opening greatly facilitates the extraction of stones, debris, and pus from the common bile duct (CBD) and pancreatic duct (PD). The risks of endoscopic sphincterotomy include hemorrhage,

From: *Clinical Gastroenterology: Diagnostic and Therapeutic Procedures in Gastroenterology*,
Edited by: G. Y. Wu, S. Sridhar, DOI 10.1007/978-1-59745-044-7_11,

retroperitoneal perforation, and acute pancreatitis. The risks of ERCP can be graded using a standardized scale (Table 1) (Cotton et al. 1991). In the USA, significant bleeding (i.e., requiring hospitalization and/or blood transfusion) occurs after 1–2% of sphincterotomies (Freeman et al. 1996; Vandervoort et al. 2002). Post-ERCP pancreatitis rates vary widely from study to study and between procedures (1–40+% of procedures), with the vast majority being "mild." The best estimate of the incidence for "all comers" is 5–10% for average-risk patients (Freeman et al. 1996; Frank and Adler 2006). Despite these risks, endoscopic sphincterotomy is central to therapeutic ERCP practice and must be mastered by those endeavoring to become skilled in this specialty.

The significant cost of ERCP accessories – and dwindling reimbursement from third-party payers – requires that ERCP endoscopists choose their cannulation tool with care. Most choose a biliary sphincterotome (papillotome) with a preloaded guide wire as their "weapon" of choice. The majority of successful sphincterotomies require deep cannulation of the desired duct as a prelude. A large number of guide wires are available on the market. The previous "default" guide wire, 0.035″ in diameter, has been superseded by guide wires of 0.021″ and 0.025″ diameter. (The 0.018″ diameter wire is too flimsy for routine use in the biliary tree and pancreas). Once the duodenoscope is passed and the papilla is targeted in the so-called "short" (60 cm) position, the sphincterotome is passed through the working channel of the scope. The "elevator" should be kept maximally elevated to prevent free passage of the catheter into the lumen, risking inadvertent trauma to the wall of the duodenum. The sphincterotome can be safely advanced by lowering the elevator and cautiously pushing the tip a few centimeters into the duodenum. Advancing the tip of the catheter into the duodenal papilla for selective cannulation is achieved by a combination of small movements employing torque of the shaft of the endoscope from the control section, up-down and lateral deviation of the scope tip, insertion and withdrawal of the endoscope shaft, manipulation of the elevator "bridge" and flexion/relaxation of the sphincterotome tip itself.

Table 1
Consensus grading of post-ERCP complications (Adapted from Cotton et al. 1991)

	Mild	*Moderate*	*Severe*
Bleeding	Clinical (not just endoscopic) evidence of bleeding, hemoglobin drop <3 g, and no need for transfusion	Transfusion (4 units or less), no angiographic intervention or surgery	Transfusion, 5 units or more, or intervention (angiographic or surgical)
Pancreatitis	Clinical pancreatitis, Amylase at least three times normal at more than 24 h after the procedure, requiring admission or prolongation of planned admission to 2–3 days	Hospitalization of 4–10 days	Hospitalization of more than 10 days, hemorrhagic pancreatitis, phlegmon or pseudocyst, or intervention (Drainage or surgery)

The sphincterotome should be inserted at an upward angle with a slight deviation towards the 11 o'clock position to facilitate preferential cannulation of the common bile duct. Successful cannulation is confirmed by fluoroscopy, or, in the case of the bile duct, by aspiration of bile-stained fluid.

After successful cannulation, the decision to perform sphincterotomy is determined by a combination of preprocedural and procedural factors, including endoscopic findings, laboratory data, prior cross-sectional imaging, and symptoms. To perform the cut, the sphincterotome wire should be positioned in the 11–1 o'clock position. Mild flexion of the cutting wire, controlled from the device handle, brings it into contact with the mucosal surface (Fig. 1). Individual cutting technique varies greatly. The senior author (JB) starts with pure cutting current to perform the first 5 mm or so of the sphincterotomy. This is done in the belief that this reduces the risk of post-ERCP pancreatitis by keeping coagulating current away from the pancreatic duct orifice. Thereafter, the cut is extended using blended cutting and coagulation current to reduce bleeding. Many ERCP endoscopists now use the ERBE™ generator (ERBE USA Marietta, GA) for this purpose; it employs feedback to regulate current density throughout the cut, greatly reducing the risk of an uncontrolled incision (the so-called "zipper" cut) (Slivka et al. 2003). If pure current is used for the entire incision, bleeding is more likely, as susceptible blood vessels are not coagulated as they are cut. The authors recommend that "pure coagulation" current should never be used for endoscopic sphincterotomy, given its association with post-ERCP pancreatitis. In general, the data point to the superiority of "pure cut" and "two-staged cut" for avoiding pancreatitis; however, published studies are mixed (Norton et al. 2005; Macintosh et al. 2004; Gorelick et al. 2001; Elta et al. 1998). Fortunately, pancreatic stenting has been proven to be effective in preventing severe post-ERCP pancreatitis in high-risk settings, such as precut papillotomy and sphincterotomy for sphincter of Oddi dysfunction (SOD) (Fazel et al. 2003; Freeman 2007).

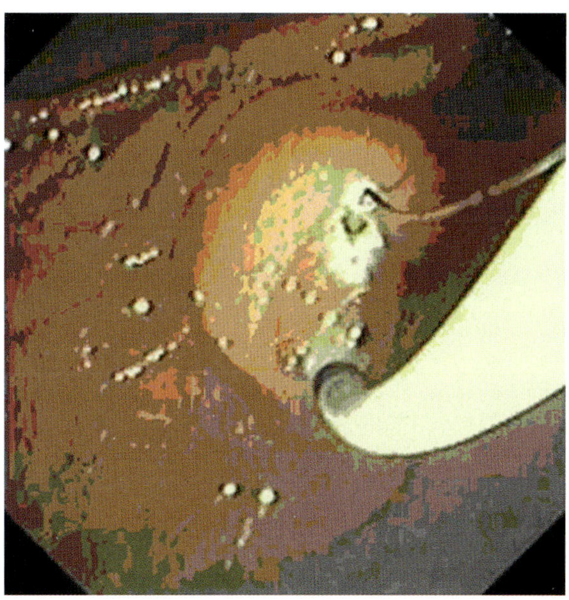

Fig. 1. An endoscopic view of biliary sphincterotomy with a standard "pull" sphincterotome (Mini-DASH™, Cook, Inc., Winston-Salem, NC).

If post-sphincterotomy bleeding occurs and does not stop spontaneously – e.g., lasting longer than 5 min – epinephrine injection (0.5–4 cc of a 1:10,000 concentration), heater probe cautery, endoscopic clip (Hemoclip^{Tm}) placement, or dilute epinephrine solution washes can be employed to induce hemostasis (Lin et al. 2004; Kuran et al. 2006; Wilcox et al. 2004).As with the initial cut, unintended spread of heat applied to the sphincterotomy site to treat bleeding may increase the risk of post-ERCP pancreatitis, and is best avoided until other, nonthermal, approaches have been exhausted.

"Precutting" the biliary sphincter can simplify a difficult cannulation, but it is not an acceptable alternative to competent cannulation technique. Several studies – albeit small ones – have indicated that precutting is safe and effective in expert hands (Laohavichitra et al. 2007; Deng et al. 2007; Bruins Slot et al. 1996; Kahaleh et al. 2004). Most experts do not need to use precut papillotomy on a routine basis. Inexperienced endoscopists are often tempted to use precutting to shorten the procedure, especially when repeated attempts to cannulate in the standard fashion have failed. The consequences of a "botched" precut can include catastrophic bleeding and retroperitoneal or free peritoneal perforation. Safe precut papillotomy requires supervised training by an experienced ERCP endoscopist.

BILE DUCT STENTING

It is often desirable to leave a plastic or metal mesh stent in the bile duct or pancreatic duct during therapeutic ERCP (Fig. 2). Indications include decompression of benign and malignant tumors, maintaining ductal drainage after stone removal, treating a biliary leak, following endoscopic ampullectomy, etc.

Successful duct cannulation precedes the placement of any stent. Typically, biliary and pancreatic stents are placed over a guide wire, although in certain situations they can be placed without one. The guide wire should be advanced deep into the duct, carefully avoiding trauma to small side branches in the pancreas and the tertiary intrahepatic bile ducts within the liver. Placement is greatly assisted by fluoroscopy, although stents can be placed without it. Knowing that the duodenoscope is 9 mm in diameter, the dimensions of the bile

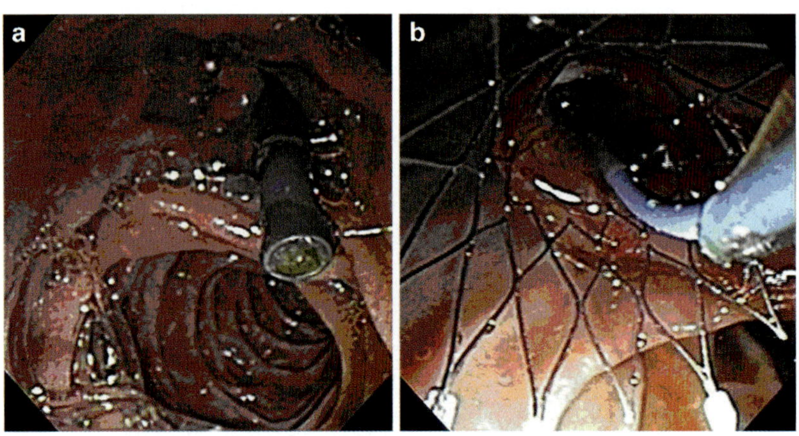

Fig. 2 Endoscopic views of (**a**) Plastic biliary stent (CLSO™ biliary stent, Cook, Inc, Winston-Salem, NC); (**b**) Uncoated metal mesh biliary stent (Flexxus™, ConMed, Billerica, MA) for pancreatic adenocarcinoma.

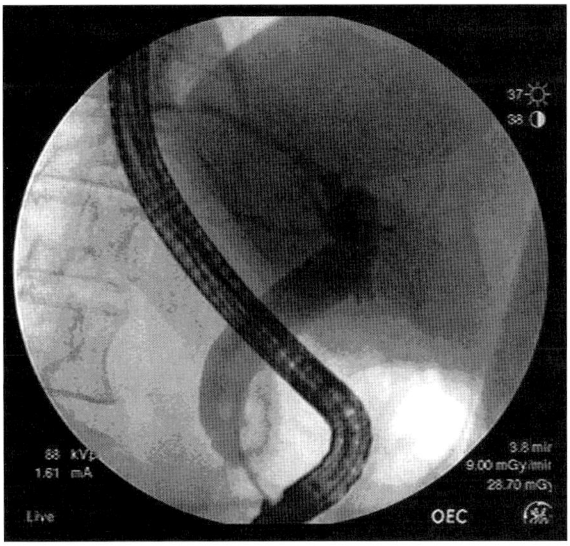

Fig. 3. Fluoroscopic ERCP image of a dilated common bile duct secondary to papillary stenosis. Note that the width of the bile duct approximates that of the duodenoscope (9 mm).

duct and pancreatic duct can be estimated during fluoroscopy (Fig. 3). Due to their ease of removal and the lack of interference with subsequent surgical fields, plastic (usually polyethylene) biliary stents are by far the most frequently used. 10 Fr and larger biliary stents are deployed over a 6 Fr "inner catheter" inserted over a guide wire, with the assistance of a slightly larger diameter "pushing" catheter. Flanges on the proximal and distal ends of the stent prevent undesired migration.

The standard biliary stent has flaps, top and bottom, cut from the plastic to prevent migration. There are side holes at the level of these flaps, which increase sites for drainage. However, these openings are also the site of turbulent flow, and have been shown to be niduses for sludge accumulation and eventual stent occlusion (Coene et al. 1990). A plastic stent without side holes and multiple flaps top and bottom (Tannenbaum™ stent, Cook, Inc, Winston-Salem, NC.) was initially reported to have extended patency over standard plastic stents, but this was later shown not to be the case (Terruzzi et al. 2000).

Plastic stents clog periodically, requiring replacement if time, surgery, or medical intervention has not addressed the initial indication for placement. If a more durable solution is desirable, then a metallic mesh stent might be preferable. These stents typically deploy to a diameter of around 10 mm, and come in varying lengths. They can be coated or uncoated. A coated metal mesh stent has a covering of an expandable plastic that prevents ingrowth of tissue through the interstices. This tissue could be normal biliary epithelium ("epithelialization") or tumor. Ingrowth of tumor can – and often does – occlude uncoated metallic stents. However, even coated stents can occlude due to tumor overgrowing the ends, which are left uncoated. A metal mesh stent can complicate biliary and pancreatic surgery. However, if a lesion is inoperable or the patient is a poor surgical candidate, a self-expanding metal mesh stent generally provides superior palliation compared to plastic. Metal mesh stents cost at least 10- and sometimes 20-times more than plastic ones, so cost-benefit has to be considered whenever they are placed. Several studies have suggested that is it not cost-effective to place a metallic stent if the patient's expected survival is less than 2 months (Kaassis et al. 2003; Prat et al. 1998).

Self-expanding metal mesh stents are generally placed over a guide wire and should be used with care in small diameter intrahepatic bile ducts, as they require "room" to deploy. They are also prone to kinking in severely angulated strictures. The choice of metal stent tends to be a personal one for the endoscopist. In terms of cost, available biliary metal mesh stents are in a similar price range. However, they each have somewhat different deployment systems and physical characteristics. Early versions of biliary metal stents were prone to over-rapid deployment, often resulting in misplacement. They also tended to shorten as they expanded. Modern metal mesh stents tend not to shorten and have more controlled release mechanisms. It is possible to "recapture" some partially deployed metal stents for repositioning.

There is debate regarding the need for sphincterotomy prior to placing stents for malignant strictures. A moderately tight-fitting stent is desirable to resist unwanted migration. However, if the endoscopist perceives significant resistance to advancing a catheter through the stricture, a step dilator (e.g., Soehendra™ biliary dilator, Cook, Inc., Winston-Salem, NC) whose maximal diameter approximates the desired stent size (e.g., 10 Fr) can be passed initially. If the dilator goes through the stricture, it is likely that a stent of the same caliber will too. Alternatively, a small "access papillotomy" can be performed to reduce resistance at papillary level.

PANCREATIC DUCT SPHINCTEROTOMY AND STENTS

Therapeutic manipulation of the pancreatic duct is increasingly common. Often during attempted cannulation of the common bile duct, endoscopists will inadvertently access the pancreatic duct (PD) with the papillotome or guide wire. Instrumentation of the pancreatic duct, and even edema from manipulations in its vicinity, can lead to postprocedural pancreatitis (Freeman et al. 1996). Mounting data show that stenting of the pancreatic duct with short, 3–5 Fr gauge plastic stents after such manipulations significantly decreases the risk of pancreatitis (Fig. 4) (Fazel et al. 2003; Freeman 2007; Das et al. 2007; Saad et al. 2008). Although very thin (3 Fr), unflanged stents have been touted as best for this purpose, they are often difficult to position (requiring a 0.018″ guide wire) and may migrate out of the duct prematurely. We have found that short (e.g., 3 or 5 cm) single-pigtail, single-flanged, 5 Fr plastic pancreatic stents (e.g., Zimmon™ stent, Cook, Inc., Winston-Salem, NC) are easily placed, and the majority spontaneously pass out of the patient within 2 weeks, obviating the need for repeat endoscopy to retrieve them. Patients at particular risk for post-ERCP pancreatitis, including those undergoing ampullectomy, biliary or pancreatic sphincterotomy for sphincter of Oddi dysfunction (SOD), needle knife papillotomy, etc., have been shown to benefit most from prophylactic stenting, provided that the stent is placed early in the procedure (Frank and Adler 2006; Fazel et al. 2003). A pancreatic stent placed after a long procedure with extensive instrumentation is usually too little, too late.

At present, the standard, commercially available metal mesh stents should be considered permanent implants. Some can be removed, but usually with difficulty. After uncoated stents have been in place for some time, they often become tightly bound to the wall of the duct by epithelialization or tumor ingrowth. Until truly removable metal stents become widely available, they should not be used to treat benign biliary or pancreatic strictures. A group of investigators from Indiana (USA) has reported their experience of using metal

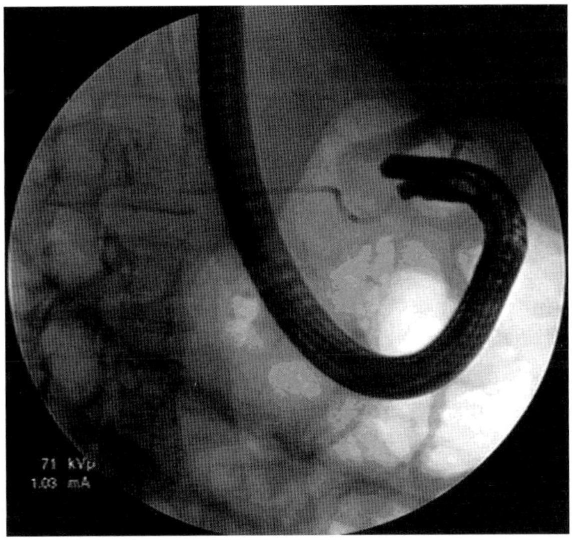

Fig. 4. A fluoroscopic image of a 5 Fr "pigtail" plastic stent being placed in an already-opacified pancreatic duct.

mesh stents in selected patients with pancreatitis in the setting of pancreas divisum to prepare them for surgical drainage (Madura et al. 2003). The metal stent expands the dorsal pancreatic duct over time until its diameter increases to a size suitable for side-to-side surgical anastomosis with a small bowel loop. This procedure remains experimental, and cannot be recommended for routine use in benign pancreatic disease.

CYSTGASTROSTOMY

The drainage of mature pseudocysts has emerged as a useful indication for the use of pancreatobiliary stents. Multiple small studies indicate that endoscopic cystgastrostomy/-enterostomy is a relatively safe and effective approach for symptom relief (Cahen et al. 2005; Cremer et al. 1989).

The "rules" guiding the management of pancreatic pseudocysts have been relaxed over the last decade. Previously, it was taught that any pseudocyst of ≥6 cm in diameter, or which had been present for more than 6 weeks, required drainage. A number of studies have shown that the majority of pseudocysts resolve without intervention although this can take up to 1 year or more (Terruzzi et al. 2000). Pancreatic pseudocysts that are symptomatic or considered to be infected require drainage. Endoscopic drainage of pseudocysts avoids the need for surgery, and is less likely to infect the cyst than percutaneous drainage. Endotherapy also eliminates the need for cumbersome external drains.

Although the procedure requires experienced hands, endoscopic cystgastrostomy or -enterostomy in the appropriate setting should be relatively straightforward. A good candidate for this type of drainage has a homogeneous fluid collection abutting the stomach or duodenum, within a cavity whose lining is not >1 cm in thickness and devoid of varices or other vascular structures. The success of the procedure is dependent on a solid "weld" between the pseudocyst and adjacent stomach or small bowel caused by inflammation.

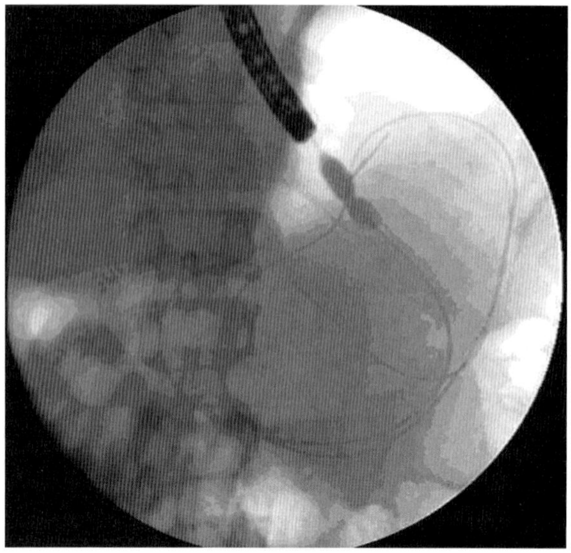

Fig. 5. A fluoroscopic image taken during a cystgastrostomy procedure, demonstrating balloon dilation of the track created through the stomach wall into the pseudocyst. A guide wire is coiled within the pseudocyst to maintain access.

This bond between structures minimizes the risk of free perforation during the procedure. Endoscopic ultrasound (EUS) is not mandatory for all such procedures; however, when available, EUS adds significantly to the accuracy and safety of the cystgastrostomy or -enterostomy (Antillon et al. 2006; Kahaleh et al. 2006). The EUS endoscopist can mark a favorable site for the ERCP endoscopist, or perform the entire procedure himself or herself under "real-time" EUS guidance. Once the transmural puncture is made with a needle knife or EUS aspiration needle, a guide wire is passed into the cyst. The track is then dilated using a balloon dilator, as extension of the opening by electrocautery risks bleeding, which is sometimes catastrophic (Fig. 5). Ideally, two 10 Fr, double-pigtail stents are then placed across the cystgastrostomy or -enterostomy fistula to ensure adequate drainage (Fig. 6). These stents are typically removed after 4–6 weeks. Failure (0–18% of cases) of the pseudocyst to resolve with this treatment may be due to the use of small caliber stents, spontaneous migration or misplacement of stents, unrecognized loculation within the cavity, or failure to separately address pancreatic ductal obstruction or communicating fistula (Cahen et al. 2005; Antillon et al. 2006; Kahaleh et al. 2006; Ahlawat et al. 2006; Baron et al. 2002; Giovannini et al. 2001; Kruger et al. 2006; Lopes et al. 2007; Lopes et al. 2008; Norton et al. 2001; Seewald et al. 2006; Voermans et al. 2007). After failure of endoscopic cystogastrostomy to resolve a pseudocyst, the treatment can sometimes repeat with success. If not, surgery or percutaneous drainage are alternatives (Nealon and Walser 2005; Aghdassi et al. 2006). Percutaneous drainage has a high success rate, but comes at the "price" of potentially infecting the pseudocyst. It is the preferred approach when dealing with a very sick patient due to an infected pseudocyst, when rapid access for decompression is the priority. Common complications of endoscopic drainage other than failure

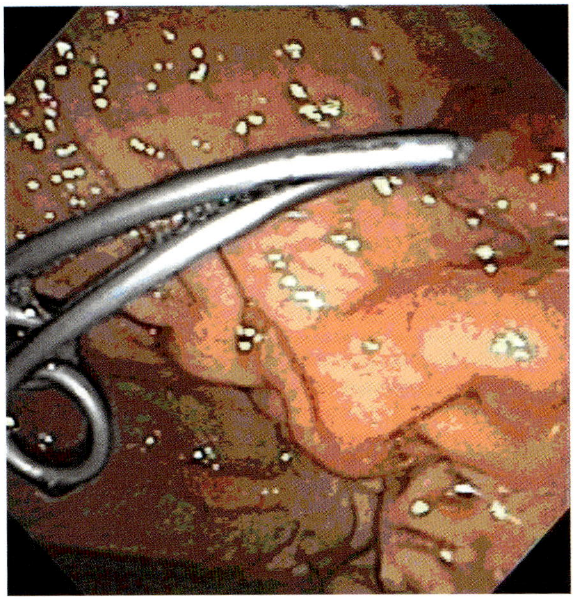

Fig. 6. An endoscopic view of two pig tail stents draining a pancreatic pseudocyst into the gastric lumen.

include bleeding, perforation, and infection. These can often be managed conservatively, but surgery or interventional radiology may be needed to address persistent sepsis and recurrent bleeding (Brandon et al. 2008).

SUMMARY OF KEY POINTS

- Endoscopic sphincterotomy is central to therapeutic ERCP practice and must be mastered by those endeavoring to become skilled in this specialty.
- Pancreatic stenting has been proven to be effective in preventing severe post-ERCP pancreatitis in high-risk settings, such as precut papillotomy and sphincterotomy for sphincter of Oddi dysfunction (SOD).
- "Pure coagulation" current should never be used for endoscopic sphincterotomy, given its association with post-ERCP pancreatitis.
- It is often desirable to leave a plastic or metal mesh stent in the bile duct or pancreatic duct during therapeutic ERCP.
- Plastic stents clog periodically, requiring replacement if time, surgery, or medical intervention has not addressed the initial indication for placement.
- It is not cost-effective to place a metallic stent if the patient's expected survival is less than 2 months.
- Endoscopic cystgastrostomy/-enterostomy is a relatively safe and effective approach for symptom relief.
- EUS adds significantly to the accuracy and safety of the cystgastrostomy or -enterostomy.
- Ideally, two 10 Fr, double-pigtail stents are then placed across the cystgastrostomy or -enterostomy fistula to ensure adequate drainage (Fig. 6). These stents are typically removed after 4–6 weeks.

REFERENCES

Aghdassi AA, Mayerle J, Kraft M, Sielenkamper AW, Heidecke CD, Lerch MM. Pancreatic pseudocysts - when and how to treat? HPB (Oxford). 2006;8(6):432–41.

Ahlawat SK, Charabaty-Pishvaian A, Jackson PG, Haddad NG. Single-step EUS-guided pancreatic pseudocyst drainage using a large channel linear array echoendoscope and cystotome: results in 11 patients. JOP. 2006;7(6):616–24.

Antillon MR, Shah RJ, Stiegmann G, Chen YK. Single-step EUS-guided transmural drainage of simple and complicated pancreatic pseudocysts. Gastrointest Endosc. May 2006;63(6):797–803.

Baron TH, Harewood GC, Morgan DE, Yates MR. Outcome differences after endoscopic drainage of pancreatic necrosis, acute pancreatic pseudocysts, and chronic pancreatic pseudocysts. Gastrointest Endosc. July 2002;56(1):7–17.

Brandon JL, Ruden NM, Turba UC, Bozlar U, Yeaton P, Hagspiel KD. Angiographic embolization of arterial hemorrhage following endoscopic US-guided cystogastrostomy for pancreatic pseudocyst drainage. Diagn Interv Radiol. Mar 2008;14(1):57–60.

Bruins Slot W, Schoeman MN, Disario JA, Wolters F, Tytgat GN, Huibregtse K. Needle-knife sphincterotomy as a precut procedure: a retrospective evaluation of efficacy and complications. Endoscopy. May 1996;28(4):334–9.

Cahen D, Rauws E, Fockens P, Weverling G, Huibregtse K, Bruno M. Endoscopic drainage of pancreatic pseudocysts: long-term outcome and procedural factors associated with safe and successful treatment. Endoscopy. Oct 2005;37(10):977–83.

Coene PP, Groen AK, Cheng J, Out MM, Tytgat GN, Huibregtse K. Clogging of biliary endoprostheses: a new perspective. Gut. Aug 1990;31(8):913–7.

Cotton PB, Lehman G, Vennes J, et al. Endoscopic sphincterotomy complications and their management: an attempt at consensus. Gastrointest Endosc. May–June 1991;37(3):383–93.

Cremer M, Deviere J, Engelholm L. Endoscopic management of cysts and pseudocysts in chronic pancreatitis: long-term follow-up after 7 years of experience. Gastrointest Endosc. Jan-Feb 1989;35(1):1–9.

Das A, Singh P, Sivak Jr MV, Chak A. Pancreatic-stent placement for prevention of post-ERCP pancreatitis: a cost-effectiveness analysis. Gastrointest Endosc. June 2007;65(7):960–8.

Deng DH, Zuo HM, Wang JF, et al. New precut sphincterotomy for endoscopic retrograde cholangiopancreatography in difficult biliary duct cannulation. World J Gastroenterol. Aug 28 2007;13(32):4385–90.

Elta GH, Barnett JL, Wille RT, Brown KA, Chey WD, Scheiman JM. Pure cut electrocautery current for sphincterotomy causes less post-procedure pancreatitis than blended current. Gastrointest Endosc. Feb 1998;47(2):149–53.

Farman J, Brunetti J, Baer JW, et al. AIDS-related cholangiopancreatographic changes. Abdom Imaging. Sept–Oct 1994;19(5):417–22.

Fazel A, Quadri A, Catalano MF, Meyerson SM, Geenen JE. Does a pancreatic duct stent prevent post-ERCP pancreatitis? A prospective randomized study. Gastrointest Endosc. Mar 2003;57(3):291–4.

Frank CD, Adler DG. Post-ERCP pancreatitis and its prevention. Nat Clin Pract Gastroenterol Hepatol. Dec 2006;3(12):680–8.

Freeman ML. Pancreatic stents for prevention of post-endoscopic retrograde cholangiopancreatography pancreatitis. Clin Gastroenterol Hepatol. Nov 2007;5(11):1354–65.

Freeman ML, Nelson DB, Sherman S, et al. Complications of endoscopic biliary sphincterotomy. N Engl J Med. Sept 26, 1996;335(13):909–18.

Giovannini M, Pesenti C, Rolland AL, Moutardier V, Delpero JR. Endoscopic ultrasound-guided drainage of pancreatic pseudocysts or pancreatic abscesses using a therapeutic echo endoscope. Endoscopy. June 2001;33(6):473–7.

Gorelick A, Cannon M, Barnett J, Chey W, Scheiman J, Elta G. First cut, then blend: an electrocautery technique affecting bleeding at sphincterotomy. Endoscopy. Nov 2001;33(11):976–80.

Kaassis M, Boyer J, Dumas R, et al. Plastic or metal stents for malignant stricture of the common bile duct? Results of a randomized prospective study. Gastrointest Endosc. Feb 2003;57(2):178–82.

Kahaleh M, Shami VM, Conaway MR, et al. Endoscopic ultrasound drainage of pancreatic pseudocyst: a prospective comparison with conventional endoscopic drainage. Endoscopy. Apr 2006;38(4):355–9.

Kahaleh M, Tokar J, Mullick T, Bickston SJ, Yeaton P. Prospective evaluation of pancreatic sphincterotomy as a precut technique for biliary cannulation. Clin Gastroenterol Hepatol. Nov 2004;2(11):971–7.

Kruger M, Schneider AS, Manns MP, Meier PN. Endoscopic management of pancreatic pseudocysts or abscesses after an EUS-guided 1-step procedure for initial access. Gastrointest Endosc. Mar 2006;63(3):409–16.

Kuran S, Parlak E, Oguz D, Cicek B, Disibeyaz S, Sahin B. Endoscopic sphincterotomy-induced hemorrhage: treatment with heat probe. Gastrointest Endosc. Mar 2006;63(3):506–11.

Laohavichitra K, Akaraviputh T, Methasate A, Leelakusolvong S, Kachintorn U. Comparison of early pre-cutting vs standard technique for biliary cannulation in endoscopic retrograde cholangiopancreatography: a personal experience. World J Gastroenterol. July 21, 2007;13(27):3734–7.

Lin LF, Siauw CP, Ho KS, Tung JN. Hemoclip treatment for post-endoscopic sphincterotomy bleeding. J Chin Med Assoc. Oct 2004;67(10):496–9.

Lopes CV, Pesenti C, Bories E, Caillol F, Giovannini M. Endoscopic-ultrasound-guided endoscopic transmural drainage of pancreatic pseudocysts and abscesses. Scand J Gastroenterol. Apr 2007;42(4):524–9.

Lopes CV, Pesenti C, Bories E, Caillol F, Giovannini M. Endoscopic ultrasound-guided endoscopic transmural drainage of pancreatic pseudocysts. Arq Gastroenterol. Jan-Mar 2008;45(1):17–21.

Macintosh DG, Love J, Abraham NS. Endoscopic sphincterotomy by using pure-cut electrosurgical current and the risk of post-ERCP pancreatitis: a prospective randomized trial. Gastrointest Endosc. Oct 2004;60(4):551–6.

Madura JA, Canal DF, Lehman GA. Wall stent-enhanced lateral pancreaticojejunostomy for small-duct pancreatitis. Arch Surg. June 2003;138(6):644–9. discussion 649–650.

Nealon WH, Walser E. Surgical management of complications associated with percutaneous and/or endoscopic management of pseudocyst of the pancreas. Ann Surg. June 2005;241(6):948–57. discussion 957–960.

Norton ID, Clain JE, Wiersema MJ, DiMagno EP, Petersen BT, Gostout CJ. Utility of endoscopic ultrasonography in endoscopic drainage of pancreatic pseudocysts in selected patients. Mayo Clin Proc. Aug 2001;76(8):794–8.

Norton ID, Petersen BT, Bosco J, et al. A randomized trial of endoscopic biliary sphincterotomy using pure-cut versus combined cut and coagulation waveforms. Clin Gastroenterol Hepatol. Oct 2005;3(10):1029–33.

Prat F, Chapat O, Ducot B, et al. A randomized trial of endoscopic drainage methods for inoperable malignant strictures of the common bile duct. Gastrointest Endosc. Jan 1998;47(1):1–7.

Saad AM, Fogel EL, McHenry L, et al. Pancreatic duct stent placement prevents post-ERCP pancreatitis in patients with suspected sphincter of Oddi dysfunction but normal manometry results. Gastrointest Endosc. Feb 2008;67(2):255–61.

Seewald S, Thonke F, Ang TL, et al. One-step, simultaneous double-wire technique facilitates pancreatic pseudocyst and abscess drainage (with videos). Gastrointest Endosc. Nov 2006;64(5):805–8.

Slivka A, Bosco JJ, Barkun AN, et al. Electrosurgical generators: MAY 2003. Gastrointest Endosc. Nov 2003;58(5):656–60.

Terruzzi V, Comin U, De Grazia F, et al. Prospective randomized trial comparing Tannenbaum Teflon and standard polyethylene stents in distal malignant biliary stenosis. Gastrointest Endosc. Jan 2000;51(1):23–7.

Vandervoort J, Soetikno RM, Tham TC, et al. Risk factors for complications after performance of ERCP. Gastrointest Endosc. Nov 2002;56(5):652–6.

Voermans RP, Veldkamp MC, Rauws EA, Bruno MJ, Fockens P. Endoscopic transmural debridement of symptomatic organized pancreatic necrosis (with videos). Gastrointest Endosc. Nov 2007;66(5):909–16.

Wilcox CM, Canakis J, Monkemuller KE, Bondora AW, Geels W. Patterns of bleeding after endoscopic sphincterotomy, the subsequent risk of bleeding, and the role of epinephrine injection. Am J Gastroenterol. Feb 2004;99(2):244–8.

12 The Use of SpyGlass Direct Visualization System in the Management of Pancreato Biliary Disease

Joel R. Judah and Peter V. Draganov

Contents

Keywords: SpyGlass, Direct, Visualization, System, Management, Pancreato, Biliary, Disease

INTRODUCTION

Intraductal endoscopy consists of the use of an endoscope to directly visualize the pancreato-biliary ductal systems. Visual inspection of the biliary tree is called cholangioscopy, and that of the pancreatic duct is termed pancreatoscopy. There have been significant technological challenges encountered in creating an endoscope that allows direct examination of these ducts. However, the recently developed SpyGlass direct visualization system (Boston Scientific Corporation, Natick, Massachusetts, USA) provides technology that promises greater opportunity to improve diagnosis and therapy.

Cholangioscopy was conceived as early as the 1950s (Roca et al. 1951). However, technology at that time caused severe limitations. Intraoperative cholangioscopy was first successfully utilized in the 1960s (Allegaert 1961; Deister 1963; Häberlin 1966). Peroral cholangioscopy was initially described in the mid-1970s. One of the first reports demonstrated that a fiberscope

From: *Clinical Gastroenterology: Diagnostic and Therapeutic Procedures in Gastroenterology*,
Edited by: G. Y. Wu, S. Sridhar, DOI 10.1007/978-1-59745-044-7_12,

8.8 mm diameter could be directly inserted through the mouth, into the biliary system after an endoscopic papillotomy, without the need of using a second scope as a guide (Urakami et al. 1977). This scope did provide a biopsy channel to obtain tissue samples. Other investigators also successfully demonstrated the use of peroral cholangioscopy to directly visualize the biliary system during this time (Nakajima et al. 1976a, b; 1978; Rösch et al. 1976; Popiela et al. 1978). The idea of guiding a small caliber "baby" cholangioscope through the channel of a "mother" duodenoscope into the common bile duct (CBD) gained acceptance (Urakami 1980; Bogardus et al. 1996; Ponsky et al. 1990). This "mother-baby" system is also known as duodenoscope-assisted cholangiopancreatoscopy. For years the "mother-baby" system was the most commonly used technology for cholangioscopy. However, use of this "mother-baby" system was difficult since optical fibers were prone to break easily and the "baby" scope had limited two-way tip deflection. Further, the procedure was time consuming, and two endoscopists were required. Multiple other small scopes have been developed in an attempt to directly visualize the biliary tree and pancreatic duct (Kozarek 1988a, 1995; Foerster et al. 1988; Bourke and Haber 1996; Neuhaus and Schumacher 1999; Soda et al. 1996; Technology Status Evaluation Report 1999; Sander and Poesl 1996; Kodama et al. 1999, 2004). An advantage of several of these scopes is that they could be advanced through a regular therapeutic duodenoscope.

Within the past few years, the SpyGlass direct visualization system has been introduced and marks a significant step forward in the ability of gastroenterologists to directly image the biliary tree and pancreatic duct (Chen 2007; Chen and Pleskow 2007). This system makes use of a reusable optical probe, a disposable access and delivery catheter (SpyScope), and disposable biopsy forceps (SpyBite). The outer diameter of the SpyScope is only 10 F.

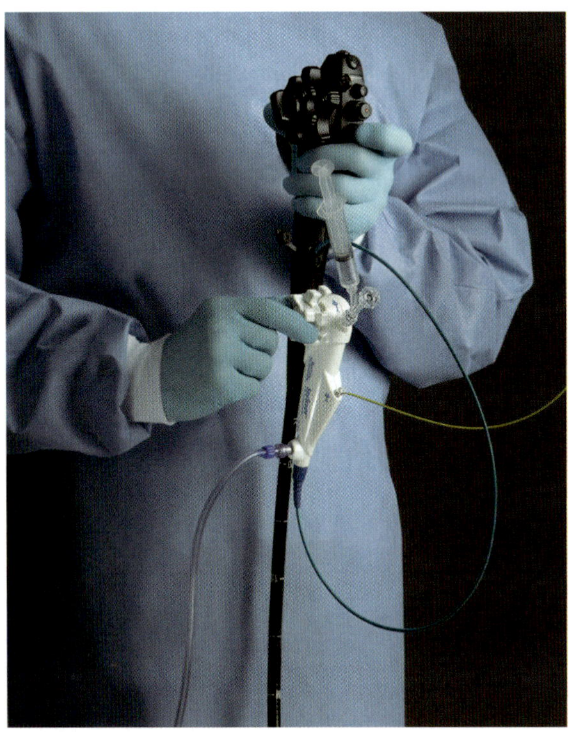

Fig. 1. SpyScope mounted to a duodenoscope.

This system offers several advantages over previous cholangioscopes. It allows for single-operator control of both the duodenoscope and the SpyScope because the SpyScope catheter is mounted on the duodenoscope by a silastic belt (Fig. 1). The endoscopist can sequentially manipulate the controls of both the duodenoscope and the SpyScope with one hand; thus, the need for two endoscopists is eliminated. This system also uses four-way tip deflection (up, down, left, and right), which allows for improved access. Further, the SpyScope incorporates two smaller dedicated irrigation channels that are separate from the 1.2 mm working channel, which allows for sustained continuous irrigation regardless of whether the working channel is in use. The working channel enables utilization of a variety of devices (i.e., guidewire, SpyBite Biopsy Forceps, laser or electrohydraulic lithotripsy probes) for diagnostic and therapeutic applications. These advances have allowed this system to be used clinically in an increasing number of endoscopy centers.

PROCEDURE DESCRIPTION

The procedure is always done in conjunction with endoscopic retrograde cholangiopancreatography (ERCP). The patient is positioned prone on an x-ray table. Peri-procedural prophylactic antibiotics are administered if clinically indicated. If sphincterotomy is anticipated, it may be necessary to hold anti-coagulants prior to the procedure after consulting with the prescribing physician. In most cases, the procedure is done with the patient under deep sedation (midazolam/fentanyl), but monitored anesthesia or general anesthesia can be used if clinically indicated. A standard therapeutic duodenoscope (ERCP scope) is inserted through the mouth and passed to the ampulla of Vater. The duct of interest is cannulated with standard ERCP techniques. A sphincterotomy is recommended to allow better access to the desired ductal system as well as to allow for drainage of the duct during irrigation. The SpyScope cholangioscope is then advanced via the cannel of the duodenoscope and into the biliary or pancreatic ductal system to allow access for direct visualization and performance of procedures (Fig. 2). As mentioned above, the SpyGlass system is mounted on the

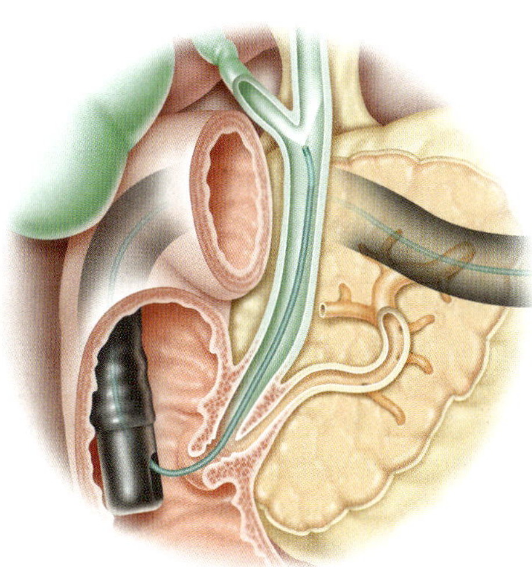

Fig. 2. Diagram of SpyScope advanced via the standard duodenoscope and then into the biliary tree.

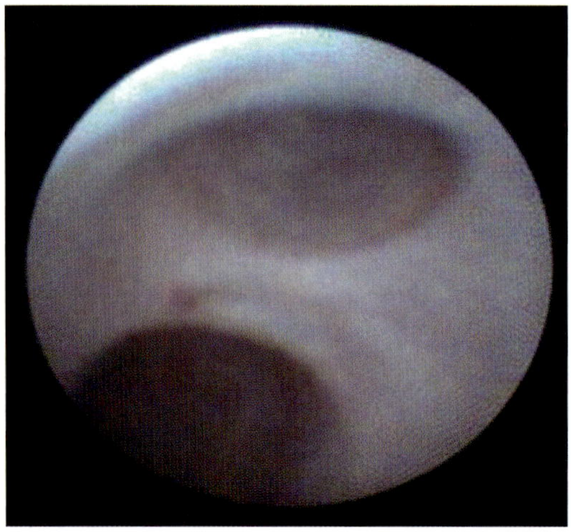

Fig. 3. Normal view of the biliary bifurcation.

duodenoscope in order to allow a single endoscopist to control both the SpyGlass system and the duodenoscope. After the SpyGlass system is introduced through the duodenoscope via the ampulla of Vater into the biliary or pancreatic ducts, these ducts are directly visualized during repeated advancement and withdrawal of the SpyScope using the four-way tip deflection (Fig. 3). It may be necessary to irrigate debris from the ducts in order to maintain adequate visualization. This is nicely facilitated by the SpyGlass independent irrigation channel. Diagnostic or therapeutic procedures, as discussed below, may be performed within the biliary tree or pancreatic duct by passing instruments through the working channel of the SpyGlass system.

INDICATIONS

Diagnostic Indications

Intraductal endoscopy, such as the SpyGlass system, may be used for multiple diagnostic indications (Table 1). Direct visualization of the ducts through various endoscopic methods has been found to increase the ability to differentiate and diagnose lesions more accurately in comparison with standard imaging and ERCP techniques. Direct visualization may provide new clinical information (Siddique et al. 1999). The visual image alone may offer information helpful in reaching a diagnosis, especially in terms of differentiating the type of biliary tumor (Seo et al. 2000; Kim et al. 2000). Intraductal endoscopy has been especially useful in differentiating an indeterminate stricture or evaluating a filling defect noted on ERCP. Direct visualization in some studies has been shown to improve diagnostic sensitivity of biliary lesions from 58% to 93% (Fukuda et al. 2005). Lesions which appear as fixed and immobile masses on cholangiogram can be shown to be bile duct stones at a glance, when directly viewed under cholangioscopy (Fig. 4).

Biliary strictures, with the exception of those clearly following surgery or trauma, are frequently of concern because of the possibility of malignancy. Obtaining adequate tissue from these biliary strictures, which can provide definitive diagnosis, is often challenging.

Table 1
Diagnostic uses of intraductal endoscopy

- Optically guided biopsies of stricture
  - Indeterminate stricture
  - Dominant stricture in primary sclerosing cholangitis
- Evaluate fixed filling defect noted on cholangiogram or other imaging
- Differentiate benign versus malignant intraductal mass
  - Optical examination yields visual clues
  - Improved yield from tissue sampling under visual guidance
- Precisely map intraductal cholangiocarcinoma prior to resection
- Collect significant fluid sample for cytology
- Visually evaluate intraductal papillary mucinous neoplasms
- Visually evaluate choledochal cyst
- Visually evaluate for post-liver transplant ductal ischemia
- Visually evaluate for intraductal spread of ampullary adenoma
- Evaluate with visual exam and tissue sampling for infection
  - Cytomegalovirus
  - Fungal infection

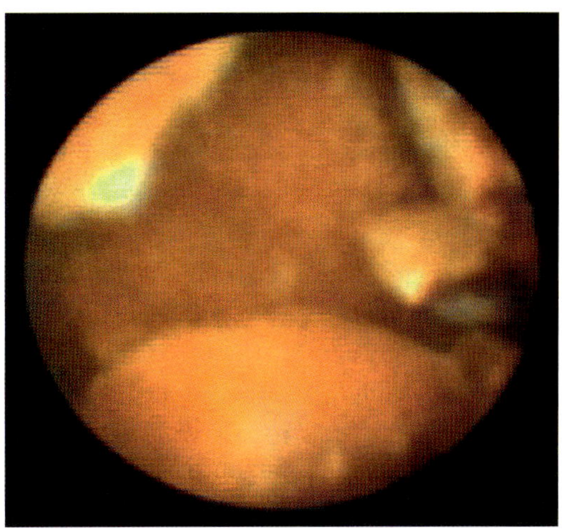

Fig. 4. Bile duct stone.

Traditionally, ERCP may be of assistance in characterizing the stricture by providing tissue sampling; however, the low yield rates of ERCP-based methods for securing the pathologic diagnosis of malignancy has been demonstrated in multiple studies. The diagnostic yield is low in the range of 35–70% (Desa et al. 1991; Foutch et al. 1991; Glasbrenner et al. 1999; Howell et al. 1996; Jailwala et al. 2000; Kurzawinski et al. 1993; Layfield et al. 1995; Lee et al. 1995; Ponchon et al. 1995; Pugliese et al. 1995; Sugiyama et al. 1996; Schoefl et al. 1997; Stewart et al. 2001). Studies using cholangioscopy techniques have

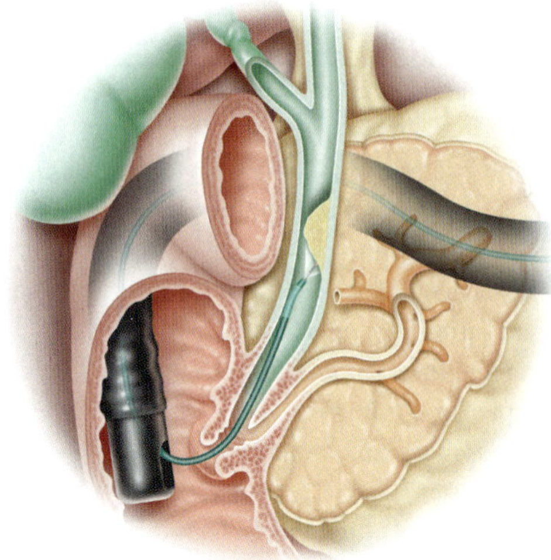

Fig. 5. SpyBite biopsy forceps used to obtain biopsy under direct visual guidance.

shown a significant increase in sensitivity and specificity when the biopsy sample is obtained under direct vision (Fig. 5). A 2006 report demonstrated biopsies obtained with the assistance of direct visualization yielded a sensitivity to detect malignancy of 89%, and specificity of 96% (Shah et al. 2006). The SpyGlass system utilized to provide optically guided biopsies demonstrated a sensitivity and specificity of 71% and 100%, respectively in evaluation of 20 patients with intraductal lesions (Chen and Pleskow 2007). In that study, the optically guided biopsies demonstrated greater success in obtaining sufficient tissue for adequate histologic evaluation, in that 95% of the biopsies yielded enough tissue for complete histologic evaluation. In two studies, utilization of SpyGlass guided biopsies has also been found to modify the pre-procedure diagnosis in a significant number of cases (Raijman et al. 2008; Loren et al. 2008). Most commonly, the diagnosis of a suspected malignant stricture was changed to a benign biliary stricture. When tumors were found within the biliary tree or pancreatic duct, precise mapping of the tumor in preparation for surgery was accomplished due to the ability to provide direct visualization (Somogyi et al. 2003). In patients with primary sclerosing cholangitis (PSC), direct visualization of dominant strictures with cholangioscopy has been found superior to ERCP in terms of detecting malignancy (Awadallah et al. 2006; Tischendorf et al. 2006).

Direct pancreatoscopy can also play a diagnostic role in differentiating pancreatic duct lesions (Tajiri et al. 1998). Pancreatoscopy can visualize chronic scarring and stenosis of the duct, pancreatic duct stones, and intraductal papillary-mucinous neoplasms (IPMNs) of the pancreas. Pancreatic juice collected during pancreatoscopy has been shown to provide a better yield for cytologic evaluation than traditional catheter collection (Uehara et al. 1997). Many other studies have shown the improved diagnostic benefits of pancreatoscopy, especially in regard to evaluating IPMNs (Kaneko et al. 1998; Kozarek 1988b; Fujita et al. 1990; Hara et al. 2002; Yamao et al. 2003; Kodama et al. 2002; Mukai et al. 1998; Yasuda et al. 2005). Recently, peroral pancreatoscopy has been combined with narrow-band imaging to emphasize certain image features often seen with IPMNs, such as mucosal structures and capillary vessels (Itoi et al. 2007).

Other diagnostic uses of intraductal endoscopy include the evaluation of choledochal cysts, (Kolodziejski et al. 2004; Scotiniotis and Kochman 2001; Huang et al. 1999) hemobilia of unknown etiology, (Kubota et al. 2000) infectious etiologies of bile duct pathology, such as cytomegalovirus (CMV) and fungal infections (Siddique et al. 1999; Prasad et al. 2005). Another proposed role for cholangioscopy is the evaluation of the biliary tree after liver transplantation. A recent report described the use of methylene blue–aided chromoendoscopy via cholangioscopy to diagnose extensive bile duct necrosis and inflammation consistent with ischemic-type biliary injury after liver transplant (Hoffman et al. 2007). Other diagnostic uses of cholangioscopy and SpyGlass in particular will become evident as better technology allows for greater use of this modality.

Therapeutic Indications

Intraductal endoscopy and the SpyGlass system are useful not only for diagnostic purposes, but they also have therapeutic applications (Table 2). Intraductal endoscopy has been frequently used to remove stones from within the ducts that cannot be removed by standard ERCP techniques, due to size, location, or adherence to biliary epithelium (Classen et al. 1988). Electrohydraulic lithotripsy (EHL) has been used in combination with cholangioscopy and pancreatoscopy in multiple reports. EHL employs the use of a bipolar electrode in an aqueous medium. The probe is placed near the surface of the stone (approximately 2–3 mm away) and directly observed using the cholangioscope. The probe emits spark discharges, which create a shock wave that fragments the stone (Wamsteker 2006). Binmoeller and colleagues reported that this technique was successful in removing stones where standard mechanical lithotripsy had failed in 64 of 65 patients (Binmoeller et al. 1993). Arya reported in 2004 on experience with 94 patients who underwent cholangioscopy combined with EHL (Arya et al. 2004). Of this group, 93 patients had failed previous standard stone extraction with ERCP. In this retrospective review, cholangioscopy combined with EHL was successful in performing stone fragmentation in 96% of cases, and stones were completely removed in 90% of cases. In both of these studies, there were no significant complications associated with the procedures. In elderly patients where biliary stone removal with traditional methods is unsuccessful, permanent biliary stenting has been attempted. However, Hui demonstrated in a prospective study of 36 high-risk patients with difficult CBD stones that cholangioscopy guided lithotripsy, when compared to insertion

Table 2
Therapeutic applications of intraductal endoscopy

- Stone extraction
  - Electrohydraulic lithotripsy (EHL)
  - Laser lithotripsy
- Argon plasma coagulation (APC)
- Photodynamic therapy
- Nd-YAG laser ablation
- Cystic duct stent placement
- Guidewire passage through strictures

of a biliary stent alone, allows for significantly less mortality and cholangitis (Hui et al. 2003). Another study reported a 100% success rate for removal of large bile duct stones after failure to remove the stone with a mechanical lithotriptor during ERCP (Farrell et al. 2005). In 2002, data from 36 patients who had strictly intrahepatic stones underwent cholangioscopy guided lithotripsy (Okugawa et al. 2002). Indeed, in these difficult cases, this form of therapy was successful in achieving complete stone removal in 64% of cases. In the initial feasibility study, the SpyGlass-directed EHL system allowed for successful biliary stone removal in five of five patients, although after the initial procedure two patients did require repeat SpyGlass-directed EHL, and one patient required repeat ERCP in order to achieve complete stone clearance (Chen and Pleskow 2007). Initial reports from an ongoing international multicenter study show that the SpyGlass system does indeed allow for safe and effective treatment of difficult-to-remove biliary stones with an overall success rate of 92% achieved in the 49 patients treated so far (Parsi et al. 2008). In a recent retrospective study, SpyGlass directed EHL was shown successful in removing pancreatic duct stones in four of five patients, although two patients did require repeat pancreatoscopy to remove residual stone material (Guda et al. 2008). The SpyGlass system has also successfully been utilized to perform peroral cholecystoscopy, in order to allow for treatment of symptomatic gallstones under direct visualization with EHL in patients with end-stage liver disease, where surgical risks were prohibitive (Chen et al. 2008a).

Standard surgical management has been difficult for patients with gallstones which erode into the common hepatic duct and form a cholecystobiliary fistula (i.e., Mirizzi syndrome types 2–4). In 25 patients (23 patients with Mirizzi syndrome type 1 and two with Mirizzi syndrome type 2), cholangioscopy combined with EHL allowed for successful treatment of the stone in all patients with type 2 Mirizzi syndrome, while it failed in both patients with type 1 Mirizzi syndrome (Tsuyuguchi et al. 2000). Thus, it was felt that cholangioscopy-guided therapy may offer a safe and effective alternative to surgery in patients with type 2 Mirizzi syndrome.

There are other therapeutic interventions which have been coupled with cholangioscopy, and as the SpyGlass technology matures it is likely that many of these techniques will be coupled with SpyGlass. Multiple reports describe the use of cholangioscopy along with laser lithotripsy (Bogardus et al. 1996; Jakobs et al. 1996; Adamek et al. 1996). Laser lithotripsy may be used under fluoroscopic or direct cholangioscopy guidance. Current evidence indicates that cholangioscopy-guided laser lithotripsy is especially preferred in cases of intrahepatic stones or in patients with stones situated proximal to a bile duct stenosis (Jakobs et al. 2007). Photodynamic therapy under peroral cholangioscopic guidance has also been utilized for patients with biliary tumors. In 1998, Ortner reported on the use of photodynamic therapy under cholangioscopic guidance to treat non-resectable Bismuth type III and IV cholangiocarcinoma (Ortner et al. 1998). In this study, therapy was successful at restoring biliary drainage, improving mortality and enhancing quality of life. In 2003, Ortner reported results of a randomized trial of cholangioscopically guided photodynamic therapy with stenting versus stenting only for non-resectable cholangiocarcinoma (Ortner et al. 2003). The improvement of survival in the group receiving photodynamic therapy was so impressive that it was considered unethical to continue with randomization after the first 39 patients. Specifically, the photodynamic therapy group had median survival to 493 days, while the stenting-only group had median survival to 98 days ($p<0.0001$). Treatment with photodynamic therapy and stenting also led to improvement of cholestasis and quality of life compared with endoscopic stenting alone. Nd-YAG laser ablation of tumor stent ingrowth and biliary angiodysplastic lesions has been also been performed in concert with cholangioscopy (Siddique et al. 1999). Most recently, a case report documented the use of the SpyGlass system in a post-transplant anastomotic stricture which could not be cannulated with a guidewire using traditional ERCP technique (Wright et al. 2008). However, the SpyGlass system allowed visualization of the stricture and facilitated easy passage of a guidewire across the stricture so it could be dilated and stented.

CONTRAINDICATIONS

The contraindications of performing intraductal endoscopy with the SpyGlass system (Table 3) include any contraindication for endoscopy in general, such as a medical status that would make the patient a poor procedural candidate. Any contraindication for ERCP would also serve as a contraindication for intraductal endoscopy. The patient must be able to tolerate sedation for the procedure. The ampulla of Vater must be accessible to the duodenoscope; therefore, in cases of proximal duodenal stricture or in patients with previous surgery (i.e., Roux-en-Y) peroral intraductal endoscopy may not be possible. Other contraindications would include recent acute pancreatitis not related to gallstones, inadequate surgical back-up, and unacceptable ranges of anticoagulation predisposing to bleeding.

COMPLICATIONS AND SAFETY

There have been no large trials specifically addressing the safety of intraductal endoscopy or the SpyGlass system. Most information regarding safety and complications comes from individual case series, often with small numbers of patients enrolled. However, intraductal endoscopy is generally believed to be a safe procedure with relatively few complications. Complications typically include minor bleeding at the time of sphincterotomy (performed to allow the scope to access the ductal systems) or lithotripsy (Tsuyuguchi et al. 2000). There was one report of bile duct perforation following cholangioscopy guided EHL in 1993 (Binmoeller et al. 1993). Obviously, the incidence of cholangitis is increased in patients with incomplete biliary drainage, from causes such as a biliary stricture or residual biliary stones; however, cholangitis has not been reported as a direct cause cholangioscopy (Tsuyuguchi et al. 2000). Pancreatitis has been reported in 2 of 52 (3.8%) of pancreatoscopy cases (Tajiri et al. 1998). In the SpyGlass feasibility study, only two patients (6%) experienced procedure-related complications, namely ascending cholangitis in one patient and cholangitis with

Table 3
Contraindications for intraductal endoscopy

- Any contraindication for endoscopy in general or ERCP
- Inadequate access to the ampulla of Vater
- Recent acute pancreatitis not related to gallstones
- Inadequate surgical back-up
- Unacceptable ranges of anticoagulation predisposing to bleeding

intrahepatic abscess in the other patient (Chen and Pleskow 2007). Both patients recovered without sequelae. The largest experience to date is an ongoing multi-center trial to evaluate the safety and effectiveness of the SpyGlass system, which has enrolled 146 patients so far (Chen et al. 2008b). It has shown no deaths directly related to the system or procedure, and only 14 serious adverse events (most commonly cholangitis, bacteremia, or abdominal pain). Complication rates will be better defined as more intraductal endoscopic procedures are performed and further prospective data is collected.

POST-PROCEDURE CARE

Intraductal endoscopy is typically performed in an outpatient setting. Unless complications occur during the procedure, the patient is expected to go home within a few hours after the procedure is completed. Post-procedure recovery is similar to that which follows any endoscopic procedure. The patient should receive monitoring of vital signs until awake. The patient should not have pain following the procedure. Thus, any pain should receive adequate evaluation to ensure there has been no perforation or post-procedure pancreatitis. Excessive insufflation may cause abdominal distension, but this discomfort should resolve when the patient passes flatus or belches. Patients should be given explicit verbal and written information following the procedure, including a 24-h contact number. A driver should accompany the patient, due to the use of intravenous sedation, and the patient should not drive or operate machinery for 24 h following the procedure. Patients usually may eat within 2 h following the procedure. The patient's medication regimen should not be altered unless sphincterotomy or other procedure with risk of bleeding has been performed, in which case it may be necessary to consider a delay in restarting the anticoagulant after consulting with the prescribing physician. Patients should call the provider for any fever, abdominal pain, persistent distension, rigors, bleeding, vomiting or other acute changes in their clinical condition.

COMPARATIVE PROCEDURES

There are two other methods which allow optical examination of the biliary ductal system. Percutaneous transhepatic cholangioscopy (PTCS), also known as percutaneous cholangioscopy, and laparoscopic choledochoscopy have both been used for diagnostic and therapeutic purposes. Percutaneous cholangioscopy is more invasive than peroral cholangioscopy. Once percutaneous access to the bile duct is achieved it allows excellent visualization, even in difficult anatomic situations where the peroral cholangioscopy technique has failed (Shim et al. 2003). Many of the same diagnostic and therapeutic techniques utilized with peroral cholangioscopy are also used with percutaneous cholangioscopy, including targeted biopsy and management of stones with lithotripsy. One unique use of percutaneous cholangioscopy was documented, where a push-type sphincterotome was used via PTCS to create a papillary sphincterotomy and allow drainage of obstructing biliary stones in three patients who each had an endoscopically inaccessible papilla (Itoi et al. 2004). There are no reports of percutaneous pancreatoscopy. There have been no significant randomized studies directly comparing percutaneous cholangioscopy versus peroral cholangioscopy. Generally, peroral cholangioscopy is preferred as the initial therapy, due to its less invasive nature.

Laparoscopic choledochoscopy has been utilized to explore the biliary tree. Frequently, this technique has been utilized at the time of laparoscopic cholecystectomy, when intra-operative cholangiogram shows concern for retained bile duct stones (Shuchleib et al. 1999). There are multiple surgical techniques which have been used to explore the bile duct, but choledochoscopy via the cystic duct appears to be the safest and most effective approach, with success rates of 90% (Lyass and Phillips 2006). A benefit of this procedure is that the papilla may be left intact without sphincterotomy (Dion et al. 1994). There is minimal experience using laparoscopic techniques to perform pancreatoscopy; however, reports do exist (Balalykin and Avaliani 1985).

COST

Early cholangioscopes cost upwards of $25,000 USD just for the scope. The processor and other equipment further increase this cost. This initial investment is compounded by the expense of repairs, due to instrument fragility. The complete capital equipment purchase for the SpyGlass direct visualization system costs around $59,000 USD; however, as previously mentioned, this system utilizes easily replaceable components, which limit the potential for repairs. Furthermore, a facility purchasing the SpyGlass system may choose to not purchase some of the items that may already by owned by the facility (i.e., monitor, irrigation pump), thus reducing the potential start-up cost. Patient costs and reimbursement vary greatly for intraductal endoscopy and depend on factors including geographic location and setting where the procedure is performed, what instrumentation (i.e., EHL, laser, etc.) is used during the case, and whether an anesthesiologist is required. Our anecdotal experience at the University of Florida shows that the reimbursements we receive make the SpyGlass system financially feasible.

SUMMARY OF KEY POINTS

- Experience with intraductal endoscopy has shown advantage over conventional ERCP with regard to the diagnosis and treatment of biliary and pancreatic disease.
- Direct optical examination may provide significant additional information about ductal lesions.
- The SpyGlass direct visualization system appears to be a substantial improvement over older technology.
- This system has shown significant promise and will likely see increasing utilization.

REFERENCES

Adamek HE, Maier M, Jakobs R, Wessbecher FR, Neuhauser T, Riemann JF. Management of retained bile duct stones: a prospective open trial comparing extracorporeal and intracorporeal lithotripsy. Gastrointest Endosc. 1996;44:40–7.

Allegaert W. Report concerning cholangioscopy, using closed-circuit television, during surgical operations on the biliary tract. Acta Gastroenterol Belg. 1961;24:599–606.

Arya N, Nelles SE, Haber GB, Kim YI, Kortan PK. Electrohydraulic lithotripsy in 111 patients: a safe and effective therapy for difficult bile duct stones. Am J Gastroenterol. 2004;99:2330–4.

Awadallah NS, Chen YK, Piraka C, Antillon MR, Shah RJ. Is there a role for cholangioscopy in patients with primary sclerosing cholangitis? Am J Gastroenterol. 2006;101:284–91.

Balalykin AS, Avaliani MV. Laparoscopic pancreatoscopy. Vestn Khir Im I I Grek. 1985;135:132–6.

Binmoeller KF, Brückner M, Thonke F, Soehendra N. Treatment of difficult bile duct stones using mechanical, electrohydraulic and extracorporeal shock wave lithotripsy. Endoscopy. 1993;25:201–6.
Bogardus ST, Hanan I, Ruchim M, Goldberg MJ. "Mother-baby" biliary endoscopy: the University of Chicago experience. Am J Gastroenterol. 1996;91:105–10.
Bourke MJ, Haber GB. Transpapillary choledochoscopy. Gastrointest Endosc Clin N Am. 1996;6:235–52.
Chen YK. Preclinical characterization of the Spyglass peroral cholangiopancreatoscopy system for direct access, visualization, and biopsy. Gastrointest Endosc. 2007;65:303–11.
Chen YK, Pleskow DK. SpyGlass single-operator peroral cholangiopancreatoscopy system for the diagnosis and therapy of bile-duct disorders: a clinical feasibility study (with video). Gastrointest Endosc. 2007;65:832–41.
Chen YK, Nichols MT, Antillon MR. Peroral cholecystoscopy with electrohydraulic lithotripsy for treatment of symptomatic cholelithiasis in end-stage liver disease (with videos). Gastrointest Endosc. 2008a;67:132–5.
Chen YK, Parsi M, Binmoeller KF, Hawes RH, Pleskow D, Slivka A, et al. Peroral cholangioscopy (PO) using a disposable steerable single operator catheter for biliary stone therapy and assessment of indeterminate strictures–a multi-center experience using spyglass. Gastrointest Endosc. 2008b;67:AB103.
Classen M, Hagenmüller F, Knyrim K, Frimberger E. Giant bile duct stones–non-surgical treatment. Endoscopy. 1988;20:21–6.
Deister J. Intraoperative cholangioscopy, an improvement in bile duct diagnosis. Langenbecks Arch Klin Chir Ver Dtsch Z Chir. 1963;303:111–22.
Desa LA, Akosa AB, Lazzara S, Domizio P, Krausz T, Benjamin IS. Cytodiagnosis in the management of extrahepatic biliary stricture. Gut. 1991;32:1188–91.
Dion YM, Ratelle R, Morin J, Gravel D. Common bile duct exploration: the place of laparoscopic choledochotomy. Surg Laparosc Endosc. 1994;4:419–24.
Farrell JJ, Bounds BC, Al-Shalabi S, Jacobson BC, Brugge WR, Schapiro RH, et al. Single-operator duodenoscope-assisted cholangioscopy is an effective alternative in the management of choledocholithiasis not removed by conventional methods, including mechanical lithotripsy. Endoscopy. 2005;37:542–7.
Foerster EC, Schneider MU, Stömmer P, Runge U, Domschke W. Miniscopes in gastroenterological endoscopy–inspection of the gallbladder and the biliary and pancreatic duct systems in autopsy specimens. Endoscopy. 1988;20:316–20.
Foutch PG, Kerr DM, Harlan JR, Kummet TD. A prospective, controlled analysis of endoscopic cytotechniques for diagnosis of malignant biliary stricture. Am J Gastroenterol. 1991;86:577–80.
Fujita N, Mochizuki F, Lee S, Kobayashi G, Kimura K, Watanabe H. Pancreatoscopy for mucus producing pancreatic tumor. Dig Endosc. 1990;2:110–5.
Fukuda Y, Tsuyuguchi T, Sakai Y, Tsuchiya S, Saisyo H. Diagnostic utility of peroral cholangioscopy for various bile-duct lesions. Gastrointest Endosc. 2005;62:374–82.
Glasbrenner B, Ardan M, Boeck W, Preclik G, Moller P, Adler G. Prospective evaluation of brush cytology of biliary strictures during endoscopic retrograde cholangiopancreatography. Endoscopy. 1999;31:712–7.
Guda NM, Geenen JE, Catalano MF. Utility of peroral cholangioscope (SpyGlass system) in treatment of stones in chronic pancreatitis. Gastrointest Endosc. 2008;67:AB228–9.
Häberlin P. Cholangioscopy. Helv Chir Acta. 1966;33:78–80.
Hara T, Yamaguchi T, Ishihara T, Tsuyuguchi T, Kondo F, Kato K, et al. Diagnosis and patients management of intraductal papillary-mucinous tumor of the pancreas by using peroral pancreatoscopy and intraductal ultrasonography. Gastroenterology. 2002;122:34–43.
Hoffman A, Kiesslich R, Moench C, Bittinger F, Otto G, Galle PR, et al. Methylene blue-aided cholangioscopy unravels the endoscopic features of ischemic-type biliary lesions after liver transplantation. Gastrointest Endosc. 2007;66:1052–8.
Howell DA, Parsons WG, Jones MA, Bosco JJ, Hanson BL. Complete tissue sampling of biliary strictures at ERCP using a new device. Gastrointest Endosc. 1996;43:498–502.
Huang SP, Wang HP, Chen JH, Wu MS, Shun CT, Lin JT. Clinical application of EUS and peroral cholangioscopy in a choledochocele with choledocholithiasis. Gastrointest Endosc. 1999;50:568–71.
Hui CK, Lai KC, Ng M, Wong WM, Yuen MF, Lam SK, et al. Retained common bile duct stones: a comparison between biliary stenting and complete clearance of stones by electrohydraulic lithotripsy. Aliment Pharmacol Ther. 2003;17:289–96.
Itoi T, Shinohara Y, Takeda K, Nakamura K, Sofuni A, Itokawa F, et al. A novel technique for endoscopic sphincterotomy when using a percutaneous transhepatic cholangioscope in patients with an endoscopically inaccessible papilla. Gastrointest Endosc. 2004;59:708–11.

Itoi T, Sofuni A, Itokawa F, Kurihara T, Tsuchiya T, Ishii K, et al. Initial experience of peroral pancreatoscopy combined with narrow-band imaging in the diagnosis of intraductal papillary mucinous neoplasms of the pancreas (with videos). Gastrointest Endosc. 2007;66:793–7.
Jailwala J, Fogel EL, Sherman S, Gottlieb K, Flueckiger J, Bucksot LG, et al. Triple-tissue sampling at ERCP in malignant biliary obstruction. Gastrointest Endosc. 2000;51:383–90.
Jakobs R, Pereira-Lima JC, Maier M, Kohler B, Benz C, Adamek HE, et al. Endoscopic laser lithotripsy for difficult calculi after unsuccessful extracorporeal shock wave lithotripsy. Arq Gastroenterol. 1996;33:145–50.
Jakobs R, Pereira-Lima JC, Schuch AW, Pereira-Lima LF, Eickhoff A, Riemann JF. Endoscopic laser lithotripsy for complicated bile duct stones: is cholangioscopic guidance necessary? Arq Gastroenterol. 2007;44:137–40.
Kaneko T, Nakao A, Nomoto S, Furukawa T, Hirooka Y, Nakashima N, et al. Intraoperative pancreatoscopy with the ultrathin pancreatoscope for mucin-producing tumors of the pancreas. Arch Surg. 1998;133:263–7.
Kim HJ, Kim MH, Lee SK, Yoo KS, Seo DW, Min YI. Tumor vessel: a valuable cholangioscopic clue of malignant biliary stricture. Gastrointest Endosc. 2000;52:635–8.
Kodama T, Sato H, Horii Y, Tatsumi Y, Uehira H, Imamura Y, et al. Pancreatoscopy for the next generation: development of the peroral electronic pancreatoscope system. Gastrointest Endosc. 1999;49:366–71.
Kodama T, Koshitani T, Sato H, Imamura Y, Kato K, Abe M, et al. Electronic pancreatoscopy for the diagnosis of pancreatic diseases. Am J Gastroenterol. 2002;97:617–22.
Kodama T, Tatsumi Y, Sato H, Imamura Y, Koshitani T, Abe M, et al. Initial experience with a new peroral electronic pancreatoscope with an accessory channel. Gastrointest Endosc. 2004;59:895–900.
Kolodziejski TR, Safadi BY, Nakanuma Y, Milkes DE, Soetikno RM. Bile duct cysts in a patient with autosomal dominant polycystic kidney disease. Gastrointest Endosc. 2004;59:140–2.
Kozarek RA. Miniscopes–a technology in search of an application. J Clin Gastroenterol. 1988a;10:475–8.
Kozarek R. Direct cholangioscopy and pancreatoscopy at time of endoscopic retrograde cholangiopancreatography. Am J Gastroenterol. 1988b;83:55–7.
Kozarek RA. Direct pancreatoscopy. Gastrointest Endosc Clin N Am. 1995;5:259–67.
Kubota H, Kageoka M, Iwasaki H, Sugimoto K, Higuchi R, Honda S, et al. A patient with undifferentiated carcinoma of gallbladder presenting with hemobilia. J Gastroenterol. 2000;35:63–8.
Kurzawinski TR, Deery A, Dooley JS, Dick R, Hobbs K, Davidson BR. A prospective study of biliary cytology in 100 patients with bile duct strictures. Hepatology. 1993;18:1399–403.
Layfield LJ, Wax TD, Lee JG, Cotton PB. Accuracy and morphologic aspects of pancreatic and biliary duct brushings. Acta Cytol. 1995;39:11–8.
Lee JG, Leung JW, Baillie J, Layfield LJ, Cotton PB. Benign, dysplastic, or malignant-making sense of endoscopic bile duct brush cytology: results in 149 consecutive patients. Am J Gastroenterol. 1995;90:722–6.
Loren D, Kowalski TE, Conn M, Singu Bheema, Haluszka O, Tokar JL, et al. Clinical applications of SpyGlass direct visualization system: a multicenter experience. Gastrointest Endosc. 2008;67:AB230.
Lyass S, Phillips EH. Laparoscopic transcystic duct common bile duct exploration. Surg Endosc. 2006;20:S441–5.
Mukai H, Yasuda K, Nakajima M. Differential diagnosis of mucinproducing tumors of the pancreas by intraductal ultrasonography and peroral pancreatoscopy. Endoscopy. 1998;30:A99–A102.
Nakajima M, Akasaka Y, Fukumoto K, Mitsuyoshi Y, Kawai K. Peroral cholangiopancreatoscopy (PCPS) under duodenoscopic guidance. Am J Gastroenterol. 1976a;66:241–7.
Nakajima M, Fukumoto K, Mitsuyoshi Y, Kato S, Aoike A. Peroral cholangiopancreatoscopy (PCPS): its development and clinical application. Nippon Shokakibyo Gakkai Zasshi. 1976b;73:1381–8.
Nakajima M, Akasaka Y, Yamaguchi K, Fujimoto S, Kawai K. Direct endoscopic visualization of the bile and pancreatic duct systems by peroral cholangiopancreatoscopy (PCPS). Gastrointest Endosc. 1978;24:141–5.
Neuhaus H, Schumacher B. Miniscopes. Baillières Best Pract Res Clin Gastroenterol. 1999;13:33–48.
Okugawa T, Tsuyuguchi T, Ando T, Ishihara T, Yamaguchi T, Yugi H, et al. Peroral cholangioscopic treatment of hepatolithiasis: long-term results. Gastrointest Endosc. 2002;56:366–71.
Ortner MA, Liebetruth J, Schreiber S, Hanft M, Wruck U, Fusco V, et al. Photodynamic therapy of nonresectable cholangiocarcinoma. Gastroenterology. 1998;114:536–42.
Ortner ME, Caca K, Berr F, Liebetruth J, Mansmann U, Huster D, et al. Successful photodynamic therapy for nonresectable cholangiocarcinoma: a randomized prospective study. Gastroenterology. 2003;125:1355–63.
Parsi MA, Neuhaus H, Pleskow D, Binmoeller KF, Hawes RH, Petersen BT, et al. Peroral cholangioscopy guided stone therapy-report of an international multicenter registry. Gastrointest Endosc. 2008;67:AB102.

Ponchon T, Gagnon P, Berger F, Labadie M, Liaras A, Chavaillon A, et al. Value of endobiliary brush cytology and biopsies for the diagnosis of malignant bile duct stenosis: results of a prospective study. Gastrointest Endosc. 1995;42:565–72.

Ponsky J, Scheeres D, Simon I. Endoscopic retrograde cholangioscopy: an adjunct to endoscopic exploration of the common bile duct. Am Surg. 1990;56:235–7.

Popiela T, Karcz D, Kulig J. Significance of intraoperative fibercholangioscopy in the diagnosis of biliary tract disorders. Endoscopy. 1978;10:275–8.

Prasad GA, Abraham SC, Baron TH, Topazian MD. Hemobilia caused by cytomegalovirus cholangiopathy. Am J Gastroenterol. 2005;100:2592–5.

Pugliese V, Conio M, Nicolo G, Saccomanno S, Gatteschi B. Endoscopic retrograde forceps biopsy and brush cytology of biliary strictures: a prospective study. Gastrointest Endosc. 1995;42:520–6.

Raijman I, Fishman DS, Tarnasky PR, Patel S. SpyGlass: experience with a new mini-endoscope in biliopancreatic disease. Gastrointest Endosc. 2008;67:AB229.

Roca J, Flichtentrei R, Parodi M. Progress in the radiologic study of the biliary tract in surgery; cholangioscopy and cholangiography; utilization of apparatus; preliminary note. Día Méd. 1951;23:3420.

Rösch W, Koch H, Demling L. Peroral cholangioscopy. Endoscopy. 1976;8:172–5.

Sander R, Poesl H. Initial experience with a new baby scope for endoscopic retrograde cholangiopancreatoscopy. Gastrointest Endosc. 1996;44:191–4.

Schoefl R, Haefner M, Wrba F, Pfeffel F, Stain C, Poetzi R, et al. Forceps biopsy and brush cytology during endoscopic retrograde cholangiopancreatography for the diagnosis of biliary stenoses. Scand J Gastroenterol. 1997;32:363–8.

Scotiniotis IA, Kochman ML. Intramural cyst of the bile duct demonstrated by cholangioscopy and intraductal US. Gastrointest Endosc. 2001;54:260–2.

Seo DW, Lee SK, Yoo KS, Kang GH, Kim MH, Suh DJ, et al. Cholangioscopic findings in bile duct tumors. Gastrointest Endosc. 2000;52:630–4.

Shah RJ, Langer DA, Antillon MR, Chen YK. Cholangioscopy and cholangioscopic forceps biopsy in patients with indeterminate pancreaticobiliary pathology. Clin Gastroenterol Hepatol. 2006;4:219–25.

Shim CS, Neuhaus H, Tamada K. Direct cholangioscopy. Endoscopy. 2003;35:752–8.

Shuchleib S, Chousleb A, Mondragon A, Torices E, Licona A, Cervantes J. Laparoscopic common bile duct exploration. World J Surg. 1999;23:698–701.

Siddique I, Galati J, Ankoma-Sey V, Wood RP, Ozaki C, Monsour H, et al. The role of choledochoscopy in the diagnosis and management of biliary tract diseases. Gastrointest Endosc. 1999;50:67–73.

Soda K, Shitou K, Yoshida Y, Yamanaka T, Kashii A, Miyata M. Peroral cholangioscopy using new fine-caliber flexible scope for detailed examination without papillotomy. Gastrointest Endosc. 1996;43:233–8.

Somogyi L, Dimashkieh H, Weber Jr FL, Buell J. Biliary intraductal papillary mucinous tumor: diagnosis and localization by endoscopic retrograde cholangioscopy. Gastrointest Endosc. 2003;57:620–2.

Stewart CJR, Mills PR, Carter R, O'Donohue J, Fullarton G, Imrie CW, et al. Brush cytology in the assessment of pancreatico-biliary strictures: a review of 406 cases. J Clin Pathol. 2001;54:449–55.

Sugiyama M, Atomi Y, Wada N, Kuroda A, Muto T. Endoscopic transpapillary bile duct biopsy without sphincterotomy for diagnosing biliary strictures: a prospective comparative study with bile and brush cytology. Am J Gastroenterol. 1996;91:465–7.

Tajiri H, Kobayashi M, Ohtsu A, Ryu M, Yoshida S. Peroral pancreatoscopy for the diagnosis of pancreatic diseases. Pancreas. 1998;16:408–12.

Technology Status Evaluation Report. Duodenoscope-assisted cholangiopancreatoscopy. Gastrointest Endosc. 1999;50:943–5.

Tischendorf JJ, Krüger M, Trautwein C, Duckstein N, Schneider A, Manns MP, et al. Cholangioscopic characterization of dominant bile duct stenoses in patients with primary sclerosing cholangitis. Endoscopy. 2006;38:665–9.

Tsuyuguchi T, Saisho H, Ishihara T, Yamaguchi T, Onuma EK. Long-term follow-up after treatment of Mirizzi syndrome by peroral cholangioscopy. Gastrointest Endosc. 2000;52:639–44.

Uehara H, Nakaizumi A, Tatsuta M, Iishi H, Kitamura T, Ohigashi H, et al. Diagnosis of carcinoma in situ of the pancreas by peroral pancreatoscopy and pancreatoscopic cytology. Cancer. 1997;79:454–61.

Urakami Y. Peroral cholangiopancreatoscopy (PCPS) and peroral direct cholangioscopy (PDCS). Endoscopy. 1980;12:30–7.

Urakami Y, Seifert E, Butke H. Peroral direct cholangioscopy (PDCS) using routine straight-view endoscope: first report. Endoscopy. 1977;9:27–30.

Wamsteker EJ. Updates in biliary endoscopy. Curr Opin Gastroenterol. 2006;22:300–4.

Wright H, Sharma S, Gurakar A, Sebastian A, Kohli V, Jabbour N. Management of biliary stricture guided by the Spyglass direct visualization system in a liver transplant recipient: an innovative approach. Gastrointest Endosc. 2008;67:1201–3.

Yamao K, Ohashi K, Nakamura T, Suzuki T, Sawaki A, Hara K, et al. Efficacy of peroral pancreatoscopy in the diagnosis of pancreatic diseases. Gastrointest Endosc. 2003;57:205–9.

Yasuda K, Sakata M, Ueda M, Uno K, Nakajima M. The use of pancreatoscopy in the diagnosis of intraductal papillary mucinous tumor lesions of the pancreas. Clin Gastroenterol Hepatol. 2005;3:S53–7.

13 Endoscopic Drainage of Pancreatic Fluid Collections

Nam Q. Nguyen and Kenneth F. Binmoeller

CONTENTS

Keywords: Endoscopic, Drainage, Pancreatic, Fluid, Collections

INTRODUCTION

Pancreatic fluid collections (PFCs) are non-epithelial-lined, cystic, fluid-filled cavities that develop as a result of inflammatory conditions of the pancreas in acute or chronic pancreatitis, pancreatic trauma, or pancreatic duct obstruction (Bollen et al. 2007). Approximately 16–50% of episodes of acute pancreatitis and 20–40% of chronic pancreatitis complicate with fluid collections (Bollen et al. 2007; Singhal et al. 2006; Giovannini 2005). The majority of PFCs are asymptomatic and resolve spontaneously (Giovannini 2005). For symptomatic PFCs, the clinical presentation is related to the location and size of the collection, and the presence of infection. Expansion of the PFC can cause abdominal pain, duodenal or biliary obstruction, vascular occlusion, or fistula formation into adjacent viscera, the pleural space, or pericardium. On rare occasions, involvement of an adjacent

From: *Clinical Gastroenterology: Diagnostic and Therapeutic Procedures in Gastroenterology*,
Edited by: G. Y. Wu, S. Sridhar, DOI 10.1007/978-1-59745-044-7_13,

vessel can lead to pseudoaneurysm formation and produce a sudden, painful expansion of the cyst or gastrointestinal bleeding due to bleeding into the pancreatic duct (Giovannini 2005; Vosoghi et al. 2002). Disruption of the pancreatic duct with fistulization to the abdomen or chest can also result in pancreatic ascites and pleural effusion (Kantharia et al. 2007). Although surgical drainage has been the mainstay of treatment for symptomatic PFCs, it is associated with a relative high morbidity and mortality (Yin 2005; Rosso et al. 2003). Thus, less invasive techniques such as ultrasound- or CT-guided needle aspiration or direct endoscopic drainage have been developed with varying success. The aims of the current chapter are to review the current endoscopic management of pancreatic fluid collections using endoscopic ultrasound (EUS).

DIAGNOSTIC WORK-UP

The diagnosis of PFCs is often made by a detailed review of the clinical history and imaging features on ultrasound or CT scan. Most of the patients with PFCs present with a recent history of acute pancreatitis or pancreatic trauma. Presentations outside such clinical context need further evaluation to exclude pancreatic cystic neoplasms and pseudoaneurysm (Rosso et al. 2003). Cystic neoplasm should be considered if there is an absence of associated inflammatory changes on CT scan and a presence of internal septae within the cyst cavity. If there is a history of unexplained gastrointestinal bleeding, sudden expansion of a PFC or an unexplained drop in hematocrit, pseudoaneurysm should be suspected and a dynamic intravenous contrast CT scan should be performed. If the diagnosis of a PFC remains in doubt, EUS- or CT- guided aspiration of cystic fluid for further analysis should be performed (Rosso et al. 2003; Vignesh and Brugge 2008). The presence of high amylase or lipase concentration without mucin in the cystic fluid should confirm the diagnosis of a PFC (Vignesh and Brugge 2008). Furthermore, the presence of infection or pancreatic abscess can be determined by the appearance and microbiological testing of the cystic fluid aspirate. When a communication between the pancreatic duct and the cyst or a presence of pancreatic duct obstruction is highly suspected, magnetic resonance cholangio-pancreatography or endoscopic retrograde pancreatography (ERP) should be performed before the drainage procedure and a transpapillary drainage approach may be preferred (Vignesh and Brugge 2008).

INDICATIONS

Conservative management is recommended within the first 4–6 weeks as most PFCs resolve spontaneously (Barthet et al. 1993). A drainage procedure is indicated for fluid collections that are symptomatic, infected, rapidly enlarging, or causing obstruction of the GI tract or neighboring structures such as the biliary tract (Barthet et al. 1993; Baron et al. 2002; Smits et al. 1995; Vitale et al. 1999). Drainage should be considered for asymptomatic fluid collections larger than 10 cm owing to an increased risk of spontaneous rupture or hemorrhage. Debridement is indicated when PFCs contain organized necrosis and nasocystic lavage when contents are infected. Contraindications for endoscopic drainage include PFCs that are multi-loculated or multi-cystic, predominantly solid with little liquefied component, or have features suspicious of neoplastic involvement (Barthet et al. 1993; Baron et al. 2002; Smits et al. 1995; Vitale et al. 1999).

PATIENT PREPARATION FOR PSEUDOCYST DRAINAGE

Meticulous care in patient preparation is essential to prevent procedure complications. It is important that all patients are given pre-procedural broad-spectrum prophylactic antibiotics (Vignesh and Brugge 2008). Normal coagulation studies (including platelet count) should be confirmed and blood type and screen obtained. Surgical backup should be available (Binmoeller and Soehendra 1995). Although the majority of endoscopic drainage procedures can be performed under conscious sedation or monitored anesthesia with propofol, general anesthesia with tracheal intubation is recommended to protect the airway from cyst fluid aspiration.

PROCEDURE

The endoscopic approaches for drainage of fluid collections are guided by the anatomic relationship of the collection to the stomach or to the duodenum, the size of the collection, and the presence of ductal communication with the pseudocyst. The three approaches to drain a PFC are: (1) transpapillary (Catalano et al. 1995); (2) transmural (Monkemuller et al. 1998); or (3) combined transpapillary and transmural (Binmoeller et al. 1995). Transpapillary drainage involves placement of a pancreatic endoprosthesis across the site of duct disruption or directly into the collection (Telford and Carr-Locke 2002). Only a minority of PFCs are candidates for a transpapillary approach, as these not only must communicate with the main pancreatic duct, but should be small (<5 cm) and the contents fully liquefied (Catalano et al. 1995; Kozarek 1990). The transmural approach involves creating a cystenterostomy by placement of one or more large-bore stents through the gastric or the duodenal wall into the cystic cavity (Smits et al. 1995; Binmoeller et al. 1995). The majority of PFC can be successfully treated with this approach. The combined approach is appropriate for large or incompletely liquified cysts known to communicate with the pancreatic duct, especially when a downstream stricture is present. A combined approach is also appropriate when drainage is incomplete using a transpapillary approach or a fluid collection recurs using a transmural approach.

Transpapillary Pseudocyst Drainage

The transpapillary approach involves identifying the communication between the collection and pancreatic duct and any downstream pancreatic duct stricture by performing a pancreatogram via ERP (Catalano et al. 1995). If a ductal stricture is present, dilatation is performed with a 4 or 6 mm dilating balloon catheter. Otherwise, a pancreatic sphincterotomy is performed and a pancreatic duct stent is placed across the site of ductal disruption, or if not possible, into the fluid collection itself (Catalano et al. 1995).

Transmural Pseudocyst Drainage

The transmural approach involves puncturing the cyst in an appropriate vessel-free window with either a 19 gauge FNA needle (e.g., EchoTIP; Cook Medical, Winston Salem NC; Fig. 1a) or an electrosurgical needle (e.g., Zimmon needle knife, Cook Medical) under real-time EUS guidance (Smits et al. 1995; Binmoeller et al. 1995) (Table 1). Color Doppler ultrasound is used to highlight vessels that may be interposed in the wall between the

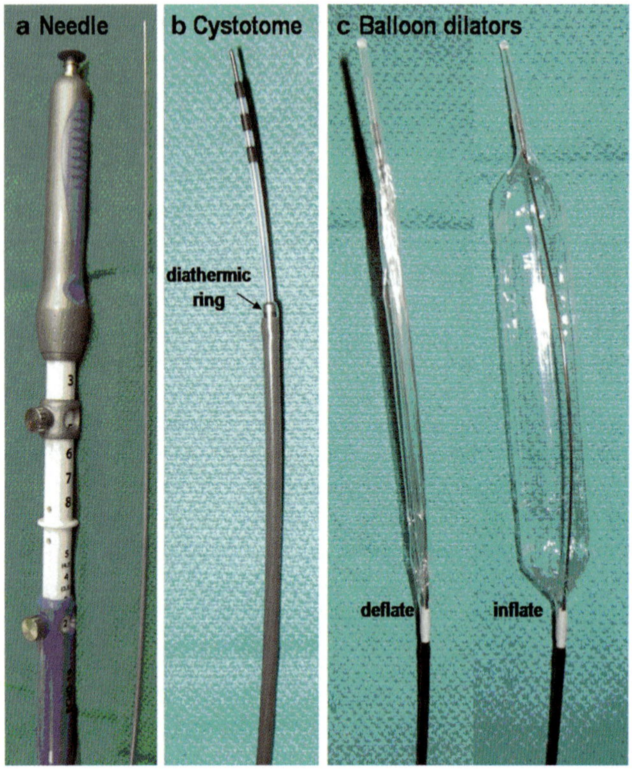

Fig. 1. Tools for endoscopic drainage of PFC: (**a**) a 19 Fr FNA puncture needle; (**b**), a cystotome with diathermic ring; and (**c**) a balloon dilator to create the gastrocystostomy tract

pseudocyst and bowel lumen. A sample of the cystic contents is aspirated for amylase, tumor markers (CEA), cytology, and culture and sensitivity. In order to evaluate for the presence of cyst communication with the pancreatic duct, a cystogram is performed by injecting contrast (Reno-30) under fluoroscopy. Under both sonographic and fluoroscopic guidance, a super stiff hydrophilic-tipped guidewire (e.g., Amplatz, 0.35/450; Boston Scientific Corp, Natick, MA) is inserted into the cyst through the needle and the wire is allowed to coil several times within the cystic cavity to stabilize the position of the guide wire (Smits et al. 1995; Binmoeller et al. 1995). The FNA needle is removed leaving the guide wire in place, and the cystenterostomy is dilated with a 6 or 8 mm balloon dilator (e.g., Hurricane; Boston Scientific Corp; Fig. 1c) placed over the guide wire. When the interposed wall is thick or fibrotic, advancement of the balloon catheter across the wall may fail. Alternative devices to "prime" the cystenterostomy include the 10 Fr Cystotome (Cook Medical; Fig. 1b) and the Soehendra Stent Retriever (Cook Medical) to burn or core a cystenterostomy path, respectively. Once primed, dilation of the cystostomy can be easily accomplished with the balloon catheter.

Cyst drainage is optimized by the placement of multiple stents that allow contents to drain through and between the stents. Stents used for cyst drainage have double pigtails for anchorage and are 3 or 4 cm long. The placement of two stents is best accomplished by initially placing two guide wires. A 9.5 Fr Cunningham-Cotton sleeve (Cook Medical) is a helpful tool to accomplish this, because the lumen is large enough to pass two 0.035 in. guide wires. Placement of a second guide wire can also be accomplished using the Cook monorail Fusion catheter (Cook Medical) (Fig. 2).

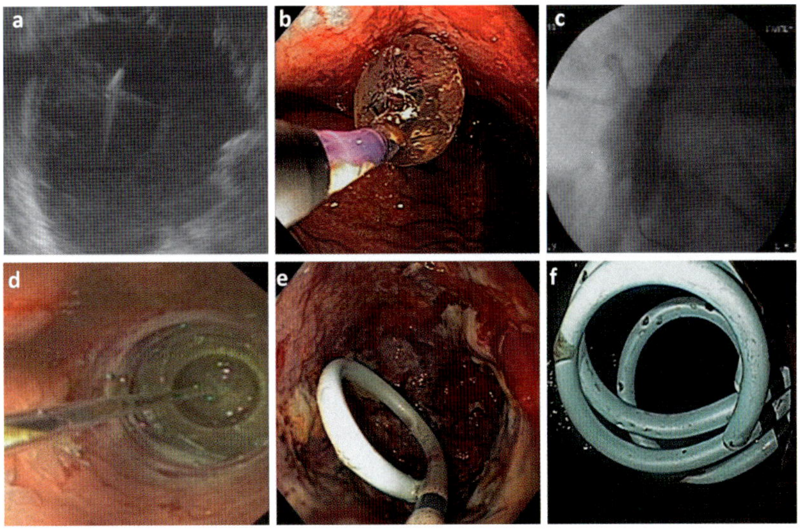

Fig. 2. Major steps involved in the endoscopic drainage of PFC. (**a**) The cyst is initially punctured with a needle (arrow) under ultrasound guidance; (**b–d**) followed by balloon dilation (arrows) of the gastrocystostomy tract; (**e** and **f**) once the tract is established, multiple stents are inserted to maintain the patency of the gastrocystostomy tract and ongoing drainage. Figure (**e**) shows cystic cavity with the insertion of a stent.

Stents often spontaneously migrate into the bowel lumen with cyst resolution, and are otherwise endoscopically removed 1–2 weeks after cyst resolution. This is shown by CT. An infected cyst/abscess requires irrigation by nasocystic catheter, inserting alongside the stents to create a "closed circuit". Continuous saline irrigation is performed for a minimum of 3 days or until aspirated content appears clear (Binmoeller and Soehendra 1995) (Table 1).

Cystoscopy-Guided Debridement

Organized pancreatic necroses (OPN) are partially liquefied and contain variable amounts of solid necrotic debris. Successful treatment of OPN requires cystoscopy-guided debridement (Fig. 3). The echoendoscope is exchanged for a large channel therapeutic gastroscope (e.g., 3.7 mm channel, Olympus GIF-1 T140). Dilation of the cystgastrostomy with larger caliber balloon dilators (15–18 mm CRE, Boston Scientific Corp., Natick MA) is performed to enable easy insertion of the gastroscope into the cyst cavity for cystoscopy. If the contents appear infected or there is necrotic debris, vigorous irrigation of the contents is performed with at least 2 L of saline (Binmoeller et al. 1995). All fluid contents within the cyst are completely aspirated (Smits et al. 1995; Binmoeller et al. 1995). Loose necrotic tissue that cannot be suctioned or flushed out with vigorous irrigation is removed using a foreign-body removal device such as a Dormia or Roth net basket (US Endoscopy, Mentor Ohio). Recently, the development of a forward viewing linear echoendoscope removes the need for scope exchange when performing cystoscopy and debridement. Preliminary data suggest that endoscopic drainage of PFC with cystoscopy and debridement can be performed successfully using this single-scope system (Kaltenbach et al. 2008).

In order to maintain drainage after cyst debridement, three 10 Fr double pigtail stents (e.g., Solace, Cook Medical) are inserted. For cysts that are infected or contain substantial

Table 1
Algorithm for endoscopic management of PFC

1. Initial stent drainage of the collection
   (a) Collection with little or no solid necrosis or debris
   - Cyst puncture with a 19-gauge needle under EUS guidance, followed by intracystic 0.035-inch guide wire
   - Cystostomy dilation with 6 or 8 mm balloon catheter
   - Multiple stents for drainage with optional naso-cystic catheter (NCC) for irrigation

   (b) Collection with visible organized necroses or debris
   - Cyst puncture with a 19-gauge needle under EUS guidance, followed by intracystic 0.035-inch guide wire
   - Cystostomy dilation with 6 or 8 mm balloon catheter
   - Exchange for therapeutic gastroscope and further cystostomy dilation up to 18 mm in diameter
   - Entry into cavity with the therapeutic gastroscope for cystoscopy and debridement.
   - Multiple stents for drainage with optional NCC for irrigation
2. Collections that fail to respond or recur after initial therapy.
   - Removal of all but one stent
   - Balloon dilation up to 18 mm alongside stent
   - Cystoscopy with aggressive and thorough debridement
   - Replacement of multiple stents followed by NCC
   - Repetition of debridement every 2–3 days as indicated until all solid necrotic material is cleared

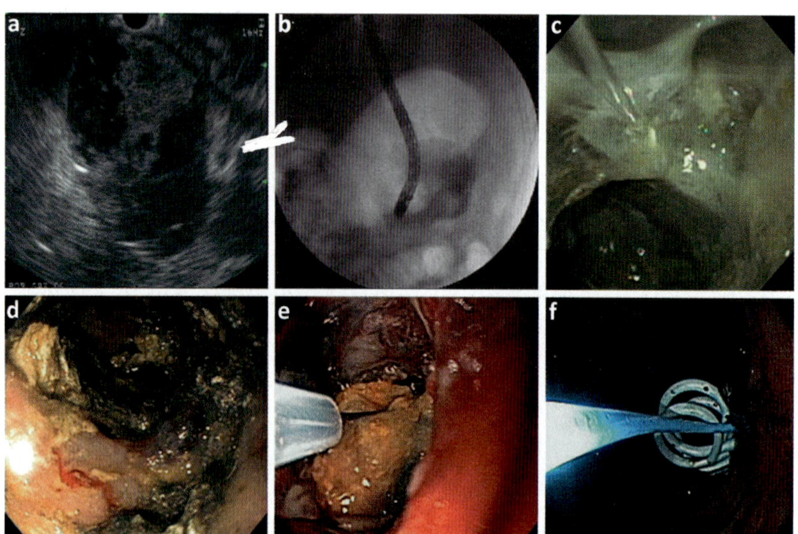

Fig. 3. (**a**) cystoscopy and debridement for PFC with solid debris or organized necrosis; (**b**) after dilatation of the gastrocystostomy tract with 15–18 mm balloon, cystoscopy is performed by inserting the therapeutic gastroscope into the cyst; (**c** and **d**) Vigorous irrigation is performed and non-adherent cyst contents aspirated; (**e**) solid debris that cannot be aspirated, is removed endoscopically using a Dormia or Roth net basket; (**f**) a nasocystic catheter may be inserted for additional irrigation of the cyst.

residual necroses after irrigation, a 7 Fr nasocystic catheter is inserted alongside the three stents for continuous irrigation, at a rate of 50 mL/h (Binmoeller et al. 1995) over a 2–3 day period.

POST-PROCEDURAL CARE

In order to reduce the risk of PFC infection, continuing broad spectrum antibiotics is recommended in all patients until the collection has resolved (Binmoeller and Soehendra 1995; Binmoeller et al. 1995). Furthermore, adjuvant acid suppression is discontinued during the duration of therapy to eliminate bacterial colonization (Binmoeller and Soehendra 1995; Binmoeller et al. 1995). For infected or heavily necrotic PFCs, the nasocystic catheter is removed after the drainage contents appear clear. Resolution of the PFC is defined as cyst size <2 cm and is monitored by interval abdominal CT scans (fortnightly in our practice). Repeat endoscopic debridement is indicated if the patient develops symptoms or signs of cyst infection, or if the cyst fails to decrease in size over a 2-week interval (Binmoeller and Soehendra 1995; Binmoeller et al. 1995). Stents that fail to spontaneously migrate after cyst resolution are removed endoscopically with a rat-tooth forceps or snare.

COMPLICATIONS AND MANAGEMENT

The rate of complications from endoscopic drainage of PFCs has been reported to be between 11% and 37%, and includes bleeding, perforation, infection, pancreatitis, pulmonary aspiration, stent migration/occlusion, pancreatic-duct damage, complications of sedation, and death (Giovannini 2005; Binmoeller et al. 1995; Kozarek et al. 1991). The complication rate is higher in patients with infected PFCs or organized pancreatic necrosis (Antillon et al. 2006).

Infectious complications are common and due to either incomplete drainage of fluid or obstructed drainage from retained solid debris. Apart from antibiotic therapy, repeat cystoscopy-guided debridement followed by nasocystic lavage is often necessary. The threshold for surgery should be low when the amount of organizing necrosis is substantial.

The most common cause of bleeding during endoscopic drainage is the inadvertent puncture of blood vessels or a pseudo-aneurysm. The judicious use of EUS with Doppler flow-directed puncture should avoid this complication. Hemostasis by injecting the bleeding site with 1:10,000 adrenaline followed by endoscopic coagulation or hemostatic clipping is usually achieved. On rare occasions, angiography and embolization or even surgery may be necessary to control bleeding (Gambiez et al. 1997). Perforation is more likely when the cyst wall is insufficiently adherent to the bowel wall. The majority of perforations, however, can be managed conservatively.

ALTERNATIVE PROCEDURES

Endoscopic drainage is widely recognized as the first-line therapy for PFC. However, surgical drainage may be preferred for PFCs that are multiple or multi-loculated or contain a large amount of organized pancreatic necroses and, therefore, unlikely to be completely drained by an endoscopic approach (Singh 2006). Fluid collections suspected to be neoplastic should also undergo surgical treatment. Percutaneous drainage of PFCs under CT or MRI guidance offers similar advantages to endoscopic drainage, but with the main drawback of harboring a significant risk of cutaneous fistula formation after drainage removal (Kariniemi et al. 2006; McFarlane 2005).

COST EFFECTIVENESS

EUS-guided drainage of PFCs should be considered a first-line treatment approach for patients because the procedure is cost saving and is associated with a shorter length of a post-procedure hospital stay when compared with surgical cyst-gastrostomy. In a retrospective case-controlled study (Varadarajulu et al. 2008), the average cost of EUS-guided transmural cyst drainage (US$9,077) is significantly lower than that of surgical approach (US$14,815), leading to a cost savings of $5,738 per patient. More importantly, current data suggest that there are no significant differences in clinical outcomes between both treatment modalities.

SUMMARY OF KEY POINTS

- Conservative management is recommended within the first 4–6 weeks as most of PFCs resolve spontaneously.
- Drainage procedure is indicated for fluid collections that are symptomatic including causing obstruction of the GI or biliary tract, greater than 10 cm in diameter, infected, rapidly enlarging, and persisting for longer than 13 weeks.
- Meticulous patient preparation is essential to prevent procedure complications. It is important that all patients are given pre-procedural broad-spectrum prophylactic antibiotics and coagulation studies (including platelet count) are normal.
- The endoscopic approaches for drainage of fluid collections are guided by the anatomic relationship of the collection to the stomach or to the duodenum, the size of the collection, and the presence of ductal communication with the pseudocyst.
- Transpapillary approach is recommended if the collection is <5 cm, fully liquid, and communicates with the main pancreatic duct, whereas transmural drainage is recommended for non-communicating PFCs that are large and/or contain necrotic material.
- Cystoscopy-guided debridement is indicated for organized pancreatic necroses.
- Repeated endoscopic debridement is required if the patient develops symptoms or signs of cyst infection, or if the cyst fails to decrease in size over a 2-week interval.
- Most complications can be managed medically or with additional endoscopic intervention.
- Endoscopic drainage of PFC is cost saving, and is associated with a shorter length of a post-procedure hospital stay when compared with surgical approach, and thus, should be considered as a first-line treatment.

REFERENCES

Bollen TL, Besselink MG, van Santvoort HC, Gooszen HG, van Leeuwen MS. Toward an update of the Atlanta classification on acute pancreatitis: review of new and abandoned terms. Pancreas. 2007;35:107–13.

Singhal D, Kakodkar R, Sud R, Chaudhary A. Issues in management of pancreatic pseudocysts. JOP. 2006;7:502–7.

Giovannini M. Endoscopic ultrasound-guided pancreatic pseudocyst drainage. Gastrointest Endosc Clin N Am. 2005;15:179–88. xi.

Vosoghi M, Sial S, Garrett B, Feng J, Lee T, Stabile BE, et al. EUS-guided pancreatic pseudocyst drainage: review and experience at Harbor-UCLA Medical Center. MedGenMed. 2002;4:2.

Kantharia CV, Prabhu RY, Dalvi AN, Raut A, Bapat RD, Supe AN. Spectrum and outcome of pancreatic trauma. Trop Gastroenterol. 2007;28:105–8.

Yin WY. The role of surgery in pancreatic pseudocyst. Hepatogastroenterology. 2005;52:1266–73.

Rosso E, Alexakis N, Ghaneh P, Lombard M, Smart HL, Evans J, et al. Pancreatic pseudocyst in chronic pancreatitis: endoscopic and surgical treatment. Dig Surg. 2003;20:397–406.

Vignesh S, Brugge WR. Endoscopic diagnosis and treatment of pancreatic cysts. J Clin Gastroenterol. 2008;42:493–506.

Barthet M, Bugallo M, Moreira LS, Bastid C, Sastre B, Sahel J. Management of cysts and pseudocysts complicating chronic pancreatitis. A retrospective study of 143 patients. Gastroentérol Clin Biol. 1993;17:270–6.

Baron TH, Harewood GC, Morgan DE, Yates MR. Outcome differences after endoscopic drainage of pancreatic necrosis, acute pancreatic pseudocysts, and chronic pancreatic pseudocysts. Gastrointest Endosc. 2002;56:7–17.

Smits ME, Rauws EA, Tytgat GN, Huibregtse K. The efficacy of endoscopic treatment of pancreatic pseudocysts. Gastrointest Endosc. 1995;42:202–7.

Vitale GC, Lawhon JC, Larson GM, Harrell DJ, Reed Jr DN, MacLeod S. Endoscopic drainage of the pancreatic pseudocyst. Surgery. 1999;126:616–21. discussion 621–3.

Binmoeller KF, Soehendra N. Endoscopic ultrasonography in the diagnosis and treatment of pancreatic pseudocysts. Gastrointest Endosc Clin N Am. 1995;5:805–16.

Catalano MF, Geenen JE, Schmalz MJ, Johnson GK, Dean RS, Hogan WJ. Treatment of pancreatic pseudocysts with ductal communication by transpapillary pancreatic duct endoprosthesis. Gastrointest Endosc. 1995;42:214–8.

Monkemuller KE, Baron TH, Morgan DE. Transmural drainage of pancreatic fluid collections without electrocautery using the Seldinger technique. Gastrointest Endosc. 1998;48:195–200.

Binmoeller KF, Seifert H, Walter A, Soehendra N. Transpapillary and transmural drainage of pancreatic pseudocysts. Gastrointest Endosc. 1995;42:219–24.

Telford JJ, Carr-Locke DL. The role of ERCP and pancreatoscopy in cystic and intraductal tumors. Gastrointest Endosc Clin N Am. 2002;12:747–57.

Kozarek RA. Pancreatic stents can induce ductal changes consistent with chronic pancreatitis. Gastrointest Endosc. 1990;36:93–5.

Kaltenbach T, De Lusong M, Soetikno RM, Shah J, Binmoeller K. Single-scope EUS guided cyst access, debridement and drainage using a novel therapeutic forward viewing echoendoscope. Gastroenterology. 2008;134:A456.

Kozarek RA, Ball TJ, Patterson DJ, Freeny PC, Ryan JA, Traverso LW. Endoscopic transpapillary therapy for disrupted pancreatic duct and peripancreatic fluid collections. Gastroenterology. 1991;100:1362–70.

Antillon MR, Shah RJ, Stiegmann G, Chen YK. Single-step EUS-guided transmural drainage of simple and complicated pancreatic pseudocysts. Gastrointest Endosc. 2006;63:797–803.

Gambiez LP, Ernst OJ, Merlier OA, Porte HL, Chambon JP, Quandalle PA. Arterial embolization for bleeding pseudocysts complicating chronic pancreatitis. Arch Surg. 1997;132:1016–21.

Singh S. Surgical management of complications associated with percutaneous and/or endoscopic management of pseudocyst of the pancreas. Ann Surg. 2006;244:630.

Kariniemi J, Sequeiros RB, Ojala R, Tervonen O. Feasibility of MR imaging-guided percutaneous drainage of pancreatic fluid collections. J Vasc Interv Radiol. 2006;17:1321–6.

McFarlane ME. The role of percutaneous drainage in the modern management of pancreatic pseudocysts. Int J Clin Pract. 2005;59:383–4.

Varadarajulu S, Lopes TL, Wilcox CM, Drelichman ER, Kilgore ML, Christein JD. EUS versus surgical cystgastrostomy for management of pancreatic pseudocysts. Gastrointest Endosc. 2008;68(4):649–55.

14 Endoscopic Management of Pancreatic Pseudocysts

Muhammad K. Hasan and Joseph Romagnuolo

CONTENTS

Keywords: Endoscopic, Management, Pancreatic, Pseudocysts, Transpapilary

INTRODUCTION

A pseudocyst is a persisting localized pancreatic or peripancreatic fluid collection that is generally rich in pancreatic enzymes. It lacks a true wall and is surrounded by a fibrous tissue wall without true epithelialization (Bradley 1993). Pseudocysts are thought to form as a result of a leak from a disrupted pancreatic duct, or more commonly a side branch, and are frequently asymptomatic. They can be sequelae of severe acute pancreatitis or of chronic pancreatitis. Symptomatic pseudocysts can be managed endoscopically, radiologically or surgically (Boerma et al. 2000). Pancreatic necrosis and cystic neoplasms can cause diagnostic dilemmas. This chapter focuses on the endoscopic management of pancreatic pseudocysts.

INCIDENCE AND ETIOLOGY OF PSEUDOCYSTS

Pseudocysts occur after an acute attack of pancreatitis in approximately 10% of cases. The incidence of pseudocysts in the general population has been reported to be 0.5–1 per 100,000 adults per year (Wade 1985). In a study of 926 patients with non-alcoholic acute pancreatitis, 5% were noted to have pseudocyst formation 6 weeks after an acute attack of

From: *Clinical Gastroenterology: Diagnostic and Therapeutic Procedures in Gastroenterology*,
Edited by: G. Y. Wu, S. Sridhar, DOI 10.1007/978-1-59745-044-7_14,

pancreatitis (Maringhini et al. 1999). In their study, Kourtesis et al. (1990) followed 128 consecutive patients with acute pancreatitis by computed tomography (CT) imaging, and 37% developed some type of acute fluid collection in the vicinity of pancreas. The majority of these acute fluid collections resolved spontaneously and only 15 (12%) patients progressed to the development of symptomatic pseudocysts. Another study has reported a 7% overall incidence of pseudocysts as a complication of acute pancreatitis (Imrie et al. 1988). The Atlanta Working Group categorizes fluid collections under 4 weeks old as "acute pancreatic fluid collections" (PFC); after 4 weeks they have generally developed a wall and so, are then referred to as "pseudocysts."

Although there is a lack of precise long term data on the incidence of pseudocyst development in patients with chronic pancreatitis, it has been reported that around 30–40% patients with chronic pancreatitis develop pseudocysts in their lifetime (Boerma et al. 2000).

Pseudocyst has been reported more commonly after alcohol-induced than after non-alcohol-related pancreatitis (Pitchumoni and Agarwal 1999). In a study of 357 patients with pancreatic pseudocysts, alcohol was reported to be a causative factor in 251 cases (70%), biliary tract disease in 28 (8%), blunt or penetrating abdominal trauma in 21 (6%), operative trauma in one case (0.3%), and idiopathic in 56 (16%) (Walt et al. 1990).

PATHOGENESIS AND CLASSIFICATION

Pseudocysts are formed due to rupture of the pancreatic duct or one of its side branches either by trauma or pancreatitis. This leads to extravasation of pancreatic juice which results in an acute fluid collection. Peripancreatic fluid can also sometimes form from edema, but usually does not result in an actual pseudocyst. Most patients with pseudocysts have demonstrable connections between the cyst and the pancreatic duct, but some lose their connection as the fibrosis walls off the area. Although necrosis is sometimes associated with these severe cases of pancreatitis, pseudocysts can occur without pancreatic necrosis; the pseudocysts themselves should have no substantial necrosis within the collection.

Liquified necrosis (post-necrotic pancreatic fluid collection, PNPFC) can mimic a pseudocyst, but generally has a different natural history, risk of infection, and different approach to management. They are usually not truly fluid-filled, but often have solid components, and a semi-solid gelatinous make-up that sometimes mimics fluid on imaging especially CT (computed tomography) (Figs. 1 and 2). PNPFCs can persist beyond a month, and evolve into "walled off pancreatic necrosis" (WOPN) – a new category in the most recent Atlanta classification, which can be confused with a pseudocyst.

In a patient with chronic pancreatitis, most often due to alcohol abuse, pseudocyst formation occurs by acute exacerbation of underlying disease (with the same mechanism as above), or by progressive ductal obstruction due to either downstream ductal stricturing or intraductal stone or protein plug formation. This prevents drainage of pancreatic juices into the small bowel. Elevation in upstream intraductal pressure predisposes to ductal leakage, with accumulation of a peripancreatic fluid.

As mentioned above, many patients develop some type of fluid collection (PFC) after acute pancreatitis and this fluid collection is termed a pseudocyst only if it persists beyond 4–6 weeks and is surrounded by a fibrous tissue without true epithelialization (Bradley 1993; Pitchumoni and Agarwal 1999). Pseudocysts can be sterile, or infected; spontaneous

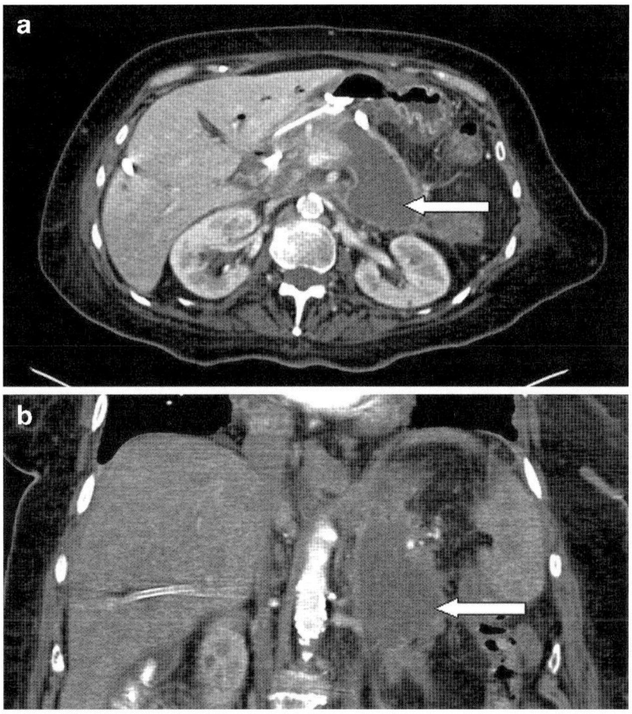

Fig. 1. CT images after endoscopic cystgastrostomy appearing to demonstrate a new or persisting collection (*arrow*) near a drained cyst. This hypodense lesion appeared to be fluid-filled on CT, surrounded by a brighter hyperdense capsule, and was reported as a "pseudocyst". It was subsequently shown by MR to be solid/semi-solid walled off pancreatic necrosis (*WOPN*). (**a**) Axial image. (**b**) Coronal image.

infection of pseudocysts is rare, and generally is either due to contamination by an intervention, or seeding from bacterial translocation or other causes of bacteremia. Infection is even rarer for acute fluid collections if not contaminated by intervention.

Pseudocysts were initially classified by D'Egidio and Schein (D'Egidio and Schein 1991) in 1991. They described three types of pseudocysts based on pancreatic duct anatomy, presence of communication between the cyst and the pancreatic duct and underlying etiology of pancreatitis (acute or chronic). Type 1 was described as one which follows an acute attack of pancreatitis and has normal duct anatomy, and only rarely communicates with the pancreatic duct. Type 2 pseudocysts follow an episode of acute-on-chronic pancreatitis, often have duct-pseudocyst communication with a diseased pancreatic duct, but the duct is not strictured. Type 3 cysts, referred to as "retention" pseudocysts, occur as a result of chronic pancreatitis and are uniformly associated with duct stricture/obstruction and pseudocyst to duct communication. This classification has variable use in practice.

To help guide decisions regarding surgical vs. non surgical therapy, Nealon and Walser (2002) classified pseudocysts based entirely on pancreatic duct anatomy. They described seven types of pseudocysts: Type 1 has normal duct with no communication with the cyst. Type 2 also has normal duct, but with duct-cyst communication. Type 3 has an otherwise normal duct, but with stricture(s) and no duct-cyst communication. Type 4 has an otherwise normal duct, with stricture(s) and duct-cyst communication. Type 5 has an otherwise normal duct but complete cut off duct with no communication with the cyst. Type 6 occurs in chronic

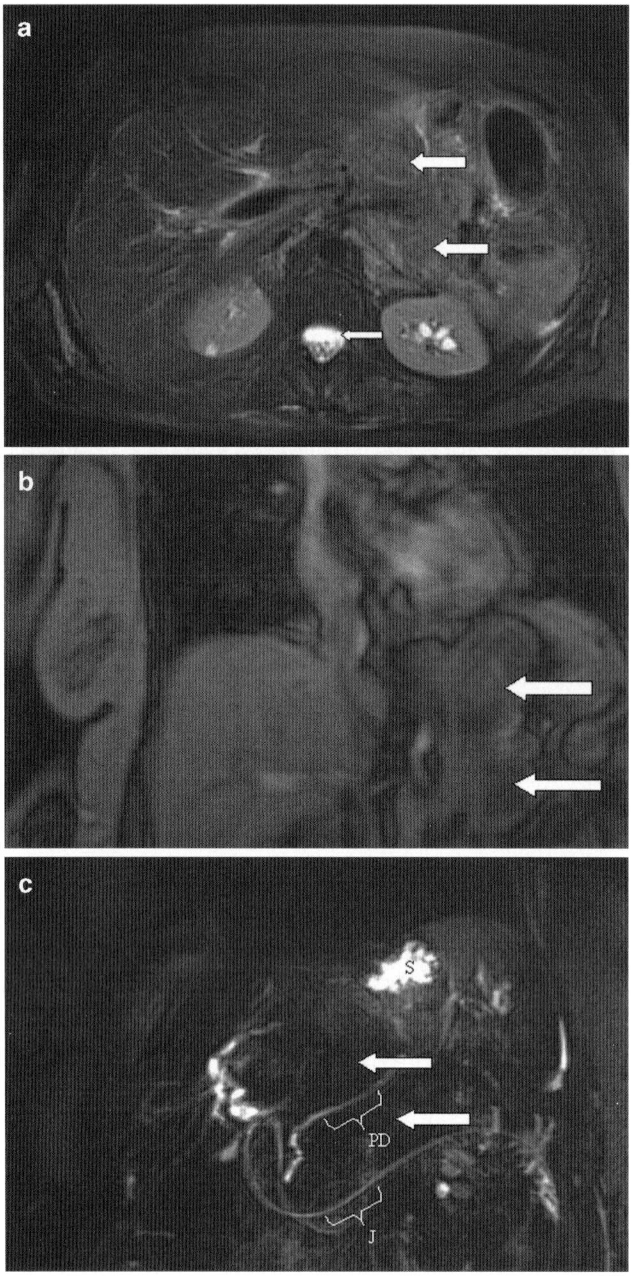

Fig. 2. T2-weighted MR images in which stagnant fluids such as ductal or luminal fluid and cerebral spinal fluid (*small arrow*) appear white (high signal) showing that the "cyst" in Fig. 1 was not fluid-filled, but rather solid/semi-solid pancreatic necrosis (mildly low signal) (*large arrows*). The heavily T-weighted MRCP shows bright fluid in the stomach (*S*), and in the pancreatic duct (*PD*), but no bright fluid at all around the pancreas. A jejunal tube is also seen (*J*). (**a**) Axial image. (**b**) Coronal image. (**c**) MRCP image.

pancreatitis, but has no duct-cyst communication. Type 7 occurs in the presence of chronic pancreatitis and has duct-cyst communication. Although helpful, ductal communication, a critical part of this classification, may be difficult to discern with non-invasive imaging. Dynamic secretin-stimulated MRCP (magnetic resonance cholangiopancreatography) and

EUS (endoscopic ultrasound) are promising, however. It is seldom necessary to use invasive studies such as endoscopic retrograde cholangiopancreatography (ERCP) for that purpose.

CLINICAL PRESENTATION AND DIAGNOSIS

A careful history of the duration of the cyst, whether pancreatitis was present and whether an etiology of the pancreatitis is known, and whether other suspicious symptoms are present (that might suggest this could be a cystic neoplasm) is very important to decide the best management.

History, Physical Examination, and Laboratory Evaluations: Narrowing the Differential

Pseudocysts can present with a wide range of clinical problems depending upon the location and size of the fluid collection, and the presence of infection. Patients with pseudocysts may be completely asymptomatic; or they can present with abdominal pain, anorexia, abdominal mass effect from a large cyst pressing on the stomach or duodenum, leading to persistent nausea/vomiting and gastric outlet obstruction, compression of the splenic vein with splenomegaly and left upper quadrant pain, or jaundice due to compression of the bile duct. Weight loss can result from nausea and pain, and can be confusing regarding the differential diagnosis of a cystic tumor. Patients also can present with other complications of pseudocysts, such as infection, bleeding into the cyst or splenic artery pseudoaneurysm, rupture of the cyst, or thrombosis of the splenic or portal vein with bleeding or non-bleeding gastric varices (Gouyon et al. 1997). Serum laboratory tests have limited utility and results depend on the clinical presentation and etiology of underlying pancreatitis. By the time a pseudocyst is found, serum pancreatic enzymes have frequently returned to normal or near-normal. A white blood count may alert one to the possibility of infection, although persistent minor elevations in the white count can be due to smoldering pancreatitis.

Pseudocysts are usually identified by cross-sectional imaging studies, such as CT done for an evaluation of the severity of an attack of pancreatitis or for persistent symptoms like fever, vomiting, or abdominal pain, after an attack. Once a pancreatic cyst is identified by an imaging modality, the most important point is to differentiate pseudocysts from necrosis, and other cystic lesions of the pancreas not related to pancreatitis (the most common of which being cystic neoplasms) and this could pose a difficult diagnostic and therapeutic dilemma for clinicians. True "simple cysts" or congenital cysts of the pancreas are thought to be rare.

Unlike in other abdominal organs, most cysts in the pancreas that are not pseudocysts are in fact cystic neoplasms, some of which have malignant potential (Fig. 3). It is crucial to differentiate pseudocysts from necrosis and other cystic lesions as management varies by the type of cystic lesion. History is often the most helpful element to help differentiate these lesions. Pseudocysts (and PNPFCs or WOPN) usually follow an acute attack of pancreatitis, can present at any age, and can be located evenly throughout the pancreas or its vicinity. When they occur in the setting of chronic pancreatitis, there is often a heavy alcohol history in the present or past, since this is the etiology of the majority of chronic pancreatitis cases. Abdominal trauma and family history can be other clues. If the pancreatitis appears idiopathic, one must consider that the pancreatitis was secondary to the cyst rather than the cyst was due to pancreatitis – i.e., cystic tumors can rarely cause pancreatitis.

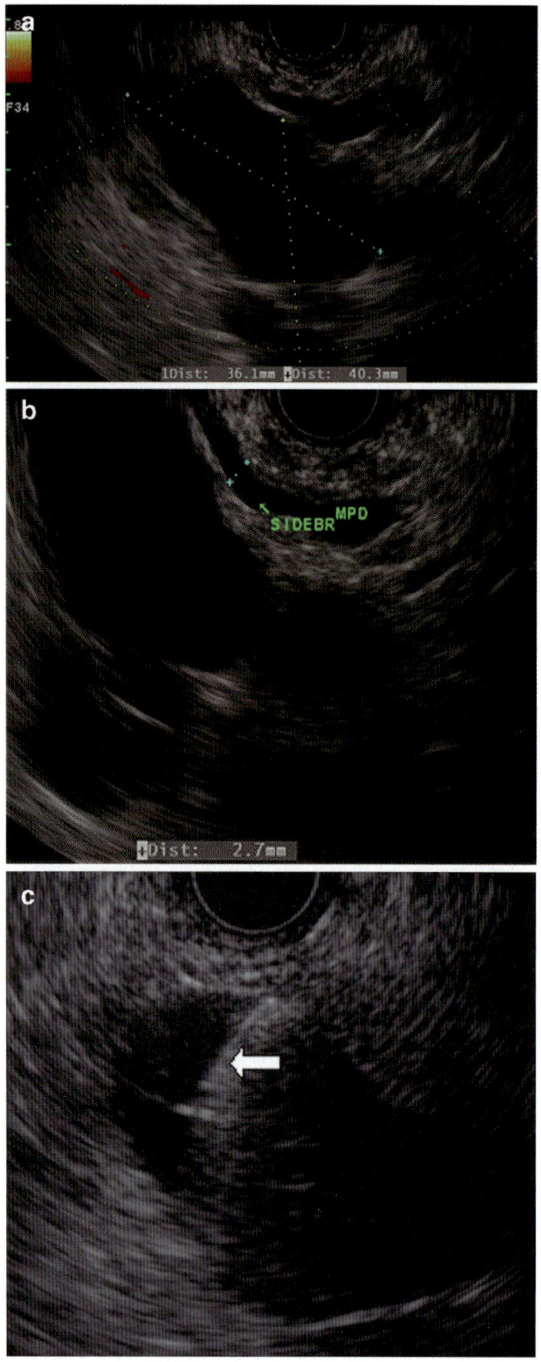

Fig. 3. Linear EUS of a slowly enlarging 3–4 cm Doppler-negative anechoic (cystic) lesion in the head of the pancreas in a middle-aged man without a history of pancreatitis. (**a**) A thin-walled cyst is seen with a dilated side branch (SIDEBR) from the main pancreatic duct (*MPD*) filling the cyst. (**b**) The lobular/tubular cyst morphology is consistent with a cluster of dilated side branches. (**c**) FNA with a 19 G needle (*arrow*) removed thick mucin consistent with a side branch variant IPMN. An intracystic brushing was obtained through the needle, but both fluid and brushing were acellular.

Imaging Studies and Possible Fluid Sampling

Different imaging modalities can be used to evaluate pseudocysts of the pancreas. The imaging studies done could be transabdominal ultrasound (US), CT, magnetic resonance imaging (MRI), ERCP and EUS. Ultrasound (regular or EUS) and T2-weighted MRI (magnetic resonance imaging; such as is used for MRCP sequences), are the best modalities for identifying solid components or refuting a suspicion of necrosis mimicking a pseudocyst (Fig. 2). Both modalities are superior to CT in distinguishing solid tissue from fluid. CT can often misdiagnose necrosis, and sometimes even a solid mass, as a pseudocyst, because the Hounsfield units can overlap (Fig. 1). CT is generally insufficient, on its own, to proceed with management. Fine needle aspiration (FNA) by CT or EUS is available for equivocal lesions, but should be avoided in classical pseudocysts to avoid the risk of infection unless therapeutic drainage is also planned; most pseudocysts do not need diagnostic aspiration.

Conventional Abdominal Ultrasound

On ultrasound, pseudocysts appear as an anechoic (black), round or oval, relatively smooth-walled and well-defined structure (although some internal irregularity of the wall is common). Conventional US has certain limitations, especially when examining a relatively small lesion in the retroperitoneum, behind the stomach, including the presence of overlying bowel gas (which can be increased if ileus or gastric obstruction accompanies the acute pancreatitis) and is operator dependent (Pitchumoni and Agarwal 1999). The patient is often in pain and because of this, the ability to press with the probe deeply on the abdomen, or roll the patient to get different views, may be limited. Generally, the sensitivity of US for the detection of moderate-sized pancreatic pseudocysts ranges from 75% to 90%, which is generally inferior to CT (sensitivity >90%). Again, US is one of the best modalities for distinguishing solid from liquid, and so significant solid debris within the cystic lesion generally implies necrosis (or more rarely, neoplasia). At the same time, US can also reliably detect cholelithiasis (arguably the best test for this) and biliary dilation, although again, the exam when the patient is in considerable pain is often a limited one; the US may need to be repeated when the pain and inflammation have settled.

CT, MRI, and ERCP

CT and MRI are very sensitive diagnostic modalities for pancreatic pseudocysts. In a patient with recent history suggestive of pancreatitis, finding a round, thick-walled, fluid filled structure in the vicinity of pancreas is very suggestive of a pseudocyst. The major limitations of CT are its poor ability to distinguish fluid from necrosis, its inability to differentiate pseudocysts from cystic neoplasm of the pancreas, and the risks of intravenous contrast (Siegelman et al. 1980). It is also poor at assessing ductal communication and pancreatic strictures or irregularity that may point to a diagnosis of chronic pancreatitis. Although not as good as EUS, it has reasonable sensitivity for pancreatic calcifications.

MRI/MRCP is superior to CT in depicting debris within pseudocysts and differentiating cysts from solid lesions (Figs. 1 and 2). Also, it can give detailed imaging of the pancreatic duct and bile duct. MRCP has some other advantages over CT including its superiority to detect choledocholithiasis (Romagnuolo et al. 2003 Oct 7), strictures, bleeding within the pseudocyst and duct to cyst communication (especially when secretin is given to stimulate pancreatic juice flow).

ERCP is not required to diagnose the pseudocyst, but it definitely has a role in the endoscopic therapy of the pseudocysts as described in the treatment section. Because of its risk of post-procedural pancreatitis, or worsening of existing pancreatitis, and the risk of contaminating the cyst with dye, which can lead to infection, it is best avoided unless therapy is planned, temporary stenting of a compressed biliary tree is needed, or removal of bile duct stones (that may have led to the attack of pancreatitis) is planned.

EUS and Possible Fine Needle Aspiration with Fluid Analysis

EUS is generally not the initial test used to diagnose pancreatic pseudocysts, but has a great role in further evaluation of cystic lesions diagnosed by other imaging modalities. It is the image modality of choice to distinguish pseudocyst from other pancreatic cystic lesions in the equivocal scenarios described above. It uses ultrasound, which is also one of the best imaging modalities to distinguish solid from liquid, and ruling out significant debris/necrosis. It is also excellent at excluding an adjacent mass if there are suspicious symptoms such as weight loss. With EUS, very high resolution images of the pancreas can be obtained due to the proximity of the pancreas to the stomach and duodenum; the proximity avoids intervening air, and allows higher frequency high-resolution probes (which have shallower depths of penetration). This allows superior ductal and parenchymal imaging; the latter is really unmatched by other imaging choices.

For cystic lesions that are thought to possibly represent cystic neoplasms, including cases wherein the cyst may have preceded the pancreatitis, cases involving elderly patients or unexplained pancreatitis, constitutional symptoms such as weight loss, and cases without a clear history of pancreatitis, EUS can be helpful. EUS can look at cyst morphology, duct communication and is very sensitive for picking up underlying chronic pancreatitis in those without a clear pancreatitis history.

A principal advantage of EUS as compared to MRI or CT is its capability of adding real-time EUS-guided FNA. In equivocal cases, cases involving a cyst without a clear attack of pancreatitis, or cysts associated with a solid mass, EUS-guided fine needle aspiration (of the cyst or mass) may be needed. In contrast, if the cystic lesion has a pseudocyst-like morphology on EUS and is in the setting of explained (e.g., alcoholic) pancreatitis, FNA is not needed, and should be avoided as it can cause infection.

Cyst morphology and fluid analysis (amylase, mucin, carcinoembryonic antigen [CEA] and cytology) are used to further clarify cystic lesions that are equivocal; generally, the latter is more helpful. Cysts with little or no malignant potential include pseudocysts and serous cyst adenomas. Fluid analysis of pseudocysts classically shows low CEA levels (although there is marked overlap with neoplasia) (van der Waaij et al. 2005; Brugge et al. 2004b), high amylase (signifying ductal communication) and inflammatory cells on cytology and no mucin. Serous cystadenomas are the most common cystic neoplasms. They are most commonly seen in elderly women and make up 32–39% of all pancreatic cystic neoplasms (Brugge et al. 2004a). On EUS, these cysts appear to have a cluster of microcysts, sometimes adjacent to a larger cyst, and often have central hyperechoic scar. Fluid analysis from these type of cysts classically shows no mucin, low amylase (no duct communication) and low CEA levels, and classically, monomorphic cuboidal cells on cytology (although the fluid is unfortunately often acellular).

Cysts with malignant potential include intraductal papillary mucinous neoplasms (IPMN) and mucinous cyst neoplasms. The accuracy of EUS and MRCP for identifying side branch IPMNs solely on morphology is improving. EUS-guided FNA and fluid analysis shows high CEA (>192 ng/mL), mucin, and high amylase/lipase levels (they communicate with the duct), and cytological analysis may be positive for malignancy, but the fluid can be hypo-/acellular (Brugge et al. 2004b). Mucinous cystadenomas are most commonly seen in middle-aged women and typically have macrocysts (>2 cm) or are unilocular and generally have no communication with the pancreatic duct. Features to be suggestive of malignant potential are septations, thickened or irregular cyst walls, and the presence of mural nodules or mass. Fluid analysis shows high CEA and mucin, low amylase levels, and cytologic analysis may have atypical or neoplastic cells.

Safety of EUS-guided FNA of cysts is well-established when the cyst is accessed with a single puncture and is drained dry. The risk of pancreatitis with EUS-guided FNA is 2–3%, with infection less than 1% and hemorrhage within the cyst less than 1% (Jacobson et al. 2005; Lee et al. 2005). To decrease the risk of infection intra-procedural antibiotics are administered before or during the procedure, and then by mouth for 3–5 days of post-procedure. The risk is likely higher if FNA contaminates the cyst, but drainage is incomplete, or if debris or necrosis is present. Therefore, very large cysts, especially ones with debris, should generally not be aspirated for diagnosis unless a drain is being placed simultaneously and the need for diagnostic sampling is justified.

TREATMENT OF PANCREATIC PSEUDOCYSTS

Preprocedural Assessment

Most acute pancreatic fluid collections and pseudocysts resolve with supportive medical care which includes intravenous fluids as needed, analgesics and anti-emetics. For patients who can tolerate oral intake, a low-fat diet is suggested at least in the short-term. Pancreatic non-enteric coated enzymes (30–50,000 lipase units per meal) are likely helpful in some patients although the literature to support this is admittedly weak (Brown et al. 1997); octreotide is used very rarely to decrease pancreatic secretions in refractory ongoing leaks. For patients who cannot tolerate oral intake, nutrition can be provided via nasojejunal feeding or a percutaneous (direct or via a percutaneous gastrostomy) J-tube; the latter is generally left in for about 6–8 weeks; total parenteral nutrition (TPN) is a far inferior way of feeding in terms of metabolic and infectious risks, a concept supported by randomized trials (McClave et al. 1997; Windsor et al. 1998; Kalfarentzos et al. 1997; Hernandez-Aranda et al. 1996; Abou-Assi et al. 2001).

It is important to make sure that the pseudocyst is "mature" with a well-developed wall, generally at least 4–6 weeks old. Interventional therapies, especially endoscopic ones, have better results, and fewer complications, when this is the case. In addition, one must make sure that sufficient time has been given to allow the cyst to have a chance to spontaneously resolve, as most do. The pseudocyst should be associated with persisting symptoms. Although size does not matter, generally cysts under 4 cm in size do not cause significant symptoms (i.e., ongoing pain is more likely due to ongoing pancreatitis), unless they cyst is in the head where biliary or duodenal compression can occur with smaller, 2–4 cm cysts. However, placing a pigtail drain, by any means, into a cyst that is under 3–4 cm in size is technically difficult, and often not feasible.

For cysts that do not resolve spontaneously with supportive medical management, and become symptomatic or lead to development of a complication (gastric outlet obstruction, infection of the cyst, biliary obstruction), some type of drainage procedure will be required.

The options for drainage include surgical, percutaneous or endoscopic techniques. Before attempting any type of drainage, there are a few critical issues that need to be addressed.

First of all, it is important to consider alternative diagnoses and a cystic neoplasm should be ruled out. If the patient does not have a history of pancreatitis, the diagnosis of a pseudocyst becomes doubtful. Also, if pancreatitis has occurred, but the etiology is unclear, one must consider that the cyst (e.g., cystic neoplasm) could have caused the pancreatitis rather than the pancreatitis caused the cyst (i.e., pseudocyst).If available, prior imaging may be helpful. Otherwise, EUS with FNA and fluid analysis (CEA of fluid being most important) is probably the best modality to answer the above question.

It is also important to determine if this is really an area of necrosis or a pseudocyst. In the former, although treatment is similar to pseudocysts when asymptomatic or resolving, and not infected, and conservative treatment is generally all that is required. If complications occur, such as infection, surgical treatment may be preferred over transcutaneous or endoscopic drainage. Attempts at endoscopic drainage and endoscopic intracystic debridement can still potentially be done, selectively, especially in patients who are poor surgical candidates, but this is not standard practice for most cases. In such selected cases, the response rate is expected to be lower than in patients with sterile pseudocysts (Hookey et al. 2006; Baron et al. 2002).

It is important to exclude a pseudoaneurysm (usually of the splenic artery running near the cyst) which occurs in approximately 10% of patients with a pseudocyst (El Hamel et al. 1991; Pitkaranta et al. 1991). The presence of a pseudoaneurysm is suggested by unexplained gastrointestinal bleeding, sudden expansion of a pseudocyst, or an obscure drop in hematocrit. Severe and even fatal hemorrhage can occur following endoscopic drainage in patients with an unsuspected pseudoaneurysm. Without preprocedural arterial embolization, a pseudoaneurysm is an absolute contraindication to transluminal drainage. CT or MRI should be performed to rule out pseudoaneurysm in all cases and if a suspicion is raised, angiography should be undertaken first. In a study of 57 patients considered for endoscopic drainage of pancreatic pseudocysts, pseudoaneurysms were detected in five patients prior to the drainage procedure. These patients were treated with a multidisciplinary approach, including embolization or resection (Marshall et al. 1996).

Surgical Drainage

Surgery is usually definitive, but is not generally first-line treatment. It could be done either open or laparoscopic; open surgery carries a significant risk of morbidity and mortality (25% to 5% respectively). Surgical drainage of pseudocysts is accomplished by providing a communication between the pseudocyst cavity and the stomach or small bowel; or it can involve resecting it entirely, often including the part of the pancreas that is leaking into it. In centers with the appropriate expertise, endoscopic management of pancreatic pseudocysts is often considered first, and surgical drainage is reserved for patients not meeting criteria for endoscopic drainage, those who fail endoscopic management or have recurrence following successful endoscopic drainage, those that have a disconnected duct or tight downstream stricture, or equivocal lesions (i.e., suspicion of a cystic tumor). In a retrospective study (Adams and Anderson 1992) of 94 patients in which 42 patients underwent internal surgical drainage and 52 patients underwent percutaneous pseudocyst drainage, seven were surgically managed patients and four percutaneously treated patients had complications (16.7% vs 7.7%). A significantly higher mortality rate was associated with surgical therapy (7.1%) than with percutaneous therapy (0%) ($P<0.05$). However, subsequent operation was required in 19.2% of the percutaneous drainage group compared with only 9.5% of the surgical group ($P>0.05$).

Percutaneous Drainage

In this procedure, an external drainage is obtained by placement of drainage catheter percutaneously into the fluid cavity; this is not always feasible anatomically, especially in the head of pancreas. Ultrasound or CT is used to guide the catheter placement, and pseudocysts that may not be accessible endoscopically can be handled this way in many cases. Catheter drainage is continued until the flow rate falls to 5–10 mL/day. The mean duration of drainage can be up to 6 weeks. This technique, though usually successful, carries a high risk of infection. In one series, it was reported to occur in 48% of the patients (Adams and Anderson 1992). It can also be associated with significant patient discomfort, and the catheter can clog and may require repositioning and exchange. Percutaneous drainage is more likely to be successful in patients with normal pancreatic ducts without downstream stricture and no communication between the duct and the cyst. It should not generally be performed in patients with cysts containing bloody or solid material, unless dilation of the tract, insertion of larger bore catheters, with or without continuous irrigation, is planned.

Although second line for mature pseudocysts, percutaneous drainage is a helpful option for less well-defined early acute pancreatic fluid collections (PFCs) that are very symptomatic and cannot wait until they resolve or mature. Because they are not mature enough to be called pseudocysts, they may not be appropriate for endoscopic transluminal drainage, and large ones may not be anticipated to resolve with transpapillary drainage alone (>3–4 cm). In these cases, the drain is usually placed, and an ERCP is performed to rule out downstream ductal pathology, bridge any disruption, and place a transpapillary pancreatic stent if ductal communication with the PFC is present. Complete disruptions, or percutaneous drains that persistently drain over the coming weeks despite the above, should be referred for surgery.

Endoscopic Drainage

Pseudocysts can be managed endoscopically with transluminal drainage (cystogastrostomy, cystoduodenostomy) or by facilitating transpapillary drainage with a stent and/or pancreatic sphincterotomy. Endoscopic transluminal drainage is considered to be a preferred therapeutic approach for qualifying mature pseudocysts as it is less invasive, avoids the need to care for an external drain and also has a high long-term success rate. In patients with relatively small pseudocysts (less than 4–6 cm) communicating with the main pancreatic duct, transpapillary drainage with a temporary pancreatic stent may be tried as initial therapy, with or without a pancreatic sphincterotomy. A transluminal (transgastric or transduodenal) drainage approach is used in patients with a large, well-circumscribed, mature and symptomatic pseudocyst directly adjacent to the gastroduodenal wall (usually less than 1 cm separation between gastric and cyst lumens), without contraindications.

Efficacy and Cost-Effectiveness of Endoscopic Management

The landmark success of endoscopic transmural pseudocyst drainage in the setting of chronic pancreatitis was reported in 1989 (Cremer et al. 1989). The technical success rate of the drainage procedure has been reported to be up to 97%, with definitive resolution in almost 75%. In cases of pancreatic necrosis and solid debris, the success rate is significantly lower. However as mentioned above, in patients who are not surgical candidates, endoscopic drainage could be tried and success in drainage has been reported in this scenario (Hookey et al. 2006; Baron et al. 2002; Kruger et al. 2006). One must be aware that for this indication, several procedures are often needed, usually as an inpatient, and usually with an endoscopically placed nasocystic irrigation catheter, flushing the cyst between procedures.

Single stents through a small cystgastrostomy often results in inadequate drainage, leading to infection and a poor outcome. Failure can also occur due to untreated underlying downstream pancreatic ductal obstruction and due to unexpected necrotic debris that may otherwise have needed extensive endoscopic necrosectomy and lavage, or due to unexpected septations that do not allow drainage of some parts of the cyst.

The use of routine EUS to guide endoscopic transmural drainage for bulging (Fig. 4) pseudocysts remains controversial. A randomized trial did not show a difference in success rates or complication rates (Kahaleh et al. 2006); however, it is required in cases of non-bulging pseudocysts. EUS is also helpful in detecting solid debris, assessing the distance between the gastrointestinal lumen and the pseudocyst lumen, in determining the maturity of the pseudocyst wall and in avoiding intervening vascular structures, including gastric varices. However, except for avoiding small vessels, MR can perform most of these functions

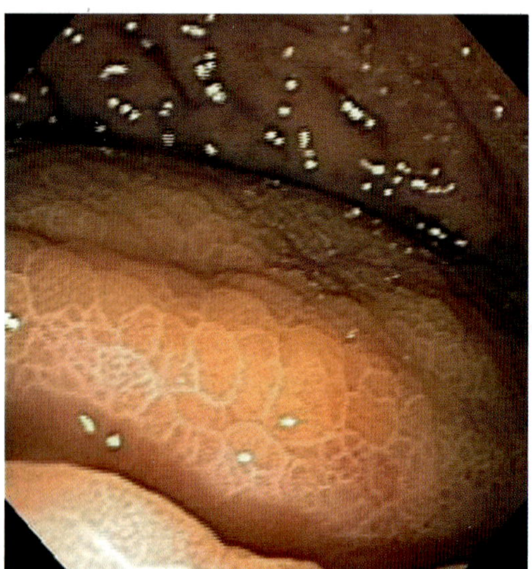

Fig. 4. An endoscopic view demonstrating a bulge in the body of the stomach from a compressing pseudocyst, with overlying congested mucosa.

very well and is more widely available. It is also likely more effective at assessing cyst contents and its relationship to other structures when the cyst is very large (>6–8 cm), as the back wall of the cyst will usually be too far away to be seen with EUS.

A retrospective study compared EUS-guided cystgastrostomy with surgery in patients with uncomplicated pancreatic pseudocysts (Varadarajulu et al. 2008). No significant differences were found in rates of treatment success (100% vs 95%, $P=0.36$), procedural complications (none in either cohort), or reinterventions (10% vs 0%, $P=0.13$) between surgery versus EUS-guided cyst-gastrostomy. The post-procedure hospital stay for EUS-guided cystgastrostomy was significantly shorter than for surgical cystgastrostomy (mean of 2.65 vs 6.5 days, $P=0.008$). The average direct cost per case for EUS-guided cystgastrostomy was significantly less than surgical cystgastrostomy ($9077 vs $14,815, $P = 0.01$; cost savings of $5738 per patient).

Technique of Cystgastrostomy/Duodenostomy

The endoscope (by visual bulge – Fig. 4) or EUS scope (by ultrasound image) is used to detect an optimal site of apposition of pseudocyst to the gastric or duodenal wall. EUS and color Doppler can be used to identify a vessel-free site for the puncture; alternatively, a miniprobe can be used to confirm that a borderline endoscopic bulge actually corresponds to an underlying cyst. The puncture is then made with either a 19 G needle (which can accommodate a guide wire) or a fine sclerotherapy needle, and a cystogram is performed under fluoroscopy. If a 19 G needle has been used, a wire can be passed through the needle and into the cyst; otherwise, a needle-knife sphincterotome or a cystotome (Fig. 5) can be used to burn a hole through the gastric wall and into the cyst cavity at the same site through which the transgastric cystography was performed, followed by a wire through the catheter. A large gauge (usually 0.035″) guide wire is generally chosen, and a generous amount of wire is curled up a few times in the cyst cavity under fluoroscopic guidance.

After wire access is achieved (Fig. 6), a dilating balloon is used to dilate the entry site (blunt dissection) (Fig. 7), or cautery can be used to enlarge the hole (regular or needle-knife

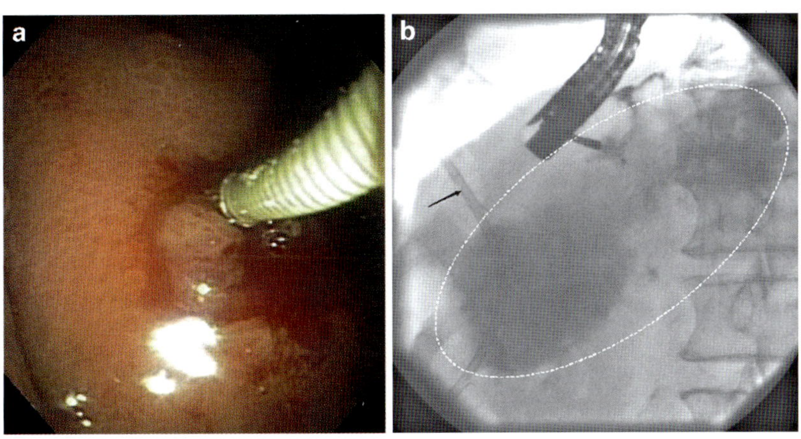

Fig. 5. A cystotome entering a pseudocyst through the gastric wall (**a**) after performing a partial transgastric cystogram (*dotted line*) using a fluoroscopically guided sclerotherapy needle inserted into the endoscopic bulge. (**b**) A biliary stent (*arrow*) had already been placed to relieve compression of the biliary tree by the cyst.

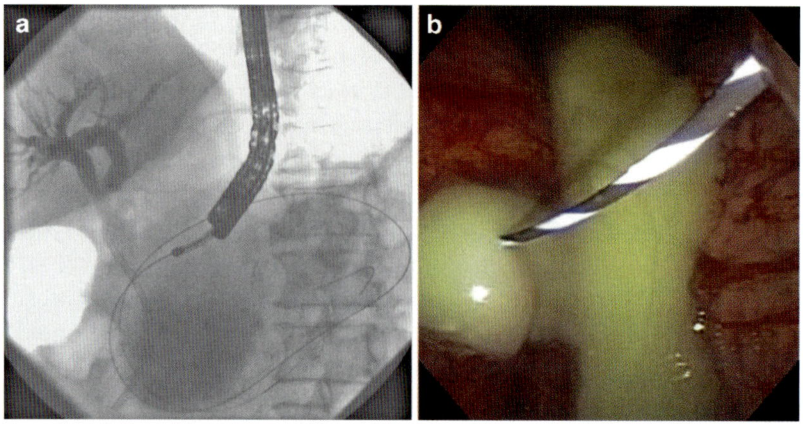

Fig. 6. Wire access to the cyst through the gastric wall. Wire coiled in the pseudocyst seen by fluoroscopy (**a**), with drainage of pseudocyst contents into the stomach around the wire seen endoscopically (**b**.)

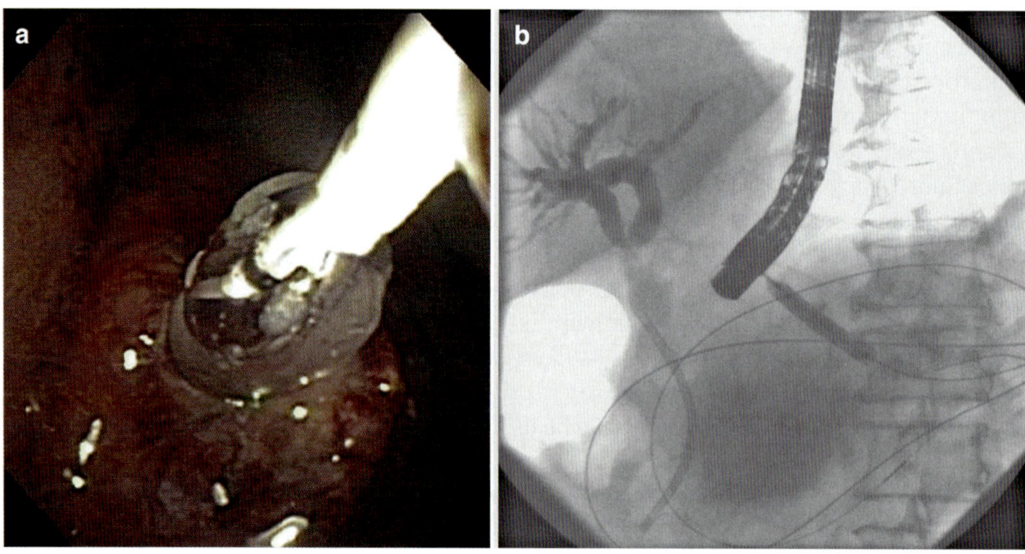

Fig. 7. An endoscopic (**a**) and fluoroscopic (**b**) view of a hydrostatic 6 mm balloon used to dilate the cystgastrostomy tract over a wire.

sphincterotome, or a cystotome); the former "cautery-free" technique may be associated with a lower bleeding risk, especially delayed bleeding (Mönkemüller et al. 1998 Aug). The size of the balloon used for dilation of the tract is based on the size of the cyst, presence of necrotic material, proximity of vessels and viscosity of the aspirated pseudocyst fluid, but is generally 6–8 mm. After dilation of the tract, a large amount of fluid can rapidly drain into the lumen, which requires aggressive prompt suctioning via the endoscope to prevent aspiration. Then, a double pigtail catheter (generally 7–10 F) is placed over the guide wire (Fig. 8), followed by recannulation alongside the first stent, replacing a wire in the cyst, and placing a second (or third) stent. If the cyst fluid appears very thick or particulate in consistency, then a nasocystic catheter to provide prolonged lavage of the cyst, for inpatients, can be considered to decrease the risk of stent/tract occlusion and infection.

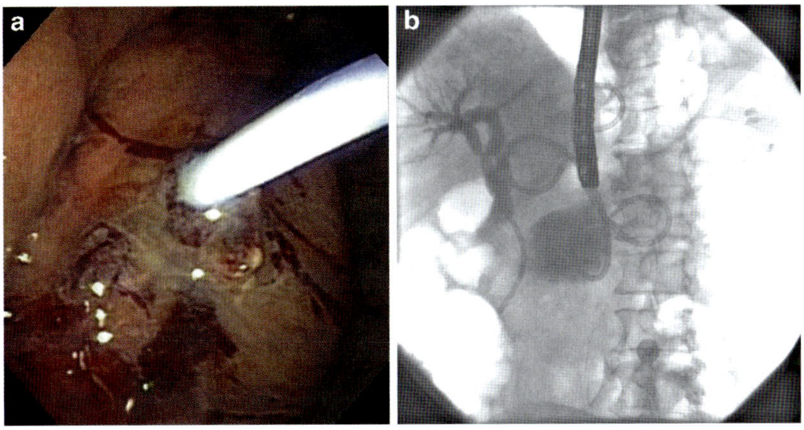

Fig. 8. A cystgastrostomy stent (**a**) was placed over the guide wire after balloon dilation, followed by placement of a double pigtail stent connecting the gastric lumen and the cyst lumen (**b**).

All patients receive a short course of antibiotics. If patients have concomitant biliary obstruction due to pseudocyst compression, they are usually treated with temporary biliary stent placement, with a subsequent repeat cholangiogram and removal of the biliary stent at a second ERCP a few months later. Although not mandatory, a pancreatogram is often helpful to exclude downstream ductal obstruction, exclude main duct disruption, and assess for a significant active duct leak in order to determine if a temporary pancreatic stent would be helpful. Recurrence is high after the transluminal stents are removed if an active leak is still present and downstream obstruction or disruption was not treated. Periampullary edema can sometimes be so severe (due to active pancreatitis or due to venous congestion from compression) that the ampulla is obscured and ERCP with selective cannulation may be difficult or impossible.

A follow-up CT scan (or EUS) in 1–2 months is then obtained, and, assuming there is no significant residual collection, the stents are removed at upper endoscopy with a snare. In patients whose pseudocysts have not resolved in 4–6 weeks, there are several options. First, one can wait. Second, one can assess the pancreatic duct for obstruction or disruption by pancreatography, with transpapillary stenting as needed. Third, one can dilate the transluminal tract and empirically replace the stents, or attempt additional transmural puncture of loculated areas. Multiple endoscopic sessions may be required in cases of persistent necrosis, with snare removal of necrotic debris under direct vision via the transluminal tract. Surgery should be considered for non-resolution of symptomatic pseudocysts, symptomatic recurrence without reversible factors, or in the presence of persistent symptomatic or infected walled off pancreatic necrosis (WOPN).

Transpapillary Drainage

For transpapillary pancreatic stent placement, a pancreatic sphincterotomy is usually performed, but is not mandatory, especially if chronic pancreatitis or intraductal stones are present. Stones are removed when possible, and strictures are dilated and stented. If there is no obstruction, but a leak is demonstrated into the cyst from the duct, a small caliber stent is reasonable as a trial. It is controversial whether the stent inner tip should be placed in the duct (as it would be for a bile duct leak), or in the cyst itself; the latter has more direct drainage, but stenting a blown-out side branch to a larger caliber duct may not be good in the long term. If the duct is partially disrupted, rejoining the duct with a stent over a wire, if the wire can bridge the disruption, is attempted (Kozarek et al. 1991; Telford et al. 2002) (Fig. 9). Prophylactic and post-procedural antibiotics are provided for a few days. The stent is generally pulled after satisfactory resolution of duct pathology on follow-up ERCP 1–2 months later.

If the cyst is accompanied by a complete main pancreatic duct disruption, it is unlikely that endoscopic therapy will ultimately succeed. Although the cyst may resolve, if one cannot reconnect the pancreas, the disconnected upstream pancreas will likely continue to cause obstructive symptoms (leak downstream from disruption) or cause the cyst to recur (leak upstream from disruption). Surgery should be strongly considered in these cases.

Complications and Their Avoidance

Complications of endoscopic pseudocyst drainage include secondary infection, bleeding, perforation, and stent migration. The frequency of these has been reported around (11–37%) in literature (Baron et al. 2002; Kahaleh et al. 2006; Antillon et al. 2006). Case selection is the key to reducing complications – not all "cysts" reported on CT can or should be treated with endoscopic drainage.

Infection is the most common complication following endoscopic drainage of pseudocysts. The infection usually develops due to malfunction or obstruction of stents or due to significant unrecognized necrosis. Use of peri- and post-procedural antibiotics can help reduce this risk. Fortunately, the majority of infectious complications can be managed endoscopically, or with percutaneous drainage of a loculated area; cases of multiloculated infected necrosis often requires surgery. Avoidance of this technique when there is significant necrosis, or in selected cases, early recognition of underlying pancreatic necrosis followed by extensive endoscopic debridement ("necrosectomy"), placement of nasal or percutaneous lavage drains, can reduce the need for surgical intervention for infection (Baron et al. 1996). As stated above, inadequate drainage from small transluminal tracts and/or single-stenting increases the risk of infection. FNA, contaminating the cyst, without complete drainage, can also lead to infection.

Significant bleeding can occur due to inadvertent puncture of a submucosal vessel or varix; this can generally be prevented by use of an EUS-guided puncture. Although rare, the presence of a pseudoaneurysm can lead to fatal hemorrhage either by guide wire trauma as it coils along the inside of the cyst, erosion of a transluminal stent, or simply due to rapid changes in size of the cyst. Preprocedure imaging can detect this. One study suggested that blunt dissection with a dilating balloon over a wire that is placed through a needle after a needle puncture (i.e., a Seldinger technique), without cautery, has a lower risk than using cautery to enter the cyst (Mönkemüller et al. 1998). However, it is not clear if the higher risk of a cautery approach still applies when the length of the cut that is made with cautery is limited (such as a small entry with a needle-knife), or when the cutting is done with a circumferential cauterizing device such as a cystotome. The Seldinger technique can be difficult with a side-viewing scope as the tip of the 19 G needle can be damaged by the elevator. Cases of needle tip fragmentation into the cyst have been reported.

Perforation has been reported to occur in about 3% of cases in the most recent series (Hookey et al. 2006; Antillon et al. 2006). Perforation is more likely to occur when the

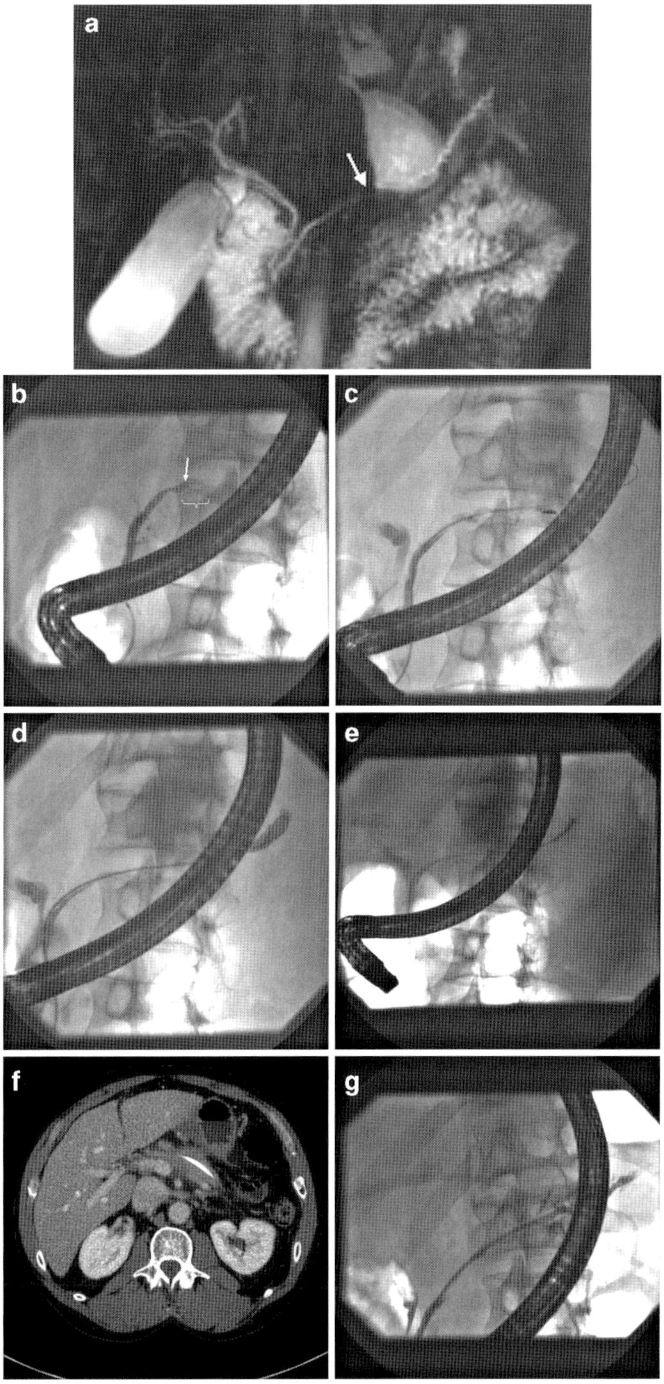

Fig. 9. A patient with alcoholic pancreatitis, persisting pseudocyst and pain. An image of a secretin-stimulated MRCP (**a**) and ERCP (**b**) leading to suspicion of a duct disruption (*small arrow*) as shown by a wisp of dye exiting from a partially cut-off pancreatogram in the body of the pancreas (*bracket*). The upstream duct (*PD*) appeared to be dilated on MRCP, and a wire was threaded across this area (**c**). Dye was injected to confirm that the wire was in the partially disconnected tail (**d**), and a stent was inserted (**e**). In follow-up, the cyst resolved on CT (**f**), and the pancreatic duct appeared to be reconnected (**g**).

pseudocyst wall is poorly defined by imaging studies, has a distance of greater than 1 cm from the intestinal lumen, or has not been present long enough to become adherent to the luminal structure into which it is being drained. Cystic tumors masquerading as pseudocysts are often not adherent to the GI lumen, as there is little or no inflammatory reaction around them, and they are more likely to be associated with perforation or free-air. Usually, free-air can be managed conservatively, with antibiotics and fasting, but emergent surgery may be required.

SUMMARY OF KEY POINTS

- Endoscopic drainage, with or without EUS-guidance, can be considered a first-line cyst drainage modality for symptomatic pseudocysts (pancreatic fluid collections (PFCs) persisting more than 4 weeks) adjacent to the gastrointestinal wall without contraindications.
- Surgery is generally reserved for salvage therapy, for complicated cysts (e.g., with infection, or significant necrosis), or those cases associated with complete duct disruptions.
- Transpapillary drainage with a pancreatic stent and/or sphincterotomy is useful for small pseudocysts with ductal communication, and is a useful adjunct to transluminal drainage when downstream ductal pathology exists.
- Acute PFCs, PNPFCs and WOPN, and cystic tumors can mimic pseudocysts, but require different interventions and have different considerations.
- Careful history-taking, waiting for cyst maturity, and US/MR/EUS imaging are key.
- Endoscopic transluminal therapy can be selectively considered for complicated pseudocysts (e.g., infected) or in symptomatic necrosis, in patients who are not good surgical candidates, but the safety and superiority over surgery is not as clear as in uncomplicated pseudocysts.
- Expertise in the technique of transluminal endoscopic debridement is limited to a very small number of endoscopists. Endoscopic approach requires inpatient lavage and generally multiple procedures.

REFERENCES

Abou-Assi S, Craig K, O'Keefe S. Prospective randomized trial of jejunal (EN) and intravenous (TPN) feeding in the management of acute pancreatitis. Gastroenterology. 2001;120:5.

Adams DB, Anderson MC. Percutaneous catheter drainage compared with internal drainage in the management of pancreatic pseudocyst. Ann Surg. 1992;215:571–8.

Antillon MR, Shah RJ, Stiegmann G, et al. Single-step EUS-guided transmural drainage of simple and complicated pancreatic pseudocysts. Gastrointest Endosc. 2006 May;63(6):797–803.

Baron TH, Thaggard WG, Morgan DE, et al. Endoscopic therapy for organized pancreatic necrosis. Gastroenterology. 1996 Sep;111(3):755–64.

Baron TH, Harewood GC, Morgan DE, et al. Outcome differences after endoscopic drainage of pancreatic necrosis, acute pancreatic pseudocysts, and chronic pancreatic pseudocysts. Gastrointest Endosc. 2002 Jul;56(1):7–17.

Boerma D, Obertop H, Gouma DJ. Pancreatic pseudocysts in chronic pancreatitis. Surgical or interventional drainage? Ann Ital Chir. 2000;71:43–50.

Bradley 3 EL. A clinically based classification system for acute pancreatitis. Summary of the International Symposium on Acute Pancreatitis, Atlanta, GA, September 11 through 13, 1992. Arch Surg. 1993;128:586–90.

Brown A, Hughes M, Tenner S, et al. Does pancreatic enzyme supplementation reduce pain in patients with chronic pancreatitis: a meta-analysis. Am J Gastroenterol. 1997 Nov;92(11):2032–5.

Brugge WR, Lauwers GY, Sahani D, et al. Cystic neoplasms of the pancreas. N Engl J Med. 2004a;351:1218–26.

Brugge WR, Lewandrowski K, Lee-Lewandrowski E, et al. Diagnosis of pancreatic cystic neoplasms: a report of the cooperative pancreatic cyst study. Gastroenterology. 2004b;126(5):1330–6.

Cahen D, Rauws E, Fockens P, et al. Endoscopic drainage of pancreatic pseudocysts: Long-term outcome and procedural factors associated with safe and successful treatment. Endoscopy. 2005;37:977–83.

Cremer M, Deviere J, Engelholm L. Endoscopic management of cysts and pseudocysts in chronic pancreatitis: long-term follow-up after 7 years of experience. Gastrointest Endosc. 1989 Jan-Feb;35(1):1–9.

D'Egidio A, Schein M. Pancreatic pseudocysts: a proposed classification and its management implications. Br J Surg. 1991;78:981–4.

El Hamel A, Parc R, Adda G, et al. Bleeding pseudocysts and pseudoaneurysms in chronic pancreatitis. Br J Surg. 1991 Sep;78(9):1059–63.

Gouyon P, Levy P, Ruszniewski P, Zins M, et al. Predictive factors in the outcome of pseudocysts complicating alcoholic chronic pancreatitis. Gut. 1997;41:821–5.

Hernandez-Aranda JC, Gallo-Chico B, Ramirez-Barba EJ. Nutrition support in severe acute pancreatitis. Controlled clinical trial. Nutr Hosp. 1996;11:160.

Hookey LC, Debroux S, Delhaye M, et al. Endoscopic drainage of pancreatic-fluid collections in 116 patients: a comparison of etiologies, drainage techniques, and outcomes. Gastrointest Endosc. 2006 Apr;63(4):635–43.

Imrie CW, Buist LJ, Shearer MG. Importance of cause in the outcome of pancreatic pseudocysts. Am J Surg. 1988;156:159–62.

Jacobson BC, Baron TH, Adler DG, et al. ASGE guideline: the role of endoscopy in the diagnosis and the management of cystic lesions and inflammatory fluid collections of the pancreas. Gastrointest Endosc. 2005;61:363–70.

Kahaleh M, Shami VM, Conaway MR, et al. Endoscopic ultrasound drainage of pancreatic pseudocyst: a prospective comparison with conventional endoscopic drainage. Endoscopy. 2006 Apr;38(4):355–9.

Kalfarentzos F, Kehagias J, Mead N, et al. Enteral nutrition is superior to parenteral nutrition in severe acute pancreatitis: results of a randomized prospective trial. Br J Surg. 1997;84:1665.

Kourtesis G, Wilson SE, Williams RA. The clinical significance of fluid collections in acute pancreatitis. Am Surg. 1990;56:796–9.

Kozarek RA, Ball TJ, Patterson DJ, et al. Endoscopic transpapillary therapy for disrupted pancreatic duct and peripancreatic fluid collections. Gastroenterology. 1991 May;100(5 Pt 1):1362–70.

Kruger M, Schneider AS, Manns MP, et al. Endoscopic management of pancreatic pseudocysts or abscesses after an EUS-guided 1-step procedure for initial access. Gastrointest Endosc. 2006 Mar;63(3):409–16.

Lee LS, Saltzman JR, Bounds BC, et al. EUS-guided fine needle aspiration of pancreatic cysts: a retrospective analysis of complications and their predictors. Clin Gastroenterol Hepatol. 2005 Mar;3(3):231–6.

Maringhini A, Uomo G, Patti R, et al. Pseudocysts in acute nonalcoholic pancreatitis: incidence and natural history. Dig Dis Sci. 1999;44:1669–73.

Marshall GT, Howell DA, Hansen BL, et al. Multidisciplinary approach to pseudoaneurysms complicating pancreatic pseudocysts. Impact of pretreatment diagnosis. Arch Surg. 1996 Mar;131(3):278–83.

McClave S, Greene L, Snider H, et al. Comparison of the safety of early enteral vs parenteral nutrition in mild acute pancreatitis. JPEN. 1997;21:14.

Mönkemüller KE, Baron TH, Morgan DE. Transmural drainage of pancreatic fluid collections without electrocautery using the Seldinger technique. Gastrointest Endosc. 1998 Aug;48(2):195–200.

Nealon WH, Walser E. Main pancreatic ductal anatomy can direct choice of modality for treating pancreatic pseudocysts (surgery versus percutaneous drainage). Ann Surg. 2002;235:751–8.

Pitchumoni CS, Agarwal N. Pancreatic pseudocysts. When and how should drainage be performed? Gastroenterol Clin North Am. 1999;28:615–39.

Pitkaranta P, Haapiainen R, Kivisaari L, et al. Diagnostic evaluation and aggressive surgical approach in bleeding pseudoaneurysms associated with pancreatic pseudocysts. Scand J Gastroenterol. 1991 Jan;26(1):58–64.

Romagnuolo J, Bardou M, Rahme E, et al. Magnetic resonance cholangiopancreatography: a meta-analysis of test performance in suspected biliary disease. Ann Intern Med. 2003 Oct 7;139(7):547–57.

Siegelman SS, Copeland BE, Saba GP, et al. CT of fluid collections associated with pancreatitis. AJR Am J Roentgenol. 1980;134:1121–32.

Telford JJ, Farrell JJ, Saltzman JR, et al. Pancreatic stent placement for duct disruption. Gastrointest Endosc. 2002 Jul;56(1):18–24.

van der Waaij LA, van Dullemen HM, Porte RJ. Cyst fluid analysis in the differential diagnosis of pancreatic cystic lesions: a pooled analysis. Gastrointest Endosc. 2005;62:383–9.

Varadarajulu S, Lopes TL, Wilcox CM, et al. EUS versus surgical cyst-gastrostomy for management of pancreatic pseudocysts. Gastrointest Endosc. 2008;68:649.

Wade JW. Twenty-five year experience with pancreatic pseudocysts. Are we making progress? Am J Surg. 1985;149:705–8.

Walt AJ, Bouwman DL, Weaver DW, Sachs RJ. The impact of technology on the management of pancreatic pseudocyst. Fifth Annual Samuel Jason Mixter Lecture. Arch Surg. 1990;125:759–63.

Windsor ACJ, Kanwar S, Li AGK, et al. Compared with parenteral nutrition, enteral feeding attenuates the acute phase response and improves disease severity in acute pancreatitis. Gut. 1998;42:431.

15 EUS-Guided Drainage of Pelvic Abscesses

Jessica Trevino and Shyam Varadarajulu

Contents

Keywords: EUS-Guided, Drainage, Pelvic, Abscesses, Transvaginal/Transrectal

INTRODUCTION

Deciding how to treat pelvic abscesses can pose a clinical dilemma. They usually occur after surgery or in patients with medical conditions such as Crohn's disease, diverticulitis, ischemic colitis, sexually transmitted diseases, or septic emboli from endocarditis. However, the anatomical challenges are what make this a clinical obstacle, with navigation needed around bony pelvis, bladder, bowel, reproductive organs in females, the prostate in men, rectum, and other neurovascular structures. Historically, pelvic abscesses necessitated surgery, ultrasound-guided transrectal or transvaginal intervention or were percutaneously drained under computed tomography (CT) guidance. Recently, there have been advances in the field of interventional endosonography that have opened a new avenue for drainage. This chapter will review the different treatment options for draining pelvic abscesses, with a focus on the technique of endoscopic ultrasound (EUS).

From: *Clinical Gastroenterology: Diagnostic and Therapeutic Procedures in Gastroenterology*,
Edited by: G. Y. Wu, S. Sridhar, DOI 10.1007/978-1-59745-044-7_15,

TRANSVAGINAL/TRANSRECTAL ULTRASOUND-GUIDED DRAINAGE

Ultrasound guidance has typically been performed using a transvaginal or transrectal approach (Sudakoff et al. 2005; Jaffe et al. 2004; Wroblicka and Kuligowska 1998; Kuligowska et al. 1995; Ryan et al. 2003). Passage through a transvaginal route was utilized because of the close proximity of the vaginal fornices to the pelvic fluid collections. In order to access the fluid collection, a catheter is attached to an endoluminal ultrasound probe which allows the passage of a needle for direct drainage. Only abscesses within the reach of the ultrasound probe can be drained using this technique. Other disadvantages with this procedure include the limitations of true sterility. Therefore, the transvaginal approach is generally limited to biopsy of solid lesions or for complete aspiration of cystic lesions (Varadarajulu 2007). Also, the procedure is associated with significant pain necessitating local infiltration with lidocaine. Attempts at transrectal drainage were evaluated in a study of 15 patients who had failed intravenous antibiotic therapy and had ill-suited collections for drainage attempts via colpotomy or transvaginal or transabdominal aspiration (Nelson et al. 2000). Out of the 15 women, 14 had return of purulent material and were successfully treated. However, some patients required an indwelling catheter for a prolonged period. Trans-rectal and trans-vaginal drainage remains limited by (1) the distance of the abscess from the ultrasound probe, (2) the inability to deploy stents for continued drainage, and (3) patient discomfort.

CT GUIDED DRAINAGE

Percutaneous abscess drainage was first introduced in the 1980s (Golfieri and Cappelli 2007). CT-guided drainage of pelvic abscesses utilizes a trans-gluteal approach if the abscess is posterior, and a transabdominal approach if located anterior (Jaffe et al. 2004). The initial step in all attempts at drainage should be needle aspiration to determine the nature of the collection and establish a differential diagnosis (Golfieri and Cappelli 2007). For collections smaller than 3 cm, simple aspiration usually suffices and percutaneous drainage is not necessary. Transabdominal anterior approach is the most preferred route secondary to technical ease. However, it is not always practical due to overlying bowel. If the fluid collection cannot be accessed via the anterior or lateral transabdominal approach, one can attempt to gain access through the greater sciatic foramen via the transgluteal approach while the patient is in the prone or lateral decubitus position (Golfieri and Cappelli 2007). Success rates range from 27% to 93%, with the variations caused by differing clinical characteristics, abscess location and morphology, and presence or absence of a fistula (Golfieri and Cappelli 2007). This procedure is associated with pain at the procedural site in up to 20% of patients, and limitations in ambulation and bed rest due to a catheter which protrudes through the buttocks in others (Harisinghani et al. 2003). Additional limitations include (1) possible injury to the inferior gluteal artery which may lead to hemorrhage or formation of a pseudoaneurysm in 2% of patients and, (2) an adequate window may not be identifiable at CT for placement of a drainage catheter in a substantial number of patients (Varadarajulu and Drelichman 2007; Trevino et al. 2008).

SURGERY

A large number of cases are a result of post-surgical complications. For this reason, the optimal treatment approach chosen should be the least invasive option. Initial surgical exploration and drainage should be limited to those patients who are clinically unstable with life-threatening infections. One study evaluated 500 cases of perirectal abscesses undergoing surgical drainage (Onaca et al. 2001). Of the 500 patients, 9.6% required re-intervention with four of these patients requiring a second re-intervention after initial drainage. The most common reason for re-intervention included initial inadequate drainage because of inadequate incision or premature closure.

WHY ENDOSCOPIC ULTRASOUND DRAINAGE?

The ability to visualize fluid collections that are extrinsic to the rectum extending up to the splenic flexure and intervene real-time under sonographic guidance makes EUS an ideal treatment modality for management of patients with pelvic abscesses (Varadarajulu 2007; Varadarajulu and Drelichman 2007; Trevino et al. 2008; Giovannini et al. 2003). This section will detail the procedural technique and treatment outcomes of patients who underwent EUS-guided drainage of pelvic abscesses.

PROCEDURAL TECHNIQUE

All patients should undergo a dedicated CT or MRI of the pelvis to define the anatomy and location of the abscess to ascertain if the fluid collection is amenable to transrectal EUS-guided drainage. Patients should receive prophylactic antibiotics (amoxicillin plus clavulanic acid, 2 g) and continue with antibiotics for 3 days. Prior to the procedure, patients should undergo local preparation with an enema to assist with optimal visualization and minimize contamination. It is essential that the procedure take place in a unit equipped with fluoroscopy to guide stent and drain placements within the abscess cavity. Also, patients should either void prior to the procedure or have an indwelling foley catheter to ensure that a distended bladder will not impair visualization of a small fluid collection or that the bladder is not mistaken for an abscess.

1. First, the abscess must be located using a curved linear array echoendoscope. Once located, intervening vasculature must be excluded using color Doppler. Under EUS guidance, a 19 gauge FNA needle is used to puncture the abscess cavity (Fig. 1). The stylet is removed and

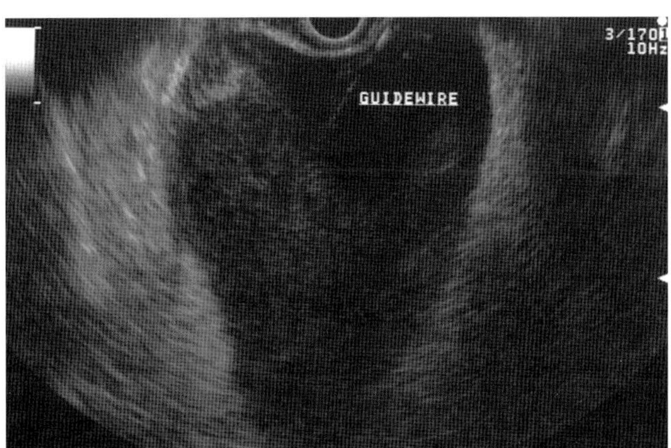

Fig. 1. A FNA needle is passed into the pelvic abscess under EUS-guidance and a guidewire is coiled within the abscess cavity.

the needle is flushed with saline and aspirated to remove as much pus as possible. At this time, a sample of purulent material can be collected for gram stain and culture.
2. With the needle in place, a 0.035 in. guidewire is passed through and coiled within the abscess. The needle is then exchanged over the guidewire for a 5Fr ERCP cannula to dilate the tract between the rectum and the abscess cavity. The tract is then further dilated using an 8-mm over the wire biliary balloon dilator (Fig. 2).
3. Once the tract is dilated, one or two 7 Fr 4 cm double pigtail trans-rectal stents are deployed (Fig. 3). The decision for one or two stents is dependent on the viscosity of the abscess contents: one is used if the fluid flows smoothly and two if the contents are thicker.

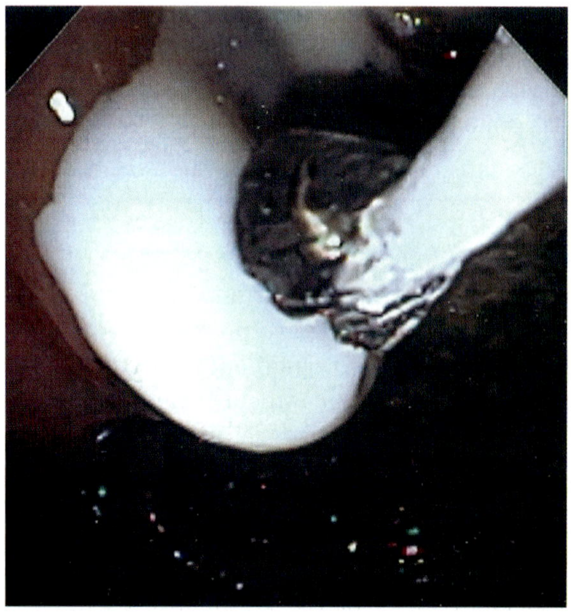

Fig. 2. The transmural tract is dilated to 8 mm with extrusion of pus.

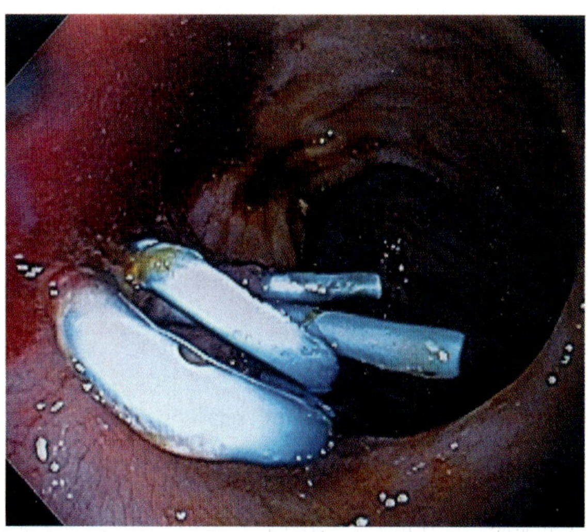

Fig. 3. Two double pigtail trans-rectal stents are deployed within the abscess cavity.

4. After the stents are deployed, the cavity is again accessed with a 5 Fr ERCP cannula to pass another 0.035 in. guidewire. A 10 Fr, 80 cm single pigtail drain is then deployed (Fig. 4). This drain will exit the anus and remain secured to the patient's gluteal region using tape. This drain is then flushed with 30 cc of normal saline every 4 h until the aspirate is clear.
5. Follow up CT should be obtained at 36–48 h to ensure the fluid collection has decreased in size. If there is greater than a 50% reduction in size of the abscess cavity, the drainage catheter can be removed and the patient discharged home.
6. The remaining stents can continue to assist with drainage and be removed in 2 weeks with sigmoidoscopy as long as a repeat CT of the pelvis shows complete abscess resolution.

TECHNICAL OUTCOMES

Three studies (Table 1) have evaluated the effectiveness of EUS for the treatment of pelvic abscesses (Varadarajulu and Drelichman 2007; Trevino et al. 2008; Giovannini et al. 2003). The first from Europe evaluated 12 patients using EUS guided trans-rectal stents (Giovannini et al. 2003). In this study, transrectal stents were deployed with a

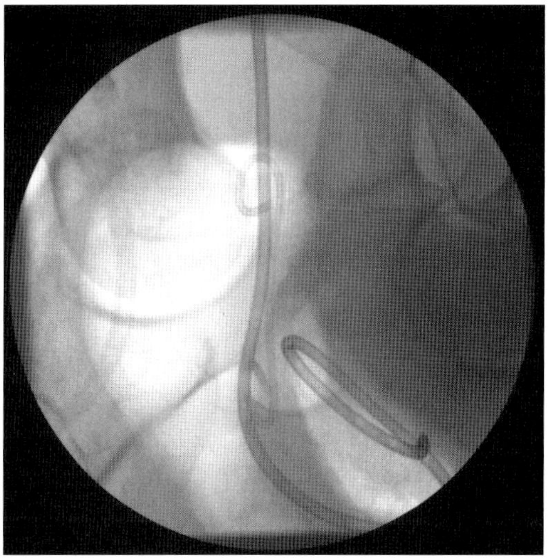

Fig. 4. A transrectal drainage catheter is seen within the pelvic abscess by fluoroscopy.

Table 1
EUS-guided drainage of pelvic abscess

Author	*No. of pts*	*Mean size (mm)*	*Drainage mode*	*Technical success rate (%)*
Giovannini et al. (2003)	12	48.9×43.4	Stent	75
Varadarajulu and Drelichman (2007)	4	68×72	Drainage catheter	100
Trevino et al. (2008)	4	93×61	Stent plus drainage catheter	100

successful clinical outcome in 8 of 12 patients (75%). The difficulty with trans-rectal stents is the high potential to clog easily, particularly by fecal matter or pus, and when left long-term can cause peri-rectal pain or migrate spontaneously. In the second study, this limitation was overcome by placement of transrectal drainage catheters in four patients (Varadarajulu and Drelichman 2007). Although the technical and treatment outcomes were successful, there was the potential for accidental dislodgement of the drainage catheter. Additionally, the need for periodic flushing and aspiration of the drainage catheter mandated a prolonged inpatient hospital stay for most patients. Therefore, a combined technique which included EUS-guided placement of a transrectal drainage catheter and stent for drainage of the pelvic abscess was adapted (Trevino et al. 2008). A short-term (36–48 h) drainage catheter provided access for continued evacuation of the abscess, while the medium-term (2 week) stent facilitated maintenance of a patent transmural tract for eventual abscess resolution. This combined therapy showed favorable outcomes for resolution of the fluid collections in all patients.

LIMITATIONS

Some limitations of EUS guided drainage include (1) multiple cavities are not be amenable to EUS-guided drainage, (2) abscesses greater than 20 mm distant from the gastrointestinal lumen preclude successful drainage, and (3) with the current limited maneuverability of echoendoscopes, accessing fluid collections which are located more proximal are not feasible.

SUMMARY OF KEY POINTS

- EUS-guided drainage is limited to those patients who have either failed US- or CT-guided drainage or those whose fluid collections are not amenable for those routes of drainage.
- Preliminary evidence reveals that EUS-guided drainage is a minimally invasive, safe and effective technique for management of patients with pelvic abscesses.
- More studies with larger numbers of patients are required to evaluate the technical and treatment outcomes of EUS-guided drainage, and cost-effectiveness studies are required comparing this technique with other modalities such as CT and ultrasound for drainage of pelvic abscesses.

REFERENCES

Giovannini M, Bories E, Moutardier V, et al. Drainage of deep pelvic abscesses using therapeutic echo endoscopy. Endoscopy. 2003;35:511–4.

Golfieri R, Cappelli A. Computed tomography-guided percutaneous abscess drainage in coloproctology: review of the literature. Tech Coloproctol. 2007;11(3):197–208.

Harisinghani MG, Gervais DA, Maher MM, et al. Transgluteal approach for percutaneous drainage of deep pelvic abscesses: 154 cases. Radiology. 2003;228:701–5.

Jaffe TA, Nelson RC, Delong DM, et al. Practice patterns in percutaneous image-guided intraabdominal abscess drainage: survey of academic and private practice centers. Radiology. 2004;233:750–56.

Kuligowska E, Keller E, Ferrucci JT. Treatment of pelvic abscesses: value of one-step sonographically guided transrectal needle aspiration and lavage. AJR Am J Roentgenol. 1995;164:201–6.

Nelson AL, Sinow RM, Olaik D. Transrectal ultrasonographically guided drainage of gynecologic pelvic abscesses. Am J Obstet Gynecol. 2000;6:1382–8.
Onaca N, Hirshberg A, Adar R. Early reoperation for perirectal abscess. Dis Colon Rectum. 2001;44:1469–73.
Ryan RS, McGrath FP, Haslam PJ, et al. Ultrasound-guided endocavitary drainage of pelvic abscesses: technique, results and complications. Clin Radiol. 2003;58:75–9.
Sudakoff GS, Lundeen SJ, Otterson MF. Transrectal and Transvaginal sonographic intervention of infected pelvic fluid collections. Ultrasound Q. 2005;21:175–85.
Trevino J, Drelichman ER, Varadarajulu S. Modified Technique for EUS-guided Drainage of Pelvic Abscess. Gastrointest Endosc. 2008 Dec;68(6):1215–9.
Varadarajulu S. EUS-Guided Drainage of Pelvic Abscess. Tech Gastrointest Endosc. 2007;9:51–4.
Varadarajulu S, Drelichman ER. EUS-guided drainage of pelvic abscess. Gastrointest Endosc. 2007;66:372–6.
Wroblicka JT, Kuligowska E. One-step needle aspiration and lavage for the treatment of abdominal and pelvic abscesses. AJR Am J Roentgenol. 1998;170(5):1197–203.

16 Technique of Endoscopic Ultrasound-Guided Fine Needle Aspiration (EUS-FNA)

Sreeram V.J. Parupudi
and Subbaramiah Sridhar

Contents

Keywords: Technique, Endoscopic, Ultrasound, Fine Needle Aspiration (EUS-FNA)

INTRODUCTION

The advent of endoscopic ultrasound (EUS) and guided fine needle aspiration (FNA) has significantly altered the management of benign and malignant gastrointestinal, biliary-pancreatic and mediastinal disorders. Over the past two decades, EUS has evolved from being a diagnostic imaging modality to an interventional modality. Several evolving therapeutic applications are paving the way to previously unimaginable procedures such as transluminal endosurgery (Giovannini 2004). The technique of EUS-guided fine needle aspiration (EUS-FNA) forms the basis for all of the more invasive applications such as

From: *Clinical Gastroenterology: Diagnostic and Therapeutic Procedures in Gastroenterology*,
Edited by: G. Y. Wu, S. Sridhar, DOI 10.1007/978-1-59745-044-7_16,

EUS-guided celiac ganglion neurolysis, pseudocyst drainage, pancreatic necrosectomy, periluminal abscess drainages, transgastric or transduodenal biliary-pancreatic drainage procedures etc (Giovannini 2004; Fritscher-ravns 2006).

The advantages of EUS-FNA are: (1) tissue diagnosis for intramural or periluminal lesions in relation to the GI tract, EUS-FNA, (2) detection and aspiration of even small sub-centimeter lymph nodes in posterior mediastinal, para-celiac and peri-portal regions for staging of malignancies, (3) access to anatomically difficult locations like aorto-pulmonary window (4) FNA of smaller lesions in pancreas, (5) in seriously ill patients such as severe necrotizing pancreatitis with fluid collections EUS guided procedures are preferable due to relatively less invasive nature of the procedure, (6) EUS guided procedures are possible even bedside in intensive care situations due to the mobility of equipment, and (7) in providing a needle access to the periluminal structures.

INDICATIONS

Diagnostic indications for US-FNA include evaluation of mediastinal and intra-abdominal lymph nodes, staging of lung cancer by evaluation of contra-lateral lymph nodes, staging of esophageal cancer by evaluation of para-celiac nodes, staging biliary-pancreatic cancers by evaluation of peri-portal/para-celiac lymph nodes, staging of ano-rectal cancers by evaluation of peri-rectal nodes. In addition, periluminal fluid collections such as small pleural effusions can be sampled, when malignancy is suspected (not accessible by US/CT guided thoracentesis), minimal ascites, when malignancy is suspected (not otherwise detected nor accessible by US/CT guided thoracentesis), peri-pancreatic fluid collection when infected pancreatic necrosis is suspected, post-surgical periluminal collections (anastomotic leaks as in peri-esophago-gastric, peri-rectal, gall bladder fossa), pseudocyst drainage, especially in the absence of a transluminal bulge or in the presence of periluminal blood vessels.

Sampling of focal lesions to exclude malignancy such as focal pancreatic lesions, suspicious biliary strictures, suspected adrenal metastases, suspected hepatic/splenic lesions, suspicious sub-mucosal lesions.

Therapeutic indications include drainage of pseudocysts, celiac ganglion neurolysis/ block, EUS-guided biliary-pancreatic drainage, drainage of abscesses (mediastinal/intra-abdominal/perirectal), and fine needle injection.

CONTRAINDICATIONS

Absolute contraindications include suspected bowel perforation, severe uncorrected coagulopathy (advanced liver disease, DIC). Relative contraindications include combative, difficult-to-sedate patient (suspect excessive alcohol use, delirium tremens or narcotic over use; preferable to proceed under general anesthesia), ongoing use anti-coagulant or anti-platelet agents, and luminal narrowing.

PRE-EVALUATION

It is preferable to pre-evaluate well in advance when consultation or referral was made for the procedure or definitely immediately prior to the procedure. Such evaluations include review of the indication, review of the available investigations, particularly any imaging (US, CT, MR) to determine the region of interest, nature of the suspected lesion and its approximate location, size, and its location vis-à-vis standard anatomical structures, if available. This greatly facilitates the rapid detection and evaluation of the lesion by EUS and potentially reduces the procedure time, and review of potential risks for sedation and safe intubation of the echoendoscope.

PREPARATION

Proper preparation is critical to optimize the safety of the procedure. Preparations should include overnight, or at least 6 h, fasting, correction of bleeding tendency, discussion and counseling of the patient regarding the details of procedure, including the need for avoiding abrupt movements during lighter planes of conscious sedation, pre-procedural antibiotics while accessing peri-luminal fluid collections, duplication cysts, cystic lesions or pseudocyst drainage, EUS-guided drainage of obstructed biliary-pancreatic system and transrectal FNA or interventions, pre-procedural benzocaine spray of posterior pharyngeal wall.

POSITION

The left lateral position of the patient is generally suitable for most indications. The left lateral semi-prone position may be useful for difficult to access lesions in the head-uncinate region of pancreas. Non-dependent gastric antral and peri-rectal lesions can be accessed in supine position. Occasionally, we have used the sitting position with a 75° back rest for mediastinal lesions in patients with severe COPD and respiratory failure or in the presence of superior vena cava syndrome.

EQUIPMENT

The Echoendoscope

Curved linear-array echoendoscopes are available from Pentax, Olympus and Toshiba-Fujinon (Table 1). While most experience is with the instruments from the former two manufacturers, for routine indication for EUS-FNA, the choice of instrument should not matter. There are differences amongst these instruments in terms of the length of the bending section of the echoendoscope, size and resolution of the transducer, length of the working channel, available diameters of the working channel, etc (Yusuf et al. 2007). Although these differences are not enormous, it helps to be familiar with the equipment if different instruments are used routinely.

The most important difference between the Olympus and the Pentax instrument that have practical implications are that in the Pentax scope, the transducer and the bending section are longer and, hence, caution is warranted while maneuvering the scope around the posterior pharyngeal curve and while intubating the duodenal bulb to enter the second part of duodenum (Fig. 1). The suction channel for the endoscope is separate from that of the balloon and it needs to be manually switched from scope (S) position to balloon (B) as desired (Fig. 2).

Another type of echoendoscope used for EUS-FNA is a mechanical linear instrument from Olympus (Fig. 3). The advantage of this scope is that it is more economical, compatible with the diagnostic radial equipment, and because it is mechanical, it does not require a dedicated US console. The main drawback is the lack of color Doppler. Currently, this model is no longer marketed.

Table 1
Curvi-linear echoendoscopes (CLE) for EUS-FNA

Instrument	*Electronic/ Mechanical*	*Working channel (mm)*	*Working length (cm)*	*Scope-balloon suction*
OLYMPUS				
GF-UMD140P	M	2.8	124.4	Dual level
GF-UC30P	E	2.8	126	Dual level
GF-UC140(P)-AL5	E	3.7 (2.8)	125	Dual level
GF-UC160(P)-OL5	E	3.7 (2.8)	125	Dual level
PENTAX				
EG-3630U	E	2.4	125	Separate
EG-3830UT	E	3.8	125	Separate

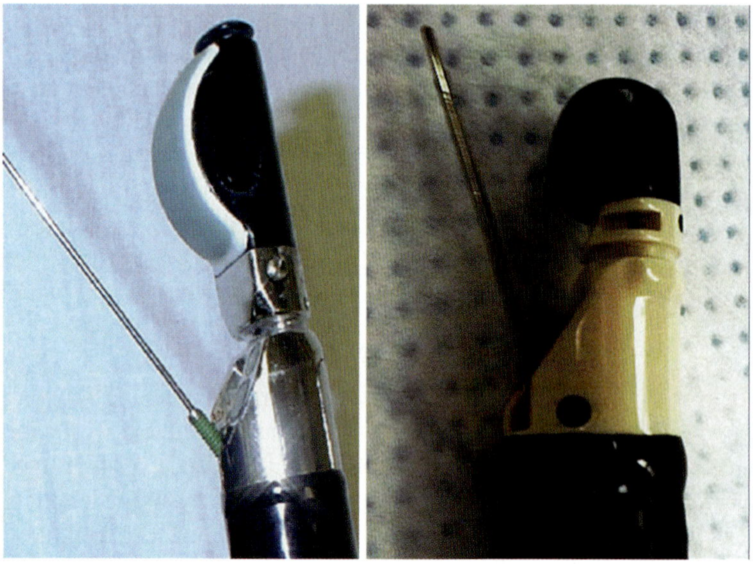

Fig. 1. Curvi-linear echoendoscopes from Olympus (*top*) and Pentax (*bottom*).

Prior Radial EUS

Although in expert hands radial EUS is not necessary when EUS-FNA is planned, in general it is a good practice to perform a quick radial EUS before proceeding for tissue diagnosis. Recent trends favor the use of linear scopes with idea of tissue acquisition (Noh et al. 2007). However, in the early phase of learning and while performing the procedure for cancer staging, it is preferable to do an initial diagnostic radial EUS to delineate the anatomy, location and echomorphology. This would greatly help with the orientation when CLE is used for EUS-FNA, and also helps in developing a plan for the puncture of the target lesions. In presence of a suspected metastasis, it is often helpful to sample the metastatic

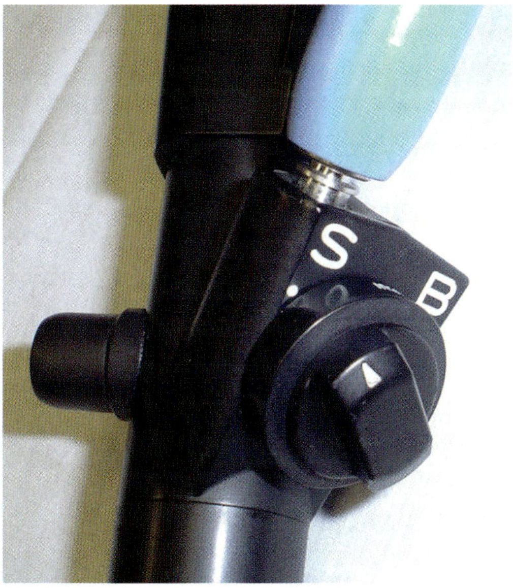

Fig. 2. Pentax instrument. The suction channel for the endoscope is different from that of the balloon and the knob has to be manually switched from scope (*S*) position to balloon (*B*) as desired.

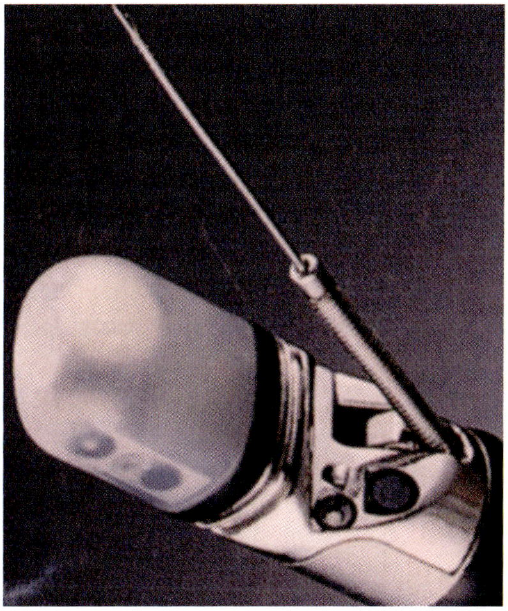

Fig. 3. Mechanical linear video echoendoscope from Olympus.

lesion before puncturing the primary tumor for tissue diagnosis to avoid using separate set of needles. If suspected metastatic lesions are present in more than one location, the farthest lesion should be sampled first, since the implications or positivity would be different in terms of staging of the lesion (such as presence of para-celiac and periportal lymph nodes in a patient with a focal pancreatic lesion in the head-uncinate region).

The Needle

Various needles are available across the world (Table 2) (Vilmann and Săftoiu 2006; Adler et al. 2007). GIP/Mediglobe needles are relatively more popular in Europe, while Wilson-Cook needles are more widely used in the US. The Cook needle systems are disposable, and are available in 25 G, 22 G and 19 G sizes besides a disposable trucut biopsy needle. Olympus makes a reusable handle and outer sheath with a disposable needle-stylet in 22 G and 25 G, and a spring-loaded biopsy needle as well. Both these needle systems have adjustable lengths of the sheath, and the needle has separate screws to maintain the selected position for use with various echoendoscopes (Fig. 4). It is important to check every time to ensure that the sheath of the needle system used is adequately exiting the working channel of the echoendoscope and its tip is visible endoscopically to avoid expensive damage to the instrument.

In general, 22 G needles are easier to handle, and the tissue sample is adequate for interpretation. The quality and quantum of the aspirate is better with 19 G, and at times it is possible to obtain tissue cores adequate for histology. However, the 19 G needle is sturdier and more difficult to maneuver while using for transduodenal indications. The main advantage of the 19 G needle is in EUS-guided interventions such as pseudocyst drainage, or transgastric or transduodenal biliary-pancreatic interventions where a 0.035″ guide wire can be deployed through the needle whereas the 22 G needle allows only a thin 0.018″ guide wire which is difficult to maintain position, and exchange accessories for further interventions. Recent studies demonstrated the non-inferiority of using 25 G needles, which may even prove to be useful in puncturing difficult pancreatic head lesions (Yusuf et al. 2009; Savides 2009).

The nature of the stylet used with the needle has an important bearing on the outcomes. Rounded tip stylets are safer in terms of avoiding accidental scope damage.

Table 2
Commonly used EUS-FNA needles

Needle	*Gauze*	*Sheath*	*Adjustable sheath*	*Disposable (D)/Reusable (R)*
Wilson-Cook				
ECHO-1–22	22G	Plastic	+	D
ECHO-19	19G	Metal spiral	+	D
ECHO-25	25G	Flexible	+	D
Olympus				
MAJ-365 (Handle)/ NA-10-J-1	22G	Metal spiral	+	Handle, sheath (R); Needle (D)
NA-200H-8022	22G	Hard plastic	–	D
Mediglobe				
Hancke-Vilman	19–22G	Metal spiral	–	R
Sonotip II	19–22G	Coated metal	+	D

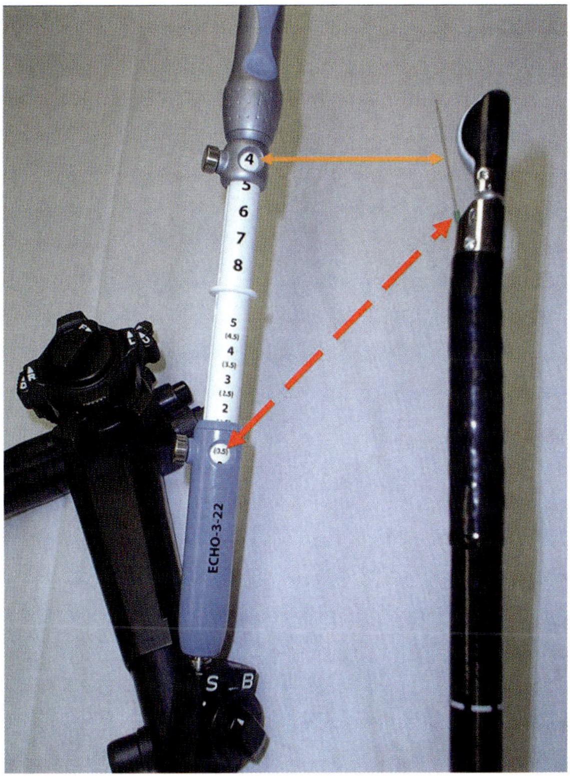

Fig. 4. Positioning the sheath and needle. The length of the sheath can be adjusted to keep it extended just beyond the bridge or elevator of the echoendoscope with a dedicated screw (*arrow with solid lines*). This can vary depending on the instrument used. The length of the needle can be separately adjusted as desired (*arrow with broken lines*).

But, they have to be withdrawn by a centimeter into the needle just before puncturing the luminal wall to allow the beveled tip of the needle to come into contact with the tissue (Fig. 5). On the other hand, while using the beveled tip stylets, one has to be obsessive to ensure that the needle is well within the channel, using the tightening screw on the handle (Fig. 4).

Suction Syringes

While most syringes use low volume suction while performing the EUS-FNA, one could sample soft, fleshy lesions that do not offer much resistance to the needle without suction, to avoid excessively bloody specimens. Some authors have demonstrated that 5–10 mL suction is better than 20 mL, and that continuous is better than intermittent suction. Unless the initial pass yields a bloody specimen, the quality of the aspirate is, in general, better by using suction (Savides 2009; Yamao et al. 2009; Puri et al. 2009). Using the special suction syringes provided with the needles is preferable. Occasionally one could improvise using a regular 10 mL syringe to apply suction by an assistant

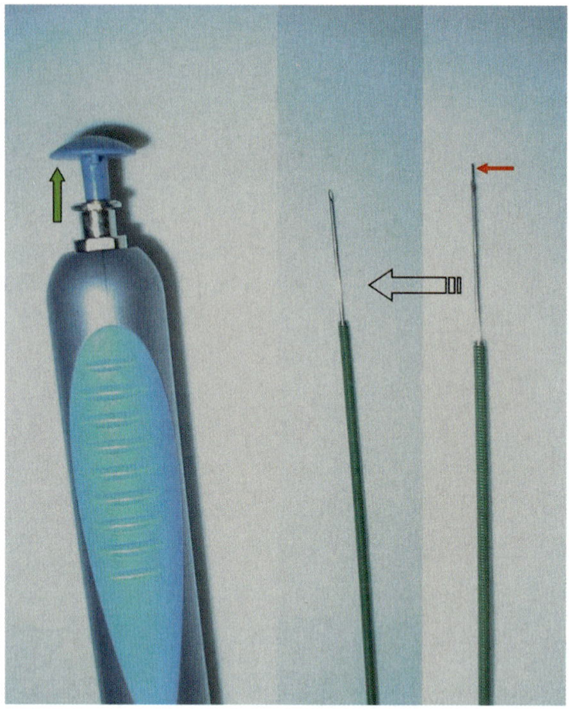

Fig. 5. Positioning the stylet. A rounded tip stylet avoids accidental scope damage, but it has to be withdrawn by a centimeter into the needle just before puncturing the luminal wall.

with a 3-way lock to maintain it. Having a 3-way attachment routinely between the suction syringe and the needle is useful to keep the syringe prepared with the suction and the 3-way in closed position. Once the needle is within the target, the nurse assistant could connect the 3-way suction syringe after removing the stylet to apply suction (Fig. 6). After 5–10 back and forth movements of the needle, depending on operator preference, the assistant or the operator releases the suction slowly while the needle tip is still within the lesion (Fig. 7). While gradually releasing the suction prior to withdrawing the needle ensures loss of aspirated material into the suction syringe, use of the 3-way attachment avoids the need to release the suction within the needle. However, one has to remember to disconnect the 3-way lock to reinsert the stylet for extracting the aspirated material from the hollow core of the needle and not try to release the 3-way lock.

TECHNIQUE

The basic technique of EUS-guided fine needle aspiration is similar across the GI tract, with certain variations according to the site (Vilmann and Săftoiu 2006; Savides 2009; Yamao et al. 2009; Erickson 2004; Fritscher-Ravens et al. 2000a, b; Binmoeller and Rathod 2002).

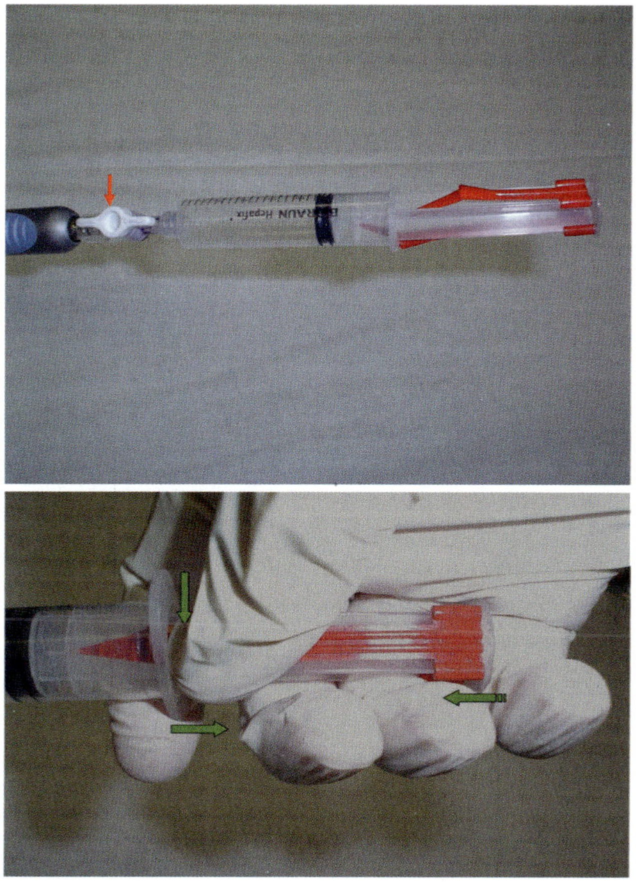

Fig. 6. (**a**) Positioning the suction syringe. When the needle is within the target and the stylet is removed, the three-way suction syringe could be attached to the needle and the three-way knob could be twisted to be in line with the needle to allow suction. (**b**) Tissue sampling. Once the lesion is sampled, while the needle tip is still within the lesion, the suction could be slowly released pressing the red stopper on the syringe with the thumb and holding the piston between the thumb and index fingers to let it slowly slide towards the syringe carefully, avoiding sudden release of suction.

The steps of the procedure are identification of the target lesion, maneuvering the echoendoscope to align the lesion in the projected path of the needle, stabilizing the transducer in the chosen position, apposing the transducer close against the GI wall, color Doppler evaluation of the projected path of the needle to insure a safe path devoid of vessels, advancing the needle out of the channel to puncture the GI wall and the lesion, sampling the targeted lesion with or without suction, withdrawal of the needle out of the lesion and removal from the scope, and transfer of the sampled tissue or fluid for cyto-pathology.

Identification/Selection of the Target Lesion

Most often, the target lesion is obvious from the pre-procedural workup. It is important to review the available imaging such as CT scans for the primary lesion, presence of

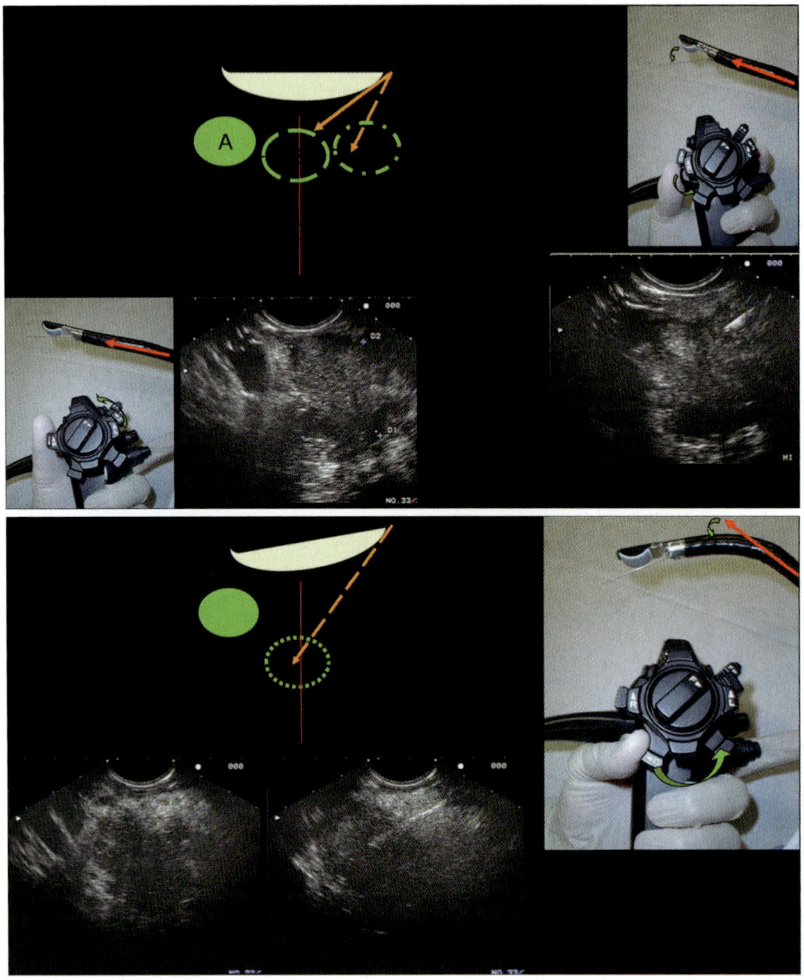

Fig. 7. (**a**) Approach to the lesion. Drawing an imaginary path of the needle, the scope is maneuvered in such way as to bring the lesion in to A, B, or C positions by either gently advancing the scope further, while maintaining the lesion within range of imaging, and by the use of elevator as demonstrated in a pancreatic head mass. (**b**) Aiming the needle. Further maneuvering to align the needle and the lesion could also be achieved by turning the big wheel upwards to change the angle of exit of the needle without straining the elevator as demonstrated in the same case as above.

enlarged regional or distant lymph nodes and for any metastatic lesions such as liver metastases or ascites. It is also important to assess the potential impact of the proposed procedure. Sampling the para-celiac nodes is important in case of distal esophageal malignancies as well as lesions in head and uncinate region of pancreas or bile duct tumors. Sampling of pleural effusion or ascites is important if minimal amounts are detected when otherwise not suspected on prior imaging. This could potentially indicate advanced stage and inoperability, if positive for malignancy. Nodal metastases could help determining the need for adjuvant chemo-radiotherapy in esophageal and rectal cancers.

Alignment of the Lesion in the Projected Path of the Needle

The side from which the needle exits on the screen is marked by a white dot outside the image indicating the oral-caudal orientation. Most Europeans orient the image with this dot on the left side, while American endosonologists use the opposite orientation. Once the needle is extended out of the channel, it is visualized as a bright linear structure. Drawing an imaginary path of the needle, the scope is maneuvered in such a way as to bring the lesion into A, B, C or D positions, as depicted in Figs. 7a and 7b, by gently advancing the scope further, all the while maintaining the lesion within range of imaging. Further maneuvering to align the needle with the lesion can be achieved by the use of an elevator or turning the big wheel upwards to change the angle of exit of the needle.

Stabilizing the Transducer

After the target lesion is aligned, the position of the transducer has to be maintained while the operator is trying to adjust the parameters on the ultrasound console, or switching on the color Doppler or performing the needle aspiration. The options available are 'fixing' the scope position by the use of "F-knob" on the big wheel (controlling the up-down movement), maintaining the direction and hand-body position of the operator (controlling the left-right movement and torque), and having an assistant to hold the scope position at the bite-guard. A combination of these maneuvers offers the best possibility to maintain the stable position of the transducer.

Apposition of the Transducer

To ensure that there is no gap between the transducer and the wall to be punctured, the position of the transducer is stabilized as described above. Gentle suction and decompression of the bowel lumen helps by removing any interfering air artifacts. At times, inflating the balloon on the transducer with water also helps achieving the best apposition and acoustic coupling to facilitate the needle puncture. If balloon inflation is used, it is advisable to extend the needle out of the channel by about 1 cm and then inflate the balloon in order to avoid puncturing the balloon.

Color Doppler Evaluation

Use of color Doppler imaging to evaluate the projected path of the needle ensures a passage devoid of large vessels. Even with Doppler scanning, most significant vessels can be detected by the appearance of anechoic linear structures that could be traced by following their course by EUS. In the event of suspicious vascular structures in the path of the needle, these can be avoided by changing the position of the transducer and the projected needle path by gently adjusting the transducer. Maintaining the hand-scope position, rotation of the scope tip by mild left or right rotation of the body of the operator can change the angle. Rarely, minimal torque on the scope by an assistant is useful to complete the procedure. When using color Doppler, it is important to adjust the noise level on the console to avoid artifacts. Microvessels within the tumor due to hypervascularity need not preclude EUS-FNA (Fig. 8). In such lesions, some amount of bloody aspirate is expected and cannot be avoided. But, this can be minimized by using less or no suction while sampling such lesions or smaller caliber needles.

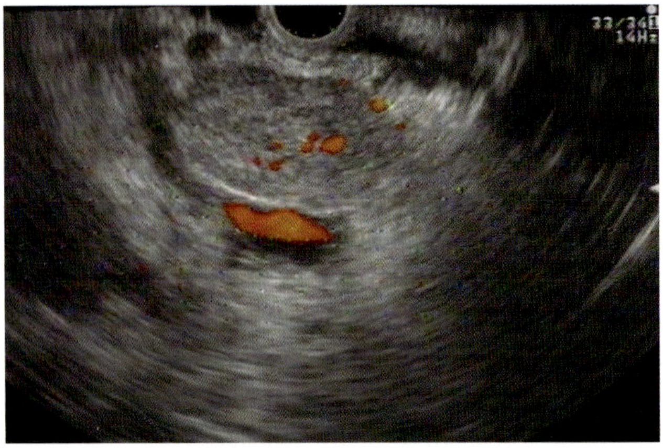

Fig. 8. Color Doppler evaluation. This is useful to avoid significant vessels in the projected path of the needle. Microvessels due to hypervascularity of the tumor need not preclude EUS-FNA.

Needle Puncture

Once the target is chosen, the transducer is positioned, the needle path is determined, measuring the distance from the center of the lesion to the site of exit of the needle provides an approximate idea of the length of needle to be extended. Accordingly, the screw on the handle of the needle is adjusted to the limit of the extended depth of penetration of the needle (Fig. 4). It is useful to allow an additional 1–2 cm to compensate for yield of the tissues or movement of the GI wall away from the transducer during puncture. Alternately, while puncturing critical areas like the aorto-pulmonary window, one could start with a shorter needle length and adjust as appropriate as the needle is advanced.

While 19 G needles come with a round-tipped stylet that extends about 1 cm beyond the beveled tip, 22 G needles have an option of a beveled stylet that is flush with the bevel of the needle or a round-tipped stylet that extends beyond the bevel. While using the needles with round tipped stylets, the stylet has to be withdrawn by 1 cm to allow the beveled needle tip to come in contact with the mucosal surface to enable puncture. Some prefer to remove the stylet altogether before the puncture. However, it is important to be aware that in the absence of the stylet, the cellular material from the tissues traversed while reaching the target lesion will be admixed with the aspirate. This could become an issue when dealing with well-differentiated malignancies (Mitsuhashi et al. 2006).

The degree of difficulty of EUS-FNA varies with location (Table 3) increasing from trans-esophageal to transduodenal to transgastric lesions by site. It is obvious that the EUS-guided therapeutic interventions are more complicated than the EUS-FNA. But, the common requirement for any advanced EUS-guided interventions is mastery of the technique of EUS-FNA. Sampling of large mediastinal masses, or enlarged mediastinal lymph nodes are the easiest and should be the first lesions to start with. Puncturing these lesions in a relatively closed space is relatively easy with the fixed structures offering counter resistance to advancement of the needle (Figs. 9 and 10).

The difficulty with the pancreatic head lesions is mostly due to the issues with positioning of the transducer, and the curvature of the bending section of the scope making it difficult to advance needle. The other issues are inherent to the nature of the lesions as in presence

Table 3
Level of difficulty in various EUS guided procedures

Level	*Location*	*Lesions*	*Unique features and tricks*
I	Mediastinum	Large tumors	Transesophageal sampling from lesions closely apposing the esophageal wall is the easiest to puncture (Fig. 9).
		Lymph nodes	• Subcarinal and lower para-esophageal are relatively easy to access (Fig. 10). • Having an assistant hold the position of the scope helps while aspirating nodes proximally located in the paratracheal and aorto-pulmonary window.
II	GE Junction	Fundal masses	• Almost similar to lower mediastinal lesions. • Apposing the transducer to the lesion or the GI wall is the key. • Diaphragm and adjacent structures offer counter resistance facilitating puncture.
	Liver	Metastases	• Accessible lesions in this large organ offer a relatively easier target
	Structures in relation to posterior gastric wall	• Paraceliac lymph nodes • Tumors of pancreatic body-tail	• Initial evaluation with radial EUS helps in orientation of the structures in relation to the vessels, pancreas and distance from the GE junction.
		• Peripancreatic lymph nodes	• Identifying the aorta, celiac and superior mesenteric vessels with the CLE and then correlating with the findings of initial radial EUS helps localizing the smaller lesions.
		• Left adrenal metastases • Fluid collections	• Position of the transducer to bring the target lesions in the imaginary path of the needle and have an assistant hold the scope orientation and position at the mouth piece. • To compensate for the yield of tissues, it is useful to allow about 1 cm longer length of needle than the estimated distance of the lesion from the scope. • Softer or easily displaced lesions are accessible by initial transgastric puncture until the lesion and subtle adjustment of position to keep the target directly in line with the tip of the needle and use a quick 'jab' movement to enter the lesion.
	Perirectal	Lymph nodes	• Access to the lower perirectal lesions is like periesophageal lesions. • The technique for the rectosigmoid lesions is similar to that described above.

Table 3 (continued)

Level	*Location*	*Lesions*	*Unique features and tricks*
III	Transduodenal	Lymph nodes in relation to pancreatic head, hepatic hilum Pancreatic head-uncinate tumors	• 19G needles are difficult to maneuver for transduodenal sampling due to multiple levels of bending of the scope.
		Biliary strictures	• Short scope position is most suitable for EUS-FNA, hence the time taken to proper positioning of the scope in relation to the lesion is well spent. • Using the big wheel to alter the direction or orientation of the needle is preferable to the use of the elevator while accessing the lesions in head and uncinate region of pancreas. • Lesions in the head-genu region are accessible through the duodenal bulb. • Distal biliary strictures are more accessible in short route along the medial duodenal wall. • Proximal biliary strictures are accessible from the duodenal bulb using torsion on the scope to change the orientation towards the superior fornix of the duodenal bulb. • Presence of biliary stent serves as an identifiable structure to trace sonologically, either proximally or distally to detect and target the lesion.
	Gastric body (anterior wall, greater curve), antrum	Intramural lesions	• Most difficult lesions to access due to the mobility of the stomach lacking any adjacent structures to offer a firm counter resistance. • The lesions get displaced as the needle is advanced and are best punctured by a 2-step method. • Initial step is to puncture the gastric wall advancing the needle tip closer to the lesion aligning it and the next step is a quick jab like movement (like *spear fishing*). • Part of the difficulty of sampling these lesions is also because of the nondependent position of the antrum making it difficult to obtain a proper acoustic coupling in left lateral position. At times, changing the patient to supine helps.
IV	EUS-guided interventions	Celiac ganglion neurolysis Pseudocyst drainage Bilioma drainage Pancreatic cyst ablation Biliary-pancreatic ductal access	

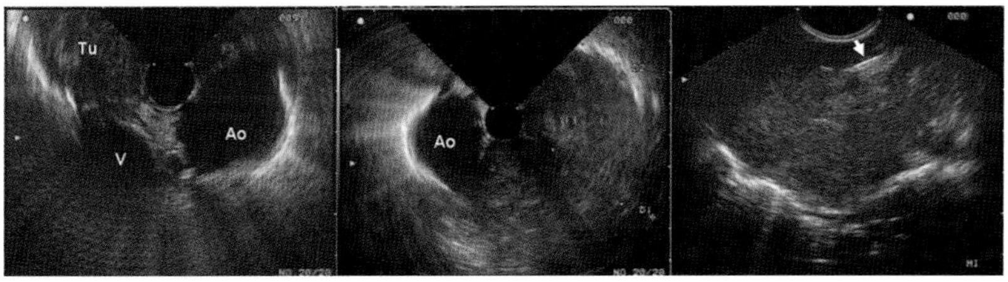

Fig. 9. Lung cancer. Large periesophageal tumor (*Tu*), predominantly in anterior location as seen on initial radial EUS (Pentax EG-3630UR) with the vertebra (*V*) at 6 o'clock, and the aorta (*Ao*) at 5 o'clock positions (*left image*). Rotating the scope by 180° brings almost the entire tumor into view (*middle image*). 19 G Fine needle (*arrow*) aspiration using Pentax EG-3630U revealed squamous cell lung cancer.

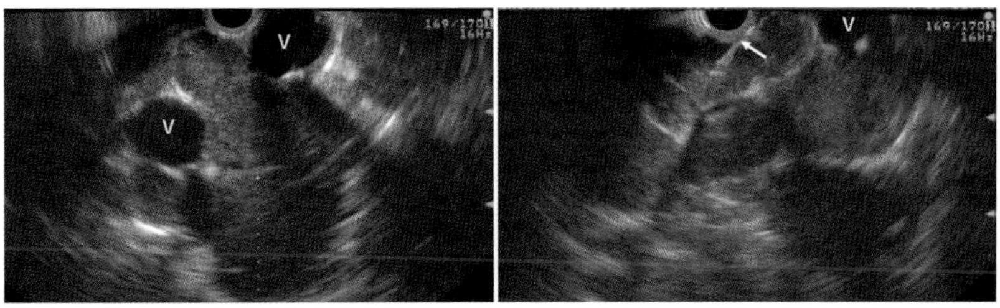

Fig. 10. Lymph nodes. Enlarged mediastinal lymph nodes in relation to vascular structures (V) using the Olympus GF-UC140P-AL5 (*left*). Advancing the scope aligns the target lesion with the needle (*arrow*) away from the vessel enabling safe puncture.

of chronic pancreatitis due to fibrosis. Whereas puncturing the lesions adjacent to or within the gastric wall are difficult due to the tremendous yield of the tissues with no counter resistance offered to allow the puncture. In such situations, it is often useful to have an extended needle length made available. Initially the advancement of the needle results in 'tenting' of the GI wall layers. At this time, a quick jab of the needle tip (spearing) rather than gentle advancement facilitates the successful puncture. It is important to develop a 'feel' for the different lesions being punctured.

Sampling the Targeted Lesion with or without Suction

Once the needle is within the lesion, the stylet is removed completely and a self-sustaining suction-syringe is attached. Due to the longer length of the stylet, as it is being removed the assistant has to carefully wind it in larger circles avoiding kinks. Some operators prefer not to use suction while some use low volume suction. In general, use of moderate suction with a 10 mL syringe provides better quality of the aspirate. However, in hypervascular lesions, excessive suction might reduce the quality of the sample due to the presence of bloody aspirate. Maintaining the suction, the needle is moved back and forth approximately 5–10 times within the lesion to disrupt the tissue and collect the cellular material.

During sampling, the material stays within the hollow needle and except while aspirating cystic lesions or fluid collection, aspirate will not be seen coming into the syringe due to the length of the needle. Detection of bloody aspirate at the level of syringe indicates puncture of a vessel. In this event, one should stop further suction and manipulation, but observe the image to determine whether there is any hypo/anechoic structure in the path of the needle. It is important to close the suction by turning the 3-way valve to the off position and withdraw the needle. If excess bleeding is noted, there is usually a change of echomorphology around the area of puncture indicating a local hematoma. Although most such events resolve spontaneously, one should use clinical judgment as to whether to continue with the procedure in such an occurrence.

Withdrawal of the Needle

Once the sample is collected within the needle, as described above, suction is released slowly in a controlled manner prior to withdrawal while the tip of the needle is still within the lesion (Fig. 6). Then, the elevator is released, the needle is drawn back in to the channel and the screw is fastened to avoid damage to the scope by extending the needle out of the channel during withdrawal. The whole needle assembly is detached and withdrawn from the scope. Then, the transducer is moved away from the bowel wall to visualize the puncture site.

Transfer of the Sampled Tissue or Fluid for Cytopathology

Extending the tip of the needle from the channel, the stylet is re-inserted slowly holding the tip of the needle over a couple of glass slides delivering a drop of the aspirate on each slide. The rest of the material is delivered into *cytolyte* solution for subsequent processing in the laboratory. The material on the glass slide is spread thin using another glass slide as shown in Fig. 11. Then, the smear is air-dried and stained to examine for adequacy by an on-site cytopathologist.

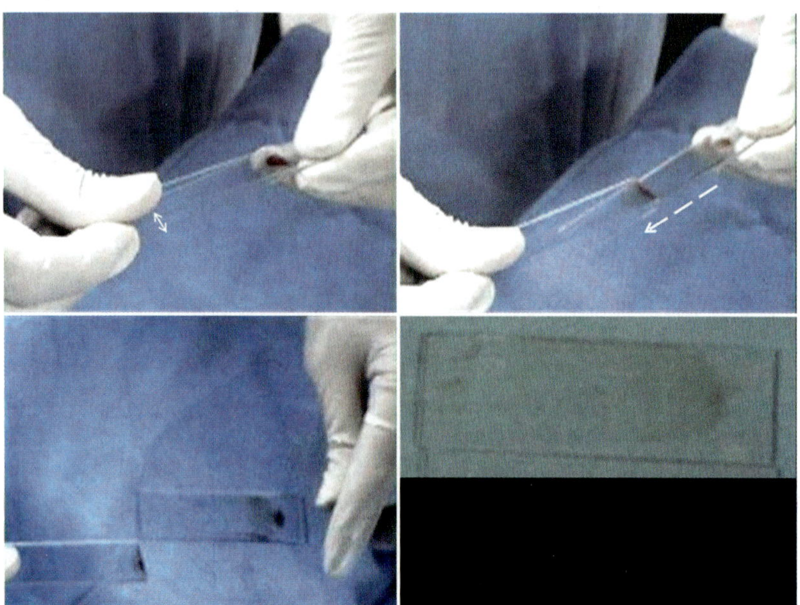

Fig. 11. A drop of the aspirate is gently expelled on to a glass slide and is smeared with the help of another glass slide placed at 10–15° angle (*top left*) and drawn down its length (*top right*), spreading the material into a thin layer (*bottom left*) that could either be air dried (*bottom right*) or stained immediately.

Alternately, the adequacy of specimen can be assessed by smearing the aspirate to prepare as many smears as possible by transferring material onto various glass slides and examining the smears for tiny particulate matter on the slides. If a good amount of particulate material is seen on at least three or four slides, the sampling will be usually adequate. Bloody specimens do not necessarily contain representative material. However, if excess blood is seen in the specimen, clots can be separated and sent to pathology in formalin solution for clot histology, which can sometimes increase the yield of the specimen. There are several studies now available highlighting the limitation of visual interpretation of endosonographer or even a technician regarding on-site evaluation of stained smears by a cytopathologist. Rapid onsite cytopathology reduces the number of passes, ensures specimen adequacy, provides definitive diagnosis, and should be used whenever available (Nguyen et al. 2009).

Once the material is collected from the needle, the stylet is re-inserted and the needle assembly is prepared for another pass. The stylets of the 22 G and 25 G needles are very thin and easily kink unless extreme care is taken while handling them. Generally, it takes one or two passes for mediastinal lesions to obtain an adequate specimen while pancreatic lesions would require 3–4 passes. The material obtained from different passes can be processed and reported together. However, when more than one lesion is punctured, it is important to use different needles, and to label the specimen for interpretation, separately. While labeling the specimens, it is important to indicate if the sampling is trans-esophageal, transgastric, or transduodenal, etc. This will help the cytopathologist to differentiate the material obtained from the lesion versus contamination from the cells of the bowel wall.

Whenever lymphoma is in the differential diagnosis of a lesion being aspirated, it is very important to send the aspirate for flow cytometry. For this purpose, every facility performing EUS-FNA should also have *RPMI* solution that preserves cellular material in the aspirate to enable flow cytometry.

When aspirating cystic lesions of the pancreas, 1–2 mL of fluid should be sent for estimation of CEA levels besides routine analysis, including cell count, amylase and lipase. Some laboratories offer cyst fluid DNA analysis in equivocal cases for excluding malignant mucinous tumors. Although routinely not available, use of molecular methods on the EUS-FNA aspirate is increasing to aid in the diagnosis of malignancy in solid tumors as well.

Examples of actual cases diagnosed by EUS-FNA are shown in Figs. 11–20.

COMPLICATIONS

Complications are uncommon with EUS as well as EUS-FNA, but are possible and have been reported. Besides sedation-related events that can occur in any endoscopic procedure, EUS is associated with two important complications, perforation and pancreatitis. In addition, EUS-FNA is also associated with bleeding and infection (Al-Haddad et al. 2008; Fisher et al. 2009; Shah and Muthusamy 2007; Al-Haddad et al. 2009).

Perforation

Although the rate of perforation for EUS-FNA is comparable to that of EGD, it is important to note the differences in conventional gastroscopes and the echoendoscopes to appreciate the higher potential for problems. Due to the presence of the transducer at the

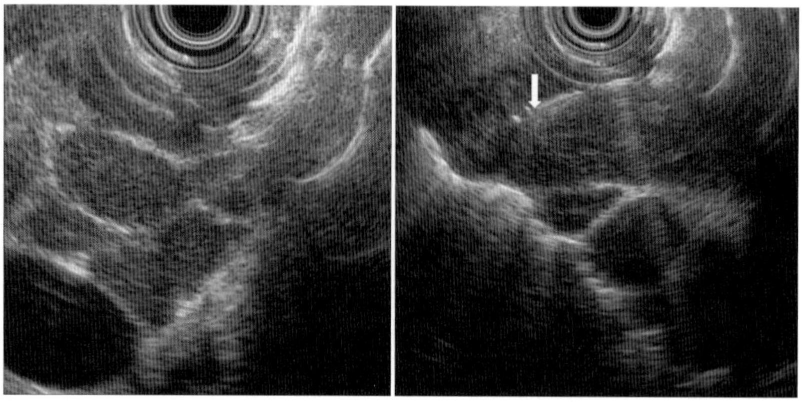

Fig. 12. Sarcoid. A 28-year-old male with dyspnea and dry cough without fever, night sweats or weight loss. Mediastinal widening was seen on chest x-ray and prominent mediastinal lymph nodes on thoracic CT. PPD negative. EUS (*left*) showed multiple paraesophageal and subcarinal enlarged coalescing lymph nodes. EUS-FNA (*right*) using a 22 G needle (*arrow*) demonstrated granulomatous inflammation without caseation or acid-fast bacilli suggesting sarcoidosis.

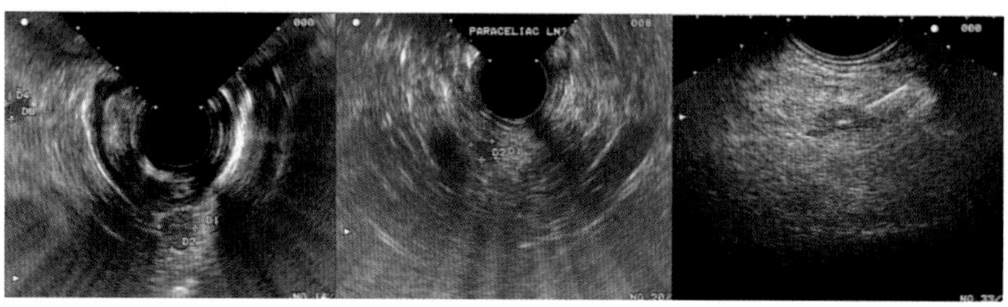

Fig. 13. Esophageal cancer. A 54-year-old male with iron deficiency anemia and no esophageal symptoms had a distal esophageal adenocarcinoma on EGD (*left*) that was staged as T2N1 (*middle*). But a 6 mm non-regional paraceliac lymph node showed metastatic disease on EUS-FNA (*right*).

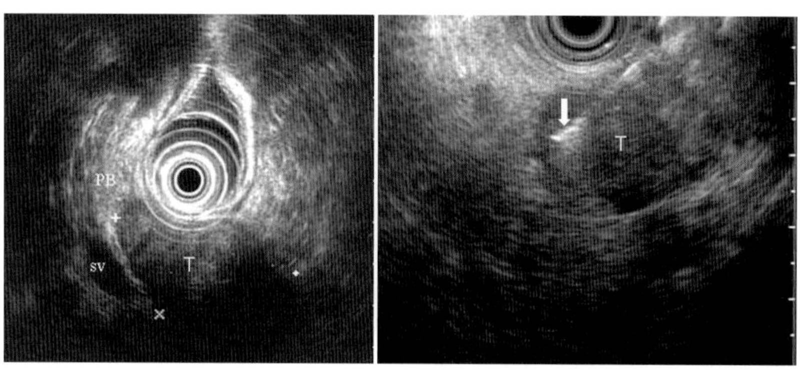

Fig. 14. Pancreatic cancer. A 62-year-old male with severe left upper quadrant pain and unexplained weight loss. Abdominal US was normal, but contrast CT showed bulky pancreatic tail. EUS showed a 3×2.5 cm hypoechoic mass (*left*) which was confirmed to be adenocarcinoma on EUS-FNA (*right*) using a 22 G needle (*arrow*) leading to a successful distal pancreatectomy. (*SV* splenic vein, *T* tumor).

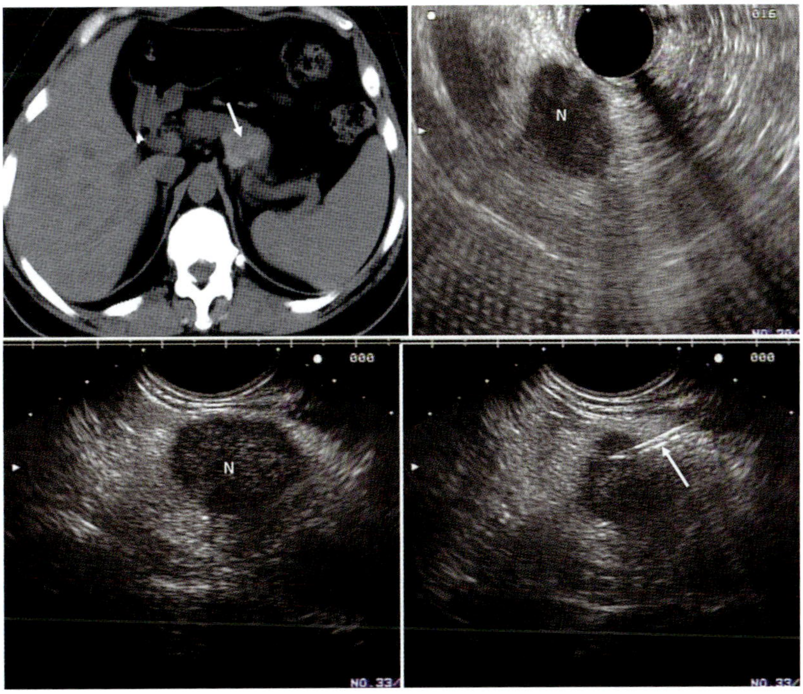

Fig. 15. Pancreatic lymphoma. Follow-up abdominal CT in a patient with large B-cell lymphoma showed a pancreatic body lesion (*arrow, top left*). He completed chemotherapy recently with excellent clinical response. CA 19–9 levels were normal. EUS was suggestive of residual peripancreatic lymph nodes (N) rather than pancreatic body mass (Radial imaging: *top right*; Linear imaging: *bottom left*). EUS-FNA using a 19 G needle (*arrow, bottom right*) showed necrotic tissue excluding residual tumor.

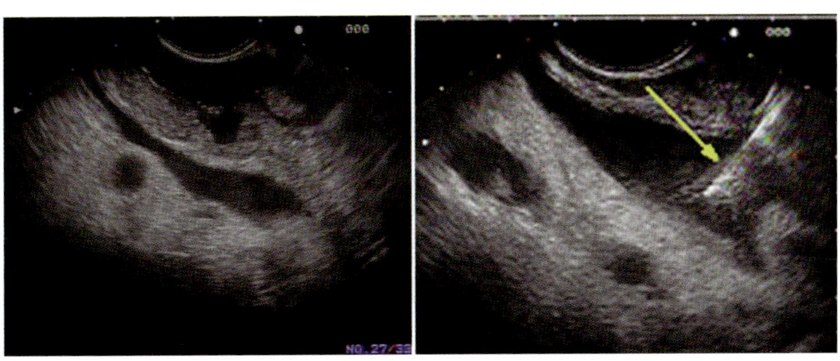

Fig. 16. Ascites in gastric cancer. A 55-year-old male with adenocarcinoma of GE junction underwent EUS for staging that showed T3N1 lesion involving the GE junction transmurally. Patient had, in addition, minimal perigastric ascites indicating peritoneal spread (*left*). EUS guided aspiration of the fluid with 22 G needle (*right*) showed metastatic disease.

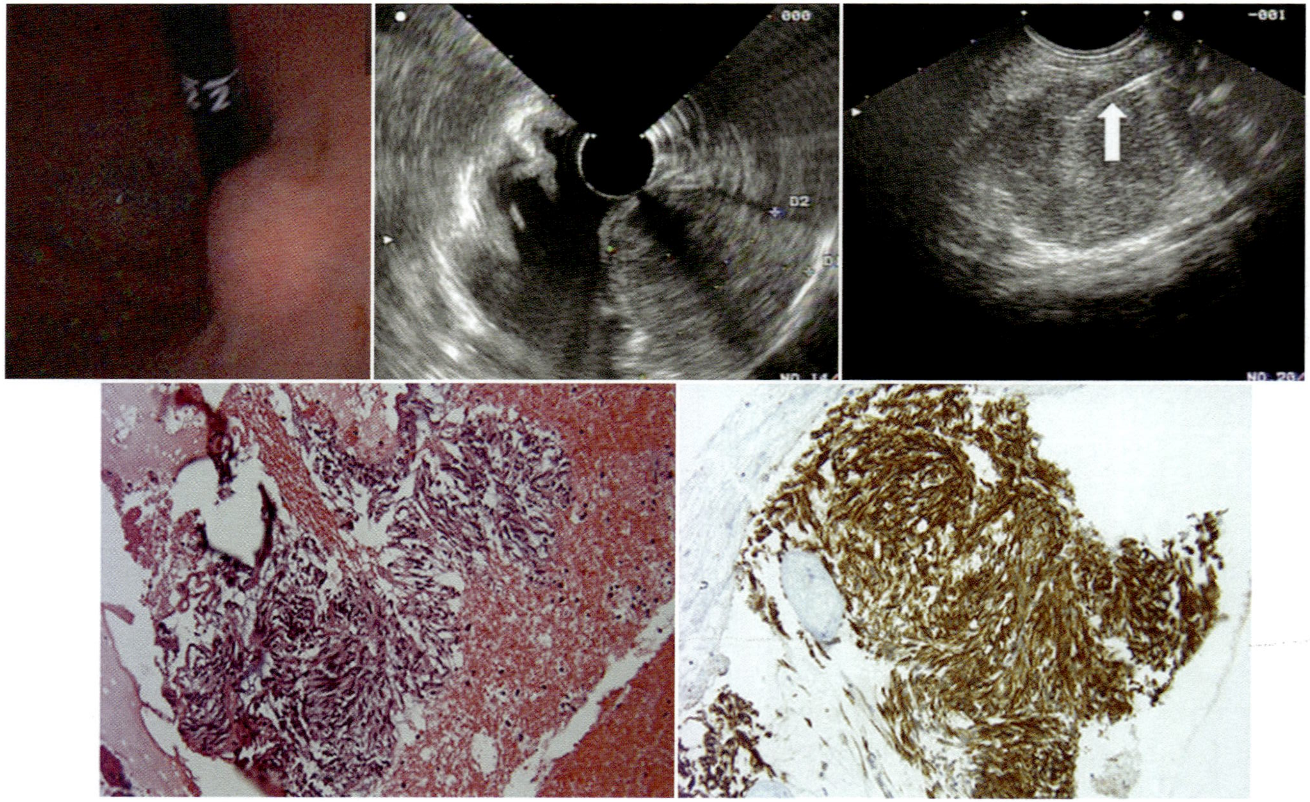

Fig. 17. Rectal stromal tumor. A distal rectal submucosal lesion (*arrow*) in retroversion (*left*) and the same on radial EUS with Pentax EG-3630UR (*middle*) suspicious for stromal tumor. EUS-FNA (*right*) using a 19 G needle (*block arrow*) provided biopsy quality material to confirm the diagnosis. Cohesive tissue fragments of the lesion described above comprised of spindle cells with fusiform nuclei on H & E (*left*). Immunohistochemistry for CD117 (c-Kit) was strongly and diffusely positive (*right*) confirming the gastrointestinal stromal tumor (*GIST*).

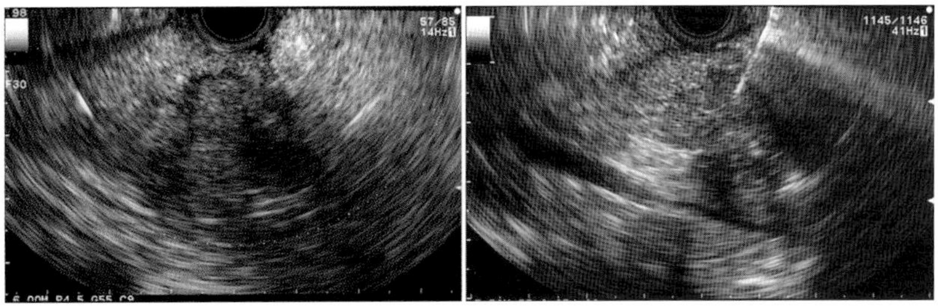

Fig. 18. Pancreatic cancer. Pancreatic head mass (*left*) imaged with the Olympus GF-UC140P-AL5. EUS-FNA using a 22 G needle (*arrow*) showed adenocarcinoma.

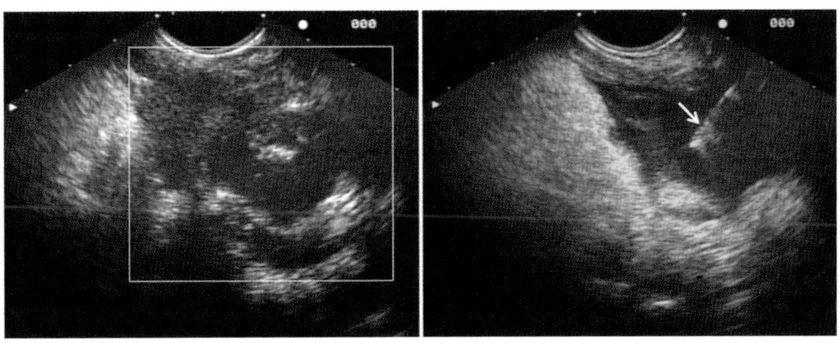

Fig. 19. Pancreatic cancer. A 36-year-old male with severe abdominal pain, vomiting and weight loss of 2 weeks duration was referred with an abdominal CT showing enlarged head of pancreas. Pancreatic enzymes and tumor markers were normal. An MRI of abdomen with contrast showed a lesion in the head of pancreas encasing the SMA (*top left*) suspicious for malignancy.

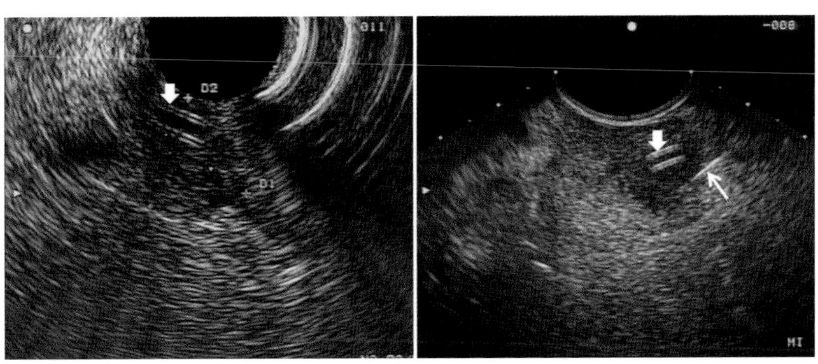

Fig. 20. Cholangiocarcinoma. A 52-year-old male admitted with painless progressive jaundice of 4 weeks duration and marked weight loss. Abdominal CT showed diffuse dilation of the intrahepatic and extrahepatic bile ducts with distal narrowing. ERCP, biliary sphincterotomy, and stenting were performed. Biliary brush cytology was inconclusive. EUS (*left*) showed distal biliary stricture seen as a thickening around the stent (*block arrow*) and EUS-FNA (*right*) using a 22 G needle (*arrow*) established cholangiocarcinoma.

tip of the echoendoscope, there is a variable length (depending on the manufacturer and the type of transducer) of a rigid segment before the bending section that makes maneuvering a little difficult during intubation across the pharyngo-esophageal junction and while negotiating the duodenal bulb into the second part of duodenum. Visual guidance and repositioning the head-neck region (neck bent forward with a backward head tilt) helps intubation across the hypopharynx. In case of intubation difficulty across the hypopharynx or when maneuvering across the duodenal bulb into the second part of duodenum, keeping the balloon around the transducer partially inflated helps to gently glide the rigid part of the echoendoscope. Another important cause of bowel wall injury is in the use of radial EUS to complete the endoscopic part of the examination, especially visualizing the proximal stomach and fundus in retroflexion. In general, it is important to keep in mind that the echoendoscopes are relatively stiffer than the conventional endoscopes. It is helpful to complete this part of the examination prior to sonological evaluation by inflating the stomach adequately for a safe retroflexion. Once this is completed, stomach can be decompressed completely and instilled with water for completing the EUS.

The rigid segment of the CLE scope is longer than the radial EUS scope and, among the two commonly used instruments, the Pentax system has a longer rigid segment. It is also important to note that the optics in the CLE is like that of a duodenoscope, and that the transducer extends up to an inch beyond the lens. Likewise, the Olympus radial instruments are oblique viewing. Hence, the axis of the tip of the echoendoscope is different from the visual axis and it is important to make the corresponding adjustments in maneuvering the big wheel to align the instrument appropriately.

Acute Pancreatitis

Acute pancreatitis has been reported with even radial EUS without FNA. This could possibly be related to the lengthy procedure during biliary pancreatic evaluation, with repeated back and forth movements of the transducer with inflated balloon along the medial aspect of the duodenum (massaging the pancreatic head and uncinate region of the gland). This is often mild and self-limiting. Occasionally, pancreatitis was reported following EUS-FNA, particularly when multiple passes had been made. In general, acute pancreatitis is not a common complication although one study reported up to 2% of the cases, and there are no predictors identified for prevention.

Bleeding

Unless repeated passes are made with a 19 G needle, mucosal bleeding is not an issue with EUS-FNA. There was an occasional report of mucosal bleeding that responded to endotherapy with epinephrine injection. Delayed bleeding is unusual and most instances of bleeding can be recognized before the echoendoscope is withdrawn from the patient. Routine use of color Doppler is important to evaluate the vascularity of the lesion and to assess the projected path of the needle. Even when dealing with an obviously safe lesion to puncture, it helps to verify the relative location of any significant vascular structures.. After completing the procedure, before the instrument is withdrawn it is always a good practice to inspect the lesion and the site of puncture, both on EUS and endoscopy for any evidence of bleeding. Local bleeding can be suspected if a solid lesion appears to have increased in size or there is excessive debris in a cystic lesion compared to before puncture. A corresponding change in hemodynamics or a drop in hematocrit >2 g/dL connotes significant bleeding and requires further measures. When significant bleeding is suspected, even in the absence of endoluminal bleeding, in-hospital observation with resuscitative measures and transfusion support may be required. It is extremely unusual to require any interventional radiology techniques for a EUS-FNA-related bleeding.

EUS-FNA is considered a high-risk procedure in the context of anticoagulant use, and it is recommended to withhold antiplatelet agents and anticoagulants 3–5 days prior to procedure, so that it can be done safely. However, in one study, the bleeding risk was not found to be increased in patients on aspirin/NSAIDs compared to controls (Kien-Fong Vu et al. 2006). However, use of prophylactic low-molecular weight heparin was still associated with a higher rate of bleeding.

Infection

Infection is a potential complication when cystic lesions are sampled, such as in mediastinum or pancreas. A routine pre-procedural prophylactic antibiotic is mandatory whenever cystic lesions, loculated collections, or necrotic tumors are punctured. In general, solid lesions are less at risk for infection following EUS-FNA, except when puncturing peri-rectal lesions, where infective complications are high and administration of antibiotics prior to procedure is recommended.

SUMMARY OF KEY POINTS

- EUS–FNA is indicated for evaluation of mediastinal and intra-abdominal lymph nodes, staging of lung, esophageal, biliary-pancreatic, ano-rectal cancers by evaluation of nodes.
- Peri-luminal fluid collections can be sampled from small pleural effusions, minimal ascites, peri-pancreatic fluid, and pseudocysts.
- Focal lesions can be sampled to exclude malignancy.
- EUS is associated with two important complications, perforation and pancreatitis, but pancreatitis, and infection can also occur.

ACKNOWLEDGMENT

I respectfully acknowledge Dr. Dharma Thiruvaiyaru, Ph.D., Dept. of Mathematics, Statistics and Computer Sciences, Augusta State University, Augusta, Georgia for critically reviewing the chapter.

REFERENCES

Adler DG, Conway JD, Coffie JM, Disario JA, Mishkin DS, Shah RJ, et al. EUS accessories. Gastrointest Endosc. 2007;66(6):1076–81.

Al-Haddad M, Wallace MB, Woodward TA, Gross SA, Hodgens CM, Toton RD, et al. The safety of fine-needle aspiration guided by endoscopic ultrasound: a prospective study. Endoscopy. 2008;40(3):204–8.

Al-Haddad M, Gill KR, Raimondo M, Woodward TA, Krishna M, Crook JE, Skarvinko LN, Jamil LH, Hasan M, Wallace MB. Safety and efficacy of cytology brushings versus standard fine-needle aspiration in evaluating cystic pancreatic lesions: a controlled study. Endoscopy 2009 Dec 7, Endoscopy. 2010;42(2):127–32.

Binmoeller KF, Rathod VD. Difficult pancreatic mass FNA: tips for success. Gastrointest Endosc. 2002;56(4 Suppl):S86–91.

Erickson RA. EUS-guided FNA. Gastrointest Endosc. 2004;60(2):267–79.

Fisher L, Segarajasingam DS, Stewart C, Deboer WB, Yusoff IF. Endoscopic ultrasound guided fine needle aspiration of solid pancreatic lesions: Performance and outcomes. J Gastroenterol Hepatol. 2009;24(1):90–6.

Fritscher-Ravens A, Brand B, Bohnacker S, Sriram P, Soehendra N. Technique of endoscopic ultrasonography-guided fine-needle aspiration of the lymph nodes. Tech Gastrointest Endosc. 2000a;2(3):142–8.

Fritscher-Ravens A, Broering DC, Sriram PV, Topalidis T, Jaeckle S, Thonke F, et al. EUS-guided fine-needle aspiration cytodiagnosis of hilar cholangiocarcinoma: a case series. Gastrointest Endosc. 2000b;52(4): 534–40.

Fritscher-ravns A. EUS-Experimental and evolving techniques. Endoscopy. 2006;38(S1):S1–4.

Giovannini M. Ultrasound-guided endoscopic surgery. Best Pract Res Clin Gastroenterol. 2004;18:183–200.

Kien-Fong Vu C, Chang F, Doig L, Meenan J. A prospective control study of the safety and cellular yield of EUS-guided FNA or Trucut biopsy in patients taking aspirin, nonsteroidal anti-inflammatory drugs, or prophylactic low molecular weight heparin. Gastrointest Endosc. 2006;63(6):808–13.

Mitsuhashi T, Ghafari S, Chang CY, Gu M. Endoscopic ultrasound-guided fine needle aspiration of the pancreas: cytomorphological evaluation with emphasis on adequacy assessment, diagnostic criteria and contamination from the gastrointestinal tract. Cytopathology. 2006;17(1):34–41.

Nguyen YP, Maple JT, Zhang Q, Ylagan LR, Zhai J, Kohlmeier C, et al. Reliability of gross visual assessment of specimen adequacy during EUS-guided FNA of pancreatic masses. Gastrointest Endosc. 2009;69(7):1264–70.

Noh KW, Woodward TA, Raimondo M, Savoy AD, Pungpapong S, Hardee JD, et al. Changing trends in endosonography: linear imaging and tissue are increasingly the issue. Dig Dis Sci. 2007;52(4):1014–8.

Puri R, Vilmann P, Săftoiu A, Skov BG, Linnemann D, Hassan H, et al. Randomized controlled trial of endoscopic ultrasound-guided fine-needle sampling with or without suction for better cytological diagnosis. Scand J Gastroenterol. 2009;44(4):499–504.

Savides TJ. Tricks for improving EUS-FNA accuracy and maximizing cellular yield. Gastrointest Endosc. 2009;69(2 Suppl):S130–3.

Shah JN, Muthusamy VR. Minimizing complications of endoscopic ultrasound and EUS-guided fine needle aspiration. Gastrointest Endosc Clin N Am. 2007;17(1):129–43. vii-viii.

Vilmann P, Săftoiu A. Endoscopic ultrasound-guided fine needle aspiration biopsy: equipment and technique. J Gastroenterol Hepatol. 2006;21(11):1646–55.

Yamao K, Mizuno N, Takagi T, Hara K. How I do it and when I use (and do not use) EUS-FNA. Gastrointest Endosc. 2009;69(2 Suppl):S134–7.

Yusuf TE, Tsutaki S, Wagh MS, Waxman I, Brugge WR. The EUS hardware store: state of the art technical review of instruments and equipment (with videos). Gastrointest Endosc. 2007;66(1):131–43.

Yusuf TE, Ho S, Pavey DA, Michael H, Gress FG. Retrospective analysis of the utility of endoscopic ultrasound-guided fine-needle aspiration (EUS-FNA) in pancreatic masses, using a 22-gauge or 25-gauge needle system: a multicenter experience. Endoscopy. 2009;41(5):445–8.

17 The Role of Endoscopic Ultrasound in Pain Management

Kamran Ayub

CONTENTS

Keywords: Endoscopic, Ultrasound, Pain, Management, Pathophysiology

INTRODUCTION

Pain is one of the most common symptoms that leads to medical evaluation. The international association for the study of pain, IASP, defines pain as "an unpleasant sensory and emotional experience associated with actual or potential tissue damage, or described in terms of such damage" (Merskey and Bogduk 1994). Numerous national and international surveys have demonstrated that 60–90% of patients with cancer develop pain in the natural history of disease. Some cancer pain syndromes tend to be intractable secondary to the nature of pain, and also due to comorbid medical as well as psychological factors associated with serious illness, terminal prognosis, and dying (Reddy and Shanti 2000).

PATHOPHYSIOLOGY

Pain is transmitted by complex neural pathways that transmit information about painful stimuli from the periphery, through the spinal cord, and to multiple areas of the brain. Modulation of nociceptive input by opioid and non-opioid mechanisms occurs in the periphery, at the dorsal horn of the spinal cord, in the brain stem, and possibly in higher centers. Pathophysiologic classification of pain forms the basis for therapeutic choices

From: *Clinical Gastroenterology: Diagnostic and Therapeutic Procedures in Gastroenterology*,
Edited by: G. Y. Wu, S. Sridhar, DOI 10.1007/978-1-59745-044-7_17,

Table 1
Neurolytic blocks of the sympathetic axis

Celiac plexus neurolysis
Superior hypogastric plexus neurolysis
Ganglion impar neurolysis

(Patt 1993). Painful states may be broadly divided into those associated with ongoing tissue damage (nociceptive), and those resulting from nervous system dysfunction (neuropathic) due to either tissue damage or, in some situations, the absence of damage.

Nociceptive pain can be of somatic or visceral type. Somatic pain results from the activation of nociceptors in cutaneous and deep tissues; it can also be described as localized aching, throbbing, and gnawing. Visceral pain is caused by activation of nociceptors resulting from distention, stretching, and inflammation of visceral organs; it is described as poorly localized, deep, aching, cramping, pressure and sometimes it is referred, e.g., pancreatic cancer pain in the abdomen referred to the back.

Neuropathic pain can attain specific characteristics based on the mechanism of the system involved. For example, compression of a plexus by a tumor may result in nociceptive nerve pain, e.g., somatic neuropathic pain, in addition to a sympathetic-mediated component. Damage to the nervous system may result in an area of reduced sensation. Such pain is typically described as burning or lancinating. Patients may offer bizarre complaints, such as painful numbness, itching or crawling sensations.

Breakthrough pain tends to be a bad prognostic factor for the successful treatment of pain. Breakthrough pain can be caused by activity or end-of-dose failure, or it can occur spontaneously. It tends to be moderate to severe, occur at a frequency of one to four episodes per day.

Management of pain requires a multidisciplinary team approach. Different modalities used in the management of pain include pharmacologic therapy, stimulation and ablation techniques, physical therapy, psychological techniques and nerve blocks. The pharmacologic therapy typically used in a step ladder approach, as described by WHO guidelines starting with non-steroidal anti-inflammatory drugs, opioid analgesics, analgesic adjuvants, including anti-depressants, steroids, anti-convulsants, and amphetamines etc. Unfortunately, most patients with cancer or other chronic conditions, e.g., chronic pancreatitis, require gradually increasing doses of narcotics; this leads to drug dependence and side effects, including narcosis, constipation, gastroparesis etc. Nerve blocks can reduce the requirement of narcotics, and in some cases ablate the pain completely. So far, three different blocks of the sympathetic axis have been described in the management of abdominal, pelvic and perineal pain, Table 1.

EUS-GUIDED CELIAC PLEXUS BLOCK AND NEUROLYSIS

Celiac plexus is located anterolateral to the aorta near the origin of celiac artery. It supplies visceral sensory fibers to the upper abdominal viscera including pancreas, liver, biliary tree and gallbladder, spleen, stomach, proximal small bowel up to transverse colon. Celiac plexus neurolysis is effective in management of pain arising from these upper abdominal viscera. See Table 2.

Table 2
Celiac plexus neurolysis: Indications

Upper abdominal pain due to carcinoma of:
Pancreas
Stomach
Gall bladder
Biliary tree
Liver metastasis
Small bowel
Chronic pancreatitis with severe pain

Celiac plexus neurolysis is an old technique. It was first described almost 100 years ago by Kappis (1914). The technique was initially performed by anesthesiologists, and surgeons. An endoscopic ultrasound-guided approach was first described in 1996. So far, the endoscopic ultrasound-guided approach has been used mostly for management of pain due to pancreatic cancer and chronic pancreatitis.

Pancreatic cancer and chronic pancreatitis are commonly associated with intense and often refractory pain (Ventafridda et al. 1990; Lankisch 2001). Celiac plexus neurolysis (CPN) with injection of absolute alcohol or in some cases, other neurolytic agents like phenol, is often used in management of patient with pancreatic cancer. Celiac plexus block (CPB) with steroids and local anesthetic is used in patients with pain due to chronic pancreatitis. Unfortunately, although CPN and CPB are considered safe, they provide limited benefit in terms of degree and duration of pain relief, and little advance has been made since Kappis first described the technique in 1914. Since then, modifications have been created in an attempt to improve the accuracy of needle placement and pain relief, while reducing procedure-related complications. These techniques differ with respect to the route of needle insertion, use of neurologic guidance versus blind procedure, and chemical composition of the injected substance. A meta-analysis by Eisenberg et al. reviewed percutaneous approaches (Eisenberg et al. 1995). They concluded that despite a few reports favoring one technique over another, the efficacy of pain relief was not influenced by the technical approach or use of radiologic guidance. Existing EUS data are limited and do not allow us to clarify whether minor technical variations, e.g., unilateral verses bilateral injection, offers an advantage in terms of efficacy and safety (Eisenberg et al. 1995; Usati et al. 2008). In addition, the lack of prospective randomized controlled trials prevent us from accurately evaluating EUS versus percutaneous approaches.

TECHNIQUES FOR PERFORMING EUS-GUIDED CPN AND CPB

Prior to performing EUS-guided celiac plexus neurolysis or block, proper patient selection is important. It should be noted that celiac neurolysis and block are effective for visceral type of pain only. Visceral pain originates from injury to sympathetically innervated organs (Newman 1974). Visceral pain is characteristically vague in distribution and quality, and is often described as deep, dull, aching, dragging, squeezing or pressure-like. When acute, it may be paroxysmal and colicky, and can be associated with nausea, vomiting, diaphoresis, and alteration in blood pressure and heart rate. Mechanisms of visceral pain include abnormal distention or contraction of smooth muscle walls (hollow viscera), rapid capsular stretch (solid viscera), ischemia of visceral muscle, serosal or mucosal irritation by analgesic substances and other chemical stimuli, traction or torsion on mesenteric attachments and vasculature, and necrosis. The viscera are, however, insensitive to simple manipulation, cutting, and burning. Visceral involvement often produces referred or "transferred" pain, a phenomenon of pain and hyperalgesia localized to superficial and or deep tissues, often distant to the source of pathology (Levy et al. 2008; Leblanc et al. 2009). A number of mechanisms have been proposed to explain the occurrence of referred pain, including presence of dual innervation of multiple structures, chemical irritation by tumor mediated by an algesic substance, central conversions of afferent impulses. Examples include back pain of pancreatic or retroperitoneal origin, abdominal wall pain and allodynia from peritoneal irritation, upper extremity pain of anginal origin, phrenic nerve-mediated shoulder pain of hepatic and gallbladder origin. Somatic pain on the other hand occurs as a result of activation of nociceptors. Nociceptors respond to a variety of stimuli, including mechanical, thermal, and biochemical stimuli. Biologic products of inflammation and tumor invasion including serotonin, bradykinin, potassium ATP, and prostaglandins are postulated to act as algesic chemical mediators serving both to produce pain by direct activation of nociceptors and to lower the threshold of their activation (sensitization). Somatic pain is typically constant and well-localized, and is frequently characterized as aching, throbbing, or gnawing. Somatic pain tends to be opioid sensitive, and amenable, at least temporarily to treatment with interruption of proximal pathway by chemical blockage or surgery.

Prior to proceeding with CPN/CPB, patients are questioned regarding allergies and use of anticoagulants. Informed consent is obtained, with specific attention to the unique complications associated with CPN/CPB. Patients are initially hydrated with 500–1,000 mL of normal saline solution to minimize the risk of orthostatic hypotension. The procedure is performed using conscious sedation and non-invasive monitoring with the patient in left lateral decubitus position.

Linear EUS imaging from the posterior lesser curvature of the gastric body allows identification of the aorta, which appears in a longitudinal plane (Figs. 1 and 2).

The aorta is traced caudally from the diaphragm to the celiac trunk, which is the first major branch of abdominal aorta below the diaphragm. The celiac plexus is not identified as a discrete structure, but is located based on its position relative to the celiac trunk. More recently, the celiac ganglion has been identified, and one study of direct celiac ganglion block has been published (Levy et al. 2008). Color Doppler can confirm the celiac artery trunk (Fig. 3).

A 22 gauge needle is primed with saline solution, and then placed through the biopsy channel and fixed to the hub. The needle is inserted under EUS guidance immediately anterior to the aorta, and superior to the level of celiac trunk, as shown in Fig. 4.

An aspiration test is performed to detect vessel penetration before each injection. For CPN in pancreatic cancer patients, 20 mL of 0.25% bupivacaine is typically injected. This is followed by 20 mL of dehydrated absolute alcohol (98%). The alcohol produces an echogenic cloud, and may lead to discomfort despite sedation. Before withdrawing the needle, it should be flushed with 3 mL of normal saline solution to prevent seeding of the needle track with alcohol. The efficacy of unilateral versus bilateral injection has been studied in few series recently, and remains controversial. Most experts tend to use a single,

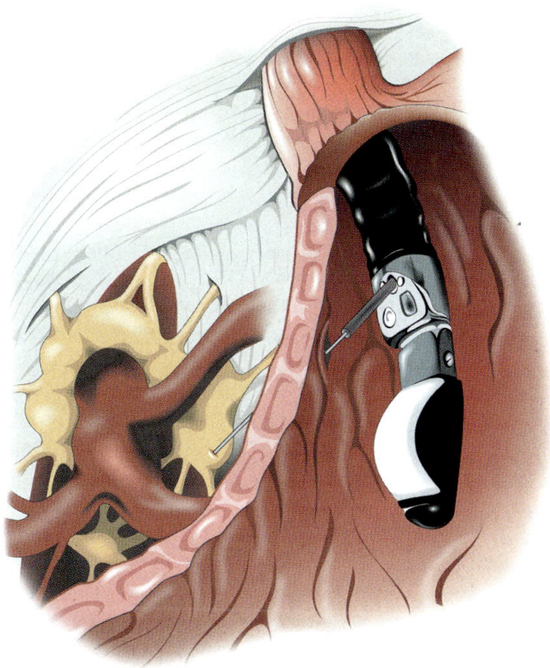

Fig. 1. Anatomy of the celiac ganglion.

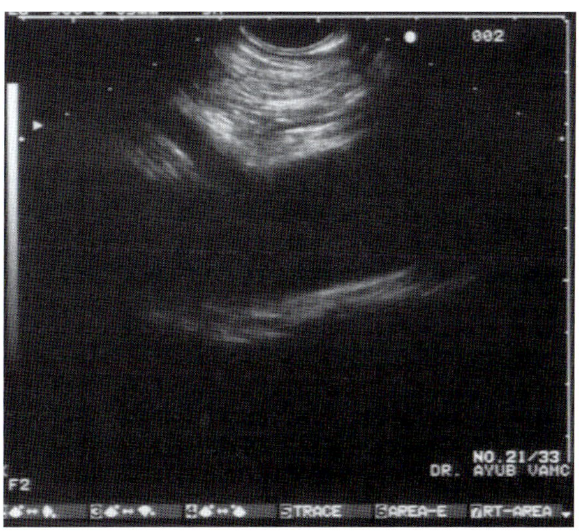

Fig. 2. Celiac artery.

midline injection technique. Recently a published paper suggested that there is no difference in duration of pain relief or onset of pain relief in subjects with chronic pancreatitis and pain, when the same amount of total medication was delivered in unilateral or bilateral injections. Both methods were safe in this study (Leblanc et al. 2009). After the procedure, the vital signs are typically monitored for 2 h. Before discharge, the blood pressure is checked both in supine and upright position to assess for orthostasis. Celiac

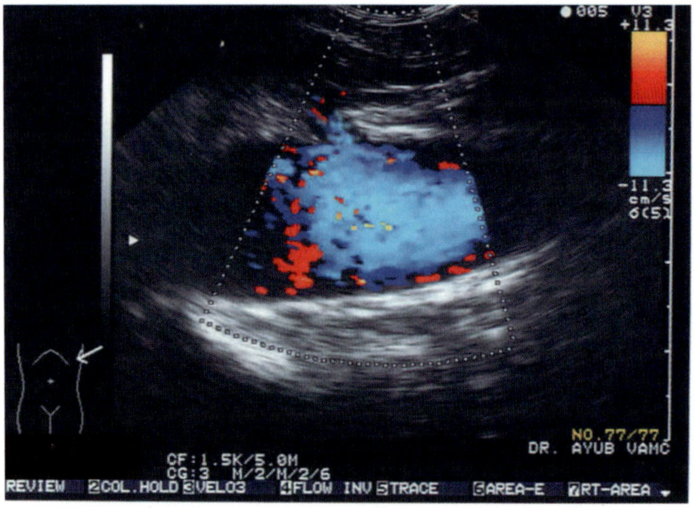

Fig. 3. Color Doppler imaging of the celiac artery.

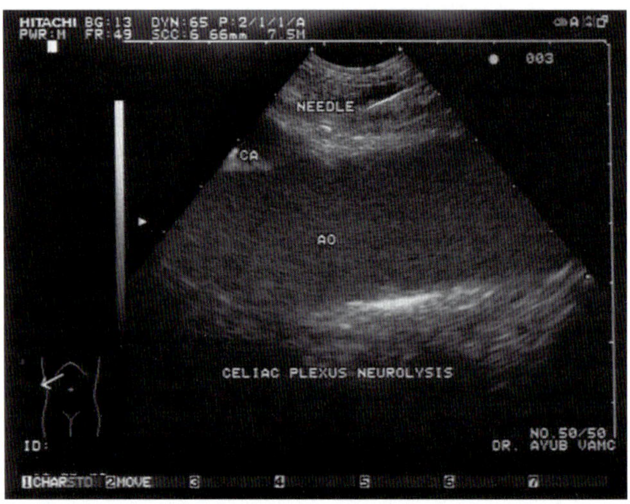

Fig. 4. Needle position for CPN/CPB.

plexus neurolysis is routinely performed as an outpatient procedure, rarely necessitating hospitalization. For CPB in patients with chronic pancreatitis, many physicians substitute a steroid, triamcinolone 80 mg, in place of alcohol. Although its use in patients with benign disease is controversial, some experts administer a small volume of alcohol, 8 mL, in addition to the steroid to increase the neurolysis. If alcohol, which is bactericidal, is not given along with the steroid, then broad spectrum antibiotics should be administered to reduce the chance retroperitoneal abscess formation, particularly if the patient is receiving acid suppressive therapy.

Wiersema et al. have studied EUS-CPN in patients with pancreatic cancer, and showed a significant reduction in pain that persisted for at least 12 weeks (Wiersema and Wiersema 1996). A subsequent prospective study by this group involved patients not only with malignancy, but also with chronic pancreatitis requiring narcotic analgesics (Wiersema et al. 1998). Initial pain scores were similar between the two patient groups. After 16 weeks of follow up, however, the pain score improvement after EUS-CPN in patients with chronic pancreatitis was not found to be significant. The malignant disease group had a mean pain score of less than base line. The estimated duration of pain control was 20 weeks for malignant group and 2 weeks for chronic pancreatitis group. Pain medication usage, decreased or stable, was similar in both groups. Gunaratnam et al. performed an updated prospective study of EUS-guided CPN for pancreatic cancer pain (Gunaratnam et al. 2001). EUS-CPN reduced pain scores in 78% of patients. The results were similar to that achieved by surgical and transcutaneous approach (Ischia et al. 1992). In malignant disease, the timing of injection may be a predictor of response. Ischia et al. found CPN to be more effective when applied soon after the diagnosis of cancer, rather than late in the course of disease (Ischia et al. 1992). This difference was postulated to be related to involvement of other visceral and somatic nerves at terminal stages. Gress et al. used injection of triamcinolone in 90 patients with chronic pancreatitis; they defined pain improvement as a decrease in pain score of greater than 3. At 8 weeks post-procedure, 55% of patients had decreased scores. This dropped off to 10% by 24 weeks. A cost comparison performed within this study demonstrated a $200 saving for the EUS-guided approach versus a CT guided approach (Gress et al. 2001). A randomized controlled trial of EUS-CPB in chronic pancreatitis patients showed this method to be more effective than CT guided CPB (Gress et al. 1999). A special needle for performing EUS guided CPN/CPB is now available. This needle is used to deliver the agent to celiac plexus, but injects from the side holes rather than the tip of the needle, thus theoretically decreasing the risk of intra-vascular injection. (ECHOTIP EUSN-20-CPN, Cook Endoscopy, Winston-Salem, NC). This is a 20 gauge needle (Fig. 5).

Complications of CPN/CPB, though rare, can be serious. Table 3 depicts the reported complications of the procedure; it should be noted that transient diarrhea, pain and hypotension have been reported in more than one-third of patients undergoing celiac plexus

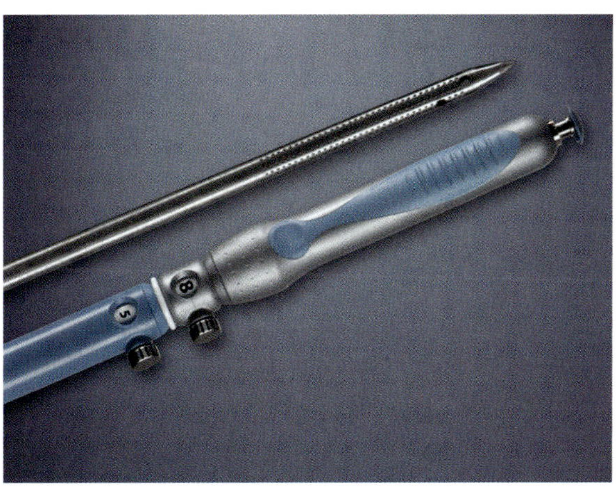

Fig. 5. A 20 gauge needle for neural block/lysis of celiac plexus, which injects from the side holes rather than the tip of the needle, theoretically decreasing the risk of intra-vascular injection (Reproduced with permission from Cook Medical Co.).

Table 3
Some side effects and complications of CPN/CPB

Hypotension
Diarrhea
Pain during and after procedure
Sub-arachnoid or epidural injection
Intravascular injection
Retroperitoneal hemorrhage
Pneumothorax[a]
Neurological deficit[a]
Parapalgia[a]
Renal puncture[a]
Abscess formation
Gastroparesis
Peritonitis

[a]Reported with posterior approach only

neurolysis, given the unopposed parasympathetic activity (Eisenberg et al. 1995; Gunaratnam et al. 2000). Severe chronic diarrhea has also been reported post-celiac plexus block and neurolysis (Chan 1996; Cataldo and Potash 1996). Potential treatments include intravenous atropine and octreotide (Mercadante 1995; Iftikhar and Loftus 1998). Transient hypotension is minimized by infusion of normal saline while the patient is recovering from conscious sedation. Transient pain has been reported, but in some studies researchers found a transient increase in pain which lasted up to 48 h. Gastroparesis has also been reported as a rare complication of celiac plexus neurolysis and block (Gress et al. 1997). The anterior approach utilized by EUS reduces the risk of major complications, such as paraplegia and pneumothorax. But, other serious complications, such as retroperitoneal hemorrhage and peripancreatic abscess formation, can still occur (Brass 1983). The risk of abscess formation has led to recommendation of antibiotic coverage prior to EUS-CPB, but its use remains operator dependent. Antibiotics are not required in CPN as the bactericidal effect of absolute alcohol seem to be adequate.

More recently, a new technique of celiac ganglion block and neurolysis has been described. In this approach, direct injection of the celiac ganglion is performed under EUS guidance (Levy et al. 2008). Further prospective trials are needed to confirm the efficacy of this new approach.

EUS-guided CPN and CPB are valuable tools for management of pain in patients with upper GI malignancy and chronic pancreatitis. In patients with pancreatic cancer, staging and fine needle aspiration can be performed at the same time as celiac plexus neurolysis, thus reducing costs and improving efficiency. The EUS-guided approach appears to be safer than the posterior percutaneous approach, and at least as effective. In future, newer techniques, including direct celiac ganglion injection and use of novel agents, might improve the safety and efficacy further.

SUPERIOR HYPOGASTRIC PLEXUS NEUROLYSIS

The pelvis contains diverse, multiple, and intricately innervated structures that are potential sources of pain, particularly when the etiologic process is gynecologic cancer, which tends to spread locally either by direct invasion or metastasis to regional lymph nodes. Pelvic pain is particularly difficult to manage because it is often vague and poorly localized, and tends to be bilateral or to cross the midline. Because of the properties of pelvic pain noted above, neurosurgical interventions generally are not applicable. The proximity of the nerves that govern bladder, bowel, and lower extremity function and those that subserve pelvic sensation make subarachnoid and epidural neurolytic injections hazardous in this region. Neurolysis of the superior hypogastric plexus has been shown to be efficacious in pelvic pain due to various malignancies and benign conditions. See Table 4.

The superior hypogastric plexus (also known as the presacral nerve) is a paired retroperitoneal structure located at the level of the lower third of the fifth lumbar vertebral body and the upper third of the first sacral vertebral body at the sacral promontory. Here, it lies in close proximity to the bifurcation of common iliac artery. It mediates painful visceral stimuli from most of the pelvic structures including descending colon, sigmoid colon, rectum, prostate, bladder, cervix, uterus, upper vagina, testicles, and seminal vesicles (Snell et al. 1988; Plancarte et al. 1990a). Superior hypogastric plexus neurolysis (SHPN) was first described by Plancarte et al. in 1990. A total of 28 patients with neoplastic involvement of pelvic viscera secondary to cervical, prostate, testicular cancer, and radiation injury were treated with superior hypogastric plexus neurolysis. Pain was significantly reduced or eliminated in all cases, and no serious complications occurred. Using visual and oral analog scales, a mean reduction in pain score of 70% was observed, and residual pain seemed generally of somatic origin. In all but two patients with pain due to neoplasm, there was no return of sympathetic-mediated pain until the patients' demise at 3 and 12 months (Plancarte et al. 1990; Waldman et al. 1991).

SHPN was found to be very successful in patients with non-oncologic pelvic pain, with the distinction that, when successful, residual pain was less common and other complementary interventions were not required.

Plancarte et al. described a two-needle approach using fluoroscopic guidance. In a modification of the technique described above, using a single needle and routine CT scanning, Waldman et al. have observed bilateral spread of contrast medium. They recommend a single injection approach (Kanazi et al. 1999; Walman et al. 1991) (Figs. 6 and 7).

Table 4
Superior hypogastric plexus neurolysis: indications

Malignant	*Benign*
Sigmoid	Endometriosis
Rectum	Pelvic inflammatory disease
Uterus	Radiation colitis
Cervix	Adhesions
Bladder	
Upper vagina	

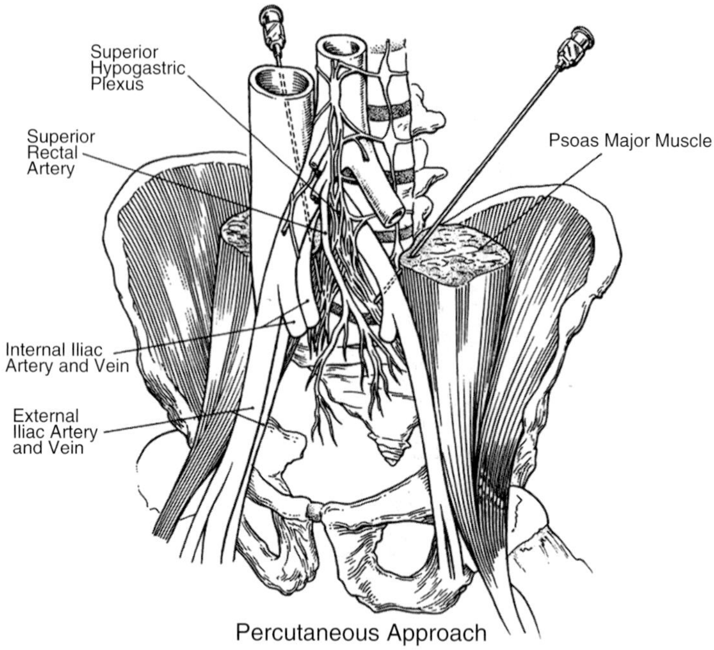

Fig. 6. Superior hypogastric plexus neurolysis: percutaneous approach.

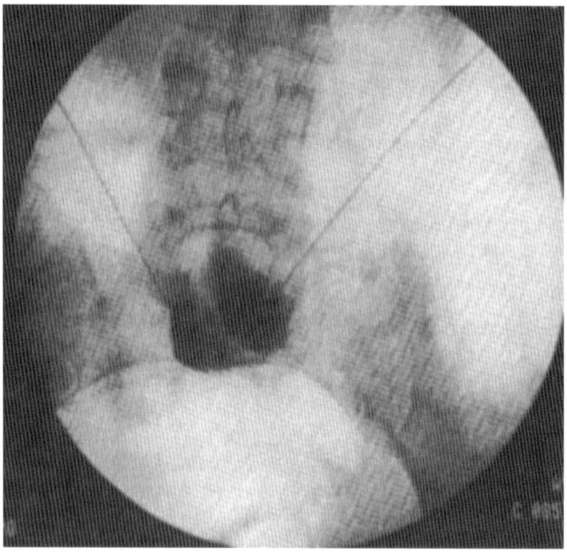

Fig. 7. Superior hypogastric plexus neurolysis: percutaneous approach with contrast injection.

The classical technique described by Plancarte et al. can be technically difficult and sometimes desired needle placement is not possible. Kanazi et al. described an anterior approach to SHPN (Kanazi et al. 1999; Ayub 2001). This approach utilized a long needle. Under biplanar fluoroscopy, the needle was inserted through the anterior abdominal wall and placed in front of sacral promontory. Once in this location, contrast was injected to confirm a retroperitoneal location of the needle tip. Then, neurolytic agent, alcohol or phenol was injected along with local anesthetic. This technique can be difficult in obese patients and in patients with other deformities of the spinal cord (Fig. 8).

An endoscopic ultrasound-guided approach to SHPN has been described (Ayub et al. 2001; Plancarte et al. 1990b). This approach utilizes a linear array echoendoscope and flouroscopy. The scope is advanced into the rectum to the level of aortic bifurcation, with the scope rotated posteriorly. It is usually easy to find the sacral promontory, as only minor adjustments in scope position are required. In the pilot study, SHPN was performed in five patients with pelvic pain due to cancer. The pain was measured before and after the procedure and weekly thereafter using a 10 point visual analog scale. In four patients, the sacral promontory was identified using fluoroscopy. In the fifth patient, fluoroscopy was not used initially. A 22 gauge needle was passed in the space posterior to the rectum between iliac artery bifurcation, and 15 mL of 0.25% bupivacaine was injected followed by 10 mL of absolute alcohol. The mean pain score was 9 before the procedure and 3 after, see Table 5. No complications were encountered in this small study. Since this study, the author has performed EUS guided SHPN in 24 patients, with similar results (unpublished data).

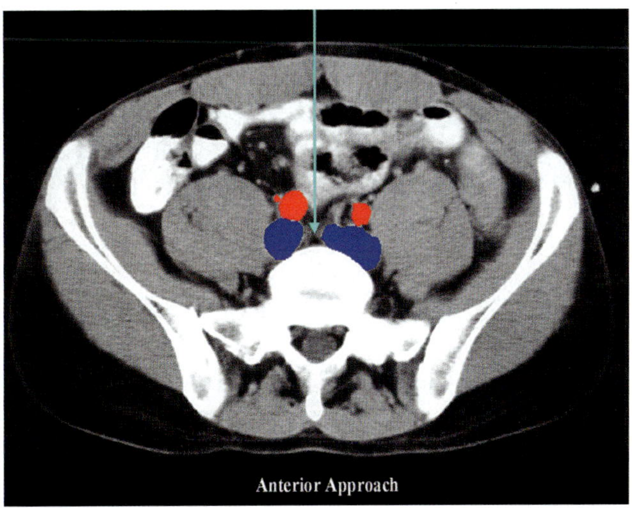

Fig. 8. SHPN anterior percutaneous approach.

Table 5
Clinical profile and results of EUS-SHPN

Number	*Diagnosis*	*Pre-VAS*	*Post-VAS*	*Duration of relief (Weeks)*
1	Rectal cancer	10	3	5
2	Prostate cancer	8	4	2
3	Rectal cancer	9	2	12
4	Rectal cancer	9	3	11
5	Rectal cancer	9	4	16

VAS Visual Analog Scale

This study concluded that EUS-guided SHPN is technically feasible and appears safe. Iliac vessels are easily identified by this approach, thus making hemorrhage an unlikely complication. Further large prospective trials are needed to study the EUS-guided approach. In patients with rectal cancer, tumor staging, neurolysis and fine needle aspiration of lymph nodes can be performed in the same session, thus saving time and cost (Figs. 9–11).

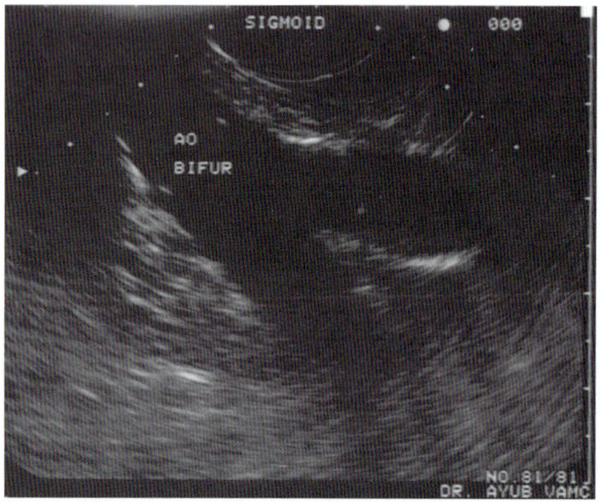

Fig. 9. Linear EUS: aortic bifurcation.

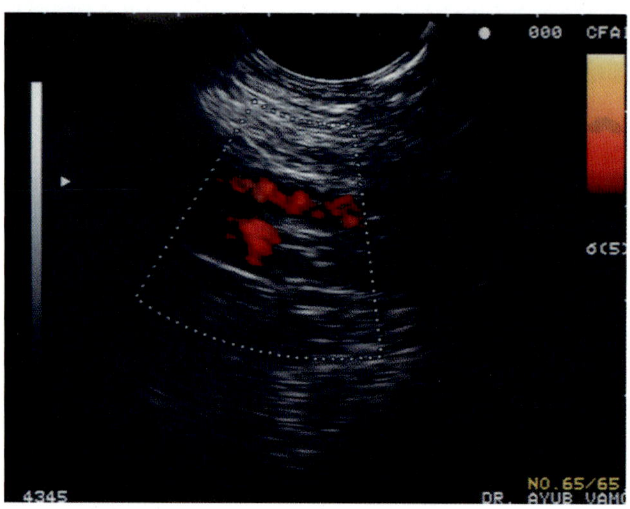

Fig. 10. Linear EUS: iliac bifurcation.

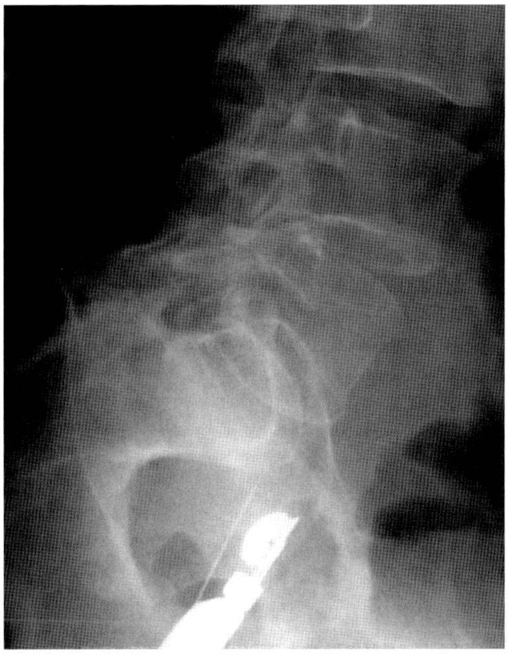

Fig. 11. EUS approach: fluoroscopy.

Table 6
Ganglion impar neurolysis: Indications

Severe or refractory perineal pain due to cancer of:
Lower rectum
Anal canal
Vagina
Urethra
Vulva
Penis
Perineum

GANGLION IMPAR NEUROLYSIS

Ganglion Impar (Ganglion of Walther) is a solitary retroperitoneal structure located anterior to sacrococcygeal junction. This unpaired ganglion marks the end of two sympathetic nerve chains. Visceral pain in the perineal area associated with malignancies may be effectively treated with neurolysis of ganglion impar. Ganglion impar transmits visceral stimuli from the lower rectum, anal canal, lower vagina, vulva, urethra, penis, perineum. Percutaneous neurolysis was first described by Plancarte et al. in 1990 (Plancarte et al. 1990; Love et al. 1998). Indications of ganglion impar neurolysis include malignant pain due to conditions shown in Table 6.

Characteristically, the sympathetic pain in the perineal region has distinct qualities. It tends to be vague and poorly localized, and is frequently accompanied by sensation of burning and urgency. The percutaneous approach to ganglion impar neurolysis used by anesthesiologists and pain physicians requires technical expertise. The patient is placed in left lateral decubitus position, and a skin weal is raised over the anococcygeal ligament and just above the anus posteriorly. Using a standard 22 gauge 3.5 in. spinal needle, the stylet is removed, and the needle is manually bent at approximately 1 in. from the hub to form a 25–30° angle (Fig. 12). This maneuver facilitates positioning of the needle tip in front of the sacrococcygeal junction. The needle is inserted through the skin weal with its concavity oriented posteriorly, and under fluoroscopic guidance, is directed anterior to the coccyx, closely approximating the anterior surface of the bone, until its tip is observed to have reached the sacrococcygeal junction under fluoroscopy.

The retroperitoneal location of the needle tip is verified by the spread of 2 mL of water soluble contrast medium, which typically assumes a smooth margined configuration resembling an apostrophe. Four milliliters of 0.25% bupivacaine is injected for diagnostic and prognostic purposes, or, alternatively, 4–6 mL of 10% phenol or absolute alcohol is injected for therapeutic neurolysis. Unless care is taken to confirm the needle's posteroanterior orientation, perforation of the rectum or periosteal injection is possible. In addition, anatomic abnormalities of the sacrococcygeal vertebral column, i.e., exaggerated anterior

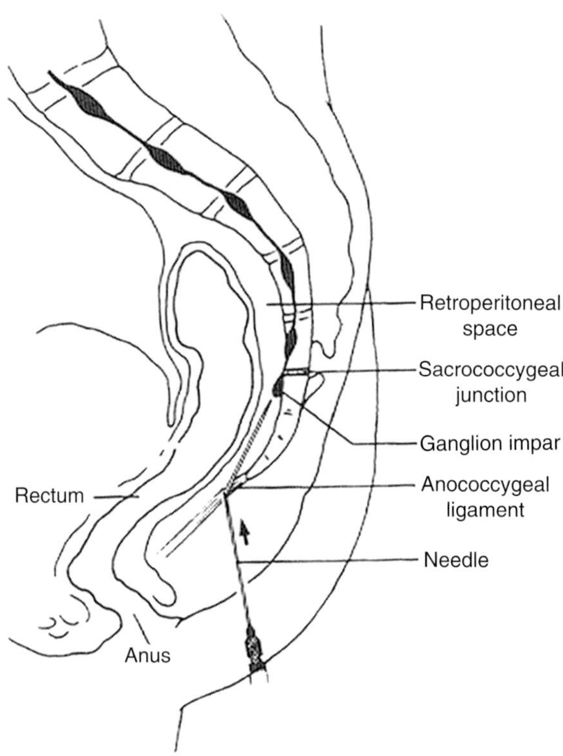

Fig. 12. Percutaneous approach.

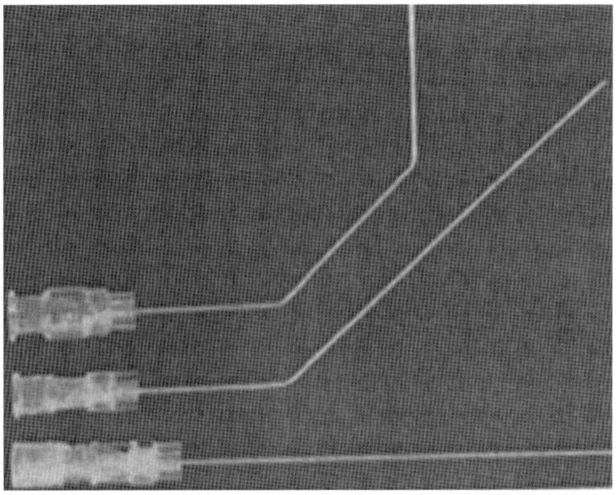

Fig. 13. Bent needle for percutaneous approach.

curvature, may inhibit access, in which case the needle may be modified further with an additional bend of 1 in. from the previous bend (Fig. 13).

As noted above, the percutaneous approach to ganglion impar neurolysis requiring a bent needle can be difficult and time consuming. Love et al. described a new approach to ganglion impar neurolysis using cryoablation, going through the sacrococcygeal junction. In this approach transsacrococcygeal puncture is utilized, and cryoablation is used as the neurolytic modality (Love et al. 1998; Toshniwal et al. 2007). Toshniwal et al. described a transsacrococcygeal approach to ganglion impar neurolysis using bupivacaine and methylprednisolone acetate in addition to 8% aqueous phenol. They performed neurolysis on 16 consecutive patients. The procedure was successful in all patients. This group also performed ganglion impar block in patients with benign pain due to proctitis, idiopathic pain in the perineum, severe coccygodynia, in addition to malignant etiologies (Ayub 2000). Although no complications were reported by this group, the potential complications include discitis, and bleeding (Toshniwal et al. 2007).

The author described a EUS-guided approach to ganglion impar neurolysis. This approach does not require a bent needle or puncture of the sacrococcygeal disc. Also, with EUS, the rectal wall and posterior space is clearly visible. Injection of contrast to confirm the needle tip position posterior to the rectal wall is not necessary. A linear echoendoscope is introduced into the rectum and rotated posteriorly. Under fluoroscopy guidance, a 22 gauge needle is placed in front of the sacrococcygeal junction, and bupivacaine and alcohol are injected. This approach is technically easy to perform and appears safe. In the pilot study, the author performed ganglion impar neurolysis in two patients (Figs. 14 and 15). The technique was successful in both patients, and no complications were noted. Further large randomized, prospective trials are needed to confirm the safety and efficacy of this approach (Ayub 2000).

In patients with lower rectal cancer, staging, neurolysis, and fine needle aspiration of relevant lymph nodes can be performed in a single setting, thus saving time and costs.

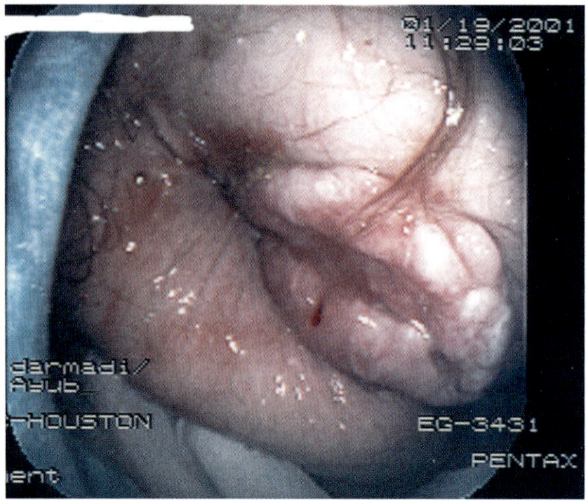

Fig. 14. Carcinoma anal canal with pain.

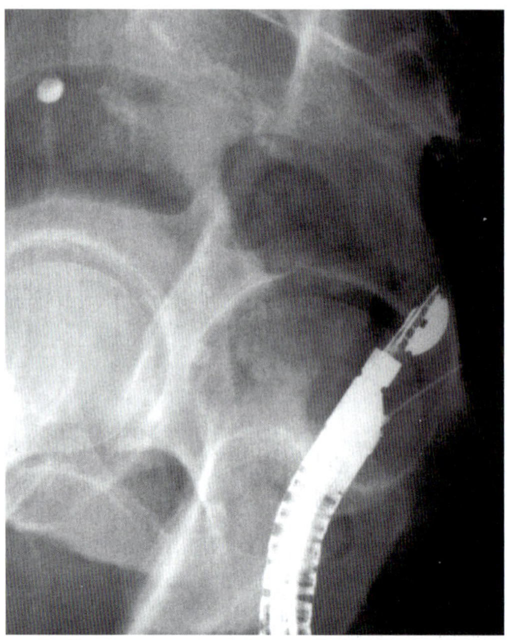

Fig. 15. EUS-guided approach.

SUMMARY OF KEY POINTS

- Chronic pain is a very common medical complaint, and is especially prevalent in patients with cancer.
- Effective nerve blocks exist for the management of abdominal, pelvic, and perineal pain in the form of neurolysis of the celiac plexus, superior hypogastric plexus and ganglion impar respectively.
- Endoscopic ultrasound guided approach to these nerve blocks appears safer and easier to perform compared to the percutaneous approach. This is because of the close

proximity of the scope to the target region and the ability to clearly visualize the blood vessels.

- In future these blocks will be performed increasingly by interventional endosonographers, thus widening the horizon of interventional endoscopy.
- Management of chronic pain requires a multidisciplinary team approach.

REFERENCES

Merskey H, Bogduk N. Classification of chronic pancreatitis. Seattle: IASP press; 1994.

Reddy SK, Shanti BF. Cancer pain: assessment and management. Prim Care Cancer. 2000;20:44–52.

Patt RB. Classification of cancer pain and cancer pain syndromes. Edited by Patt RB. Philadelphia: Lippincot-Raven Publishers; 1993. p. 3–57.

Kappis M. Erfahrungen mit local anasthesie bie bauchopertionen [German with English abstract]. Verh Dtsch Gesellsch Chir. 1914;43:87–9.

Ventafridda GV, Caraceni AT, Sbanotto AM, et al. Pain treatment in cancer of the pancreas. Eur J Surg Oncol. 1990;16:1–6.

Lankisch PG. Natural course of chronic pancreatitis. Pancreatology. 2001;1:3–14.

Eisenberg E, Carr DB, Chalmers TC. Neurolytic celiac plexus block for treatment of cancer pain: a meta-analysis. Anesth Analg. 1995;80:290–5. erratum 1995;81:213.

Usati M, Paquin SC, Dagenais M, et al. Preliminary results of a randomized, double blind, controlled trial of early EUS-guided celiac plexus neurolysis (EUS-CPN) versus conventional management for pain in patients with inoperable pancreatic cancer [abstract]. Gastrointest Endosc. 2008;68:AB211.

Newman PP. Visceral afferent functions of the nervous system. London: Arnold; 1974.

Levy MJ, Topazian MD, Wiersema MJ, et al. Initial evaluation of the efficacy and safety of endoscopic ultrasound-guided direct Ganglia neurolysis and block. Am J Gastroenterol. 2008;103:98–103.

Leblanc J, DeWitt J, Calley C, et al. A prospective randomized trial of 1 versus 2 injections during a single EUS-guided celiac plexus block for chronic pancreatitis pain. Gastrointest Endosc. 2009;69:835–42.

Wiersema MJ, Wiersema LM. Endosonography guided celiac plexus neurolysis. Gastrointest Endosc. 1996;44:656–62.

Wiersema MJ, Harada N, Wiersema LM. Endosonography guided celiac plexus neurolysis efficacy in chronic pancreatitis and malignant disease. Acta Endoscopia. 1998;28:67–79.

Gunaratnam NT, Sarma AV, Norton ID, Wiersema MJ. A prospective study of EUS-guided celiac plexus neurolysis for pancreatic cancer pain. Gastrointest Endosc. 2001;54:316–24.

Ischia S, Ischia A, Polati B, Finco G. Three posterior percutaneous celiac plexus block techniques. A prospective, randomized study in 61 patients with pancreatic cancer pain. Anesthesiology. 1992;76:534–40.

Gress F, Schmitt C, Sherman S, Ciccia D, Ikenberry S, Lehman G. Endoscopic ultrasound guided celiac plexus block for managing abdominal pain associated with chronic pancreatitis: a prospective single center experience. Am J Gastroenterol. 2001;96:409–16.

Gress F, Schmitt C, Sherman S, Ikenberry S, Lehman G. A prospective randomized comparison of endoscopic ultrasound and computed tomography-guided celiac plexus block for managing chronic pancreatitis pain. Am J Gastroenterol. 1999;94:900–5.

Gunaratnam NT, Wong GY, Wiersema MJ. EUS-guided celiac plexus block for the management of pancreatic pain. Gastrointest Endosc. 2000;52:S28–34.

Chan VW. Chronic diarrhea: an uncommon side effect of celiac plexus block. Anesth Analg. 1996;82:205–7.

Cataldo R, Potash M. Atropine as a treatment of diarrhea after celiac plexus block. Anesth Analg. 1996;83:1131–2.

Mercadante S. Octreotide in the treatment of diarrhea induced by celiac plexus block. Pain. 1995;61:345–6.

Iftikhar S, Loftus Jr EV. Gastroparesis after celiac plexus block. Am J Gastroenterol. 1998;93:2223–5.

Gress F, Ciacca D, Kiel J, Sherman S, Lehman G. Endoscopic ultrasound (EUS) guided celiac plexus block (CB) for management of pain due to chronic pancreatitis (CP): a large single center experience. Gastrointest Endosc. 1997;45:AB173.

Brass A. Anatomy and physiology: autonomic nerves and ganglia in pelvis. In: Netter FH, editor. The Ciba collection of medical illustrations, Nervous System, vol. 1. USA: Ciba Pharmaceutical Co; 1983. p. 85.

Snell RS, Katz J. Clinical anatomy for anesthesiologists. Norwalk: Appleton and Lange; 1988. p. 271.

Plancarte R, Amescua C, Patt R, et al. Superior hypogastric plexus block for pelvic cancer pain. Anesthesiology. 1990a;73:236.

Waldman SD, Wilson WL, Kreps RD. Superior hypogastric plexus block using a single needle and computed tomography guidance: description of a modified technique. Reg Anesth. 1991;16:286.

Kanazi G, Perkins FM, Thakur R, Dotson E. New technique for superior hypogastric plexus block. Reg Anesth Pain Med. 1999;24:473–6.

Ayub K. EUS guided superior hypogastric plexus neurolysis: a new technique for management of pelvic pain. Gastrointest Endosc. 2001;53:AB113.

Plancarte R, Amescua C, Patt RB, Aldrete JA. Superior hypogastric plexus block for pelvic cancer pain. Anesthesiology. 1990b;73:236–9.

Plancarte R, Amescua C, Patt RB. Presacral blockade of the ganglion of Walther (ganglion impar). Anesthesiology 1990; 73:A751.

Love MA, Varklet VL, Wilsey BL, Ferrante FM. Cryoablation: a novel approach to neurolysis of the ganglion impar block. Anesthesiology. 1998;88:1391–3.

Ayub K. A new approach to ganglion impar neurolysis using endoscopic ultrasound. Endoscopy. 2000;32 Suppl 1:244.

Toshniwal GR, Dureja GP, Prashanth SM. Transsacrococcygeal approach to ganglion impar block for management of chronic perineal pain: a prospective observational study. Pain Physician. 2007;10:661–6.

18 Colonoscopic Polypectomy

Peter H. Rubin and Jerome D. Waye

Contents

Keywords: Colonoscopic, Polypectomy, Contraindications, Procedure, Complications

INTRODUCTION

In the past three decades, flexible colonoscopy has proven to be the best tool available for the detection of both colonic polyps and cancer. The colonoscope provides not only superior diagnostic accuracy for detecting and obtaining biopsies of colonic luminal lesions, but also, in the case of polyps, the potential for simultaneous minimally invasive definitive therapy as polypectomy (Tolliver and Rex 2008).

Notwithstanding rare exceptions, the prevailing pathophysiologic dogma is that there is a polyp-cancer sequence so that that removal of colon polyps will prevent the development of colon cancer (Lofti et al. 1986; Winawer et al. 1993). Based on this, it is the prevailing practice that polyps discovered at colonoscopy should be resected. This chapter will review colonoscopic polypectomy, emphasizing technique, and placing it in the context of alternative available treatment strategies.

From: *Clinical Gastroenterology: Diagnostic and Therapeutic Procedures in Gastroenterology*,
Edited by: G. Y. Wu, S. Sridhar, DOI 10.1007/978-1-59745-044-7_18,

INDICATIONS

Most colon polyps are either hyperplastic or adenomatous. While it is true that adenomatous polyps carry a higher risk of evolving into malignancies than do hyperplastic polyps, the ability to predict accurately the pathology based on macroscopic inspection is poor. Nor is size per se a reliable criterion for determining malignant or pre-malignant pathology (Butterly et al. 2006). Therefore, all polyps detected at colonoscopy can be considered for colonoscopic removal and therapeutic polypectomy should be an intrinsic part of diagnostic colonoscopy. It is routine for colonoscopy consent forms to include polypectomy as part of the potential description of the procedure, and this should be discussed with the patient prior to the endoscopic examination.

On inspection, polyps can be classified as pedunculated or sessile (Figs. 1 and 2). Most polyps in the colon are sessile, and many of these will be located in the right colon, from

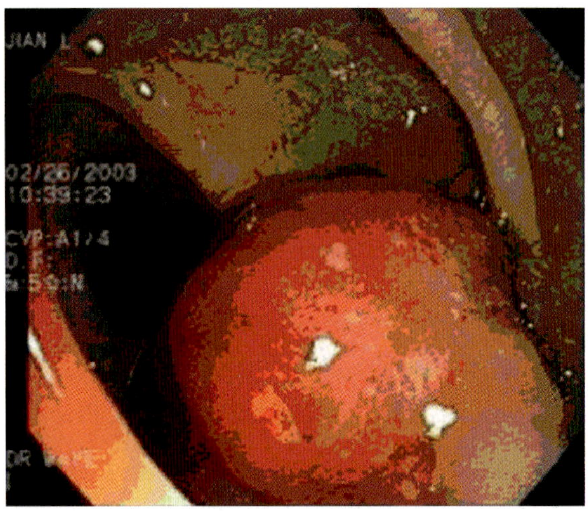

Fig. 1. Pedunculated polyp with reddish head arising from pale stalk in lower right.

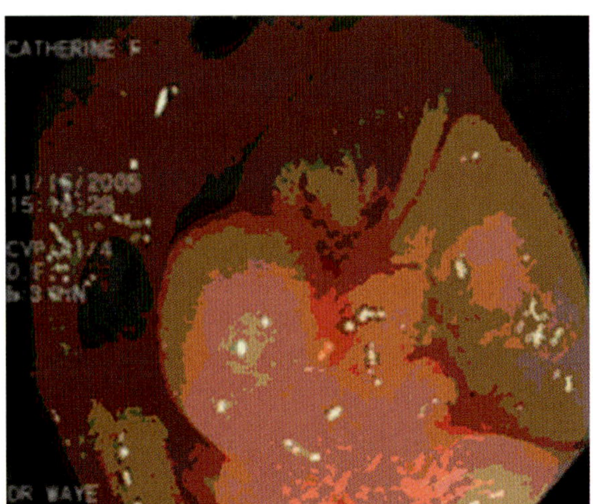

Fig. 2. Sessile polyp arising directly from the surrounding mucosa with no intervening stalk.

the hepatic flexure to the cecal caput. Pedunculated polyps have a pedicle of mucosa and submucosa that is thought to be generated by the persistent action of colonic peristalsis to evacuate the polyp. They are usually located in the sigmoid colon. In spite of the contractility of the rectum, large sessile polyps may grow in the rectum without a pedicle. The "ideal" polyp for colonoscopic resection is the pedunculated variety since the stalk separates the head of the polyp from the surrounding colon mucosa and thereby virtually assures complete removal of the polyp and minimizes the risk of thermal injury to the adjacent tissue. Nevertheless, most sessile polyps also can be safely and successfully removed by colonoscopy.

CONTRAINDICATIONS

Colonoscopic polypectomy cannot be performed adequately in a poorly cleansed colon. Residual fecal matter not only obscures the discovery and removal of smaller polyps, but also makes it more difficult to recover resected polyps, and increases the chance of explosion due to the presence of methane gas during electrocautery. Similarly, a poorly cooperative patient who is not able to follow instructions for the pre-procedure preparation or the post-polypectomy period, such as withholding anticoagulants, aspirin, and nonsteroidal anti-inflammatory medications, poses a relative contraindication.

As colonoscopic polypectomy is more invasive than purely diagnostic examinations, it is imperative that the patient does not have an underlying or medically-induced coagulopathy, and that anticoagulants be withheld during and immediately following the procedure (Hui et al. 2004; Friedland and Soetikno 2006). Anticoagulants such as warfarin usually are withheld for three or more days prior to colonoscopic polypectomy, usually in consultation with the patient's internist or cardiologist. In cases of artificial cardiac valves or other conditions in which anticoagulation must be continuous, enoxaparin or heparin is employed after stopping warfarin.

Not all colon polypoid lesions can be removed colonoscopically. A broad-based sessile polyp arising from more than one-half of the luminal circumference is a challenging task for all but the most proficient colonoscopist, although partial snare polypectomy can be performed to provide the pathologist with larger and deeper specimens for analysis. When a polyp is suspicious for invasive carcinoma or judged by the endoscopist to be unresectable colonoscopically, the site can be marked with an injected solution of carbon particles to aid the endoscopist in locating the polypectomy site at follow-up colonoscopic examination or for the surgeon to locate the site for resection, when approaching it from the serosal side of the colon (Fig. 3).

In placing the marker, it is important to ensure the carbon particles are deposited into the submucosal space, resulting in a visible elevated blue/black bleb under the mucosa. Sometimes the needle is inserted into the colon wall and the injected solution flows out through the needle tract back into the lumen instead of remaining in the submucosa which does not result in a permanent stain. If this happens, no mark is identifiable by the endoscopist or surgeon.

Other polyps that are unlikely to be removed successfully are those that traverse more than two adjacent haustral folds, encircle the base of the appendix, or form a flat, carpet-like expanse of polypoid tissue. Polyps that cross over two haustral folds usually cannot be cleared from the depressed area between the folds. Polyps that surround and go into the

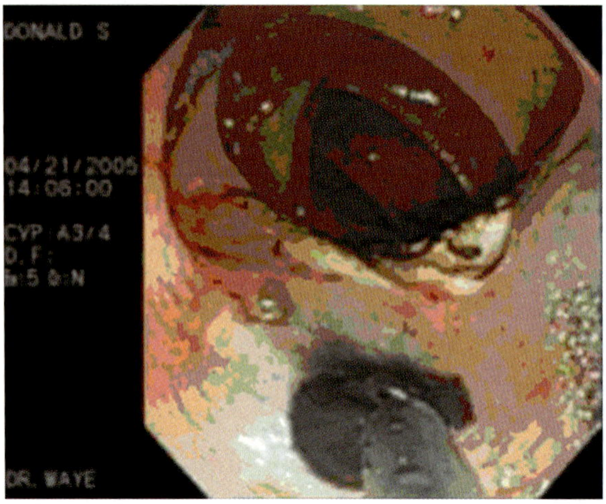

Fig. 3. Intramucosal injection of carbon particle solution to mark the polypectomy site. Some of the solution has leaked back into the lumen, but the pigmented blebs remain on the bottom and right side. It is best to mark all four quadrants for identification of the site if surgery is likely.

appendiceal base may be impossible to completely remove from the narrow appendix. A carpet-like polyp which extends over several centimeters may not be amenable to complete endoscopic resection and may require surgical extirpation by segmental resection. An attempt can be made to fulgurate the surface of such polyps with an argon plasma coagulator, the shank of the monopolar biopsy forceps, or a Bicap probe. However, it is unusual to be able to eradicate these lesions completely because of the superficial depth of tissue injury by these thermal probes. Furthermore, the tissue destroyed by thermal modalities is not available for pathology analysis.

The size of the polyp per se does not preclude polypectomy. Large polyps, however, may require special techniques for removal, as will be described below (Doniec et al. 2003; Boix et al. 2007).

Patients with implanted cardiac defibrillators pose a relative contraindication if electrocoagulation is to be employed for polypectomy because of concern for inducing a cardiac arrhythmia. Implanted defibrillators should be inactivated for the duration of the polypectomy using monopolar electric current, and reactivated when no further electrosurgical equipment is being employed. However, pacemakers pose no problem for electrosurgery since the electrical circuit is from the intestinal tract to the grounding pad and does not flow through the area of the pacemaker.

PROCEDURE SITE

Colonoscopic polypectomy can be performed as an outpatient in a hospital or in an office-based or ambulatory surgical center endoscopy suite. The rate of immediate complication is so low in colonic polypectomy, even for removal of large polyps, that usually it is unnecessary to hospitalize patients for removal of polyps. The literature supports the concept that all polyps that are endoscopically resectable can be successfully managed in an office situation (remote from the hospital).

Special situations such as antibiotic prophylaxis, anticoagulation, and implanted cardiac defibrillators also can be handled on an outpatient basis, often in consultation with the patient's general physician or cardiologist.

Hospitalization may be necessary when the patient's co-morbidities and special related needs make ambulatory colonoscopy a significant risk. These would include advanced neurologic, pulmonary, or renal disease.

PROCEDURE DESCRIPTION

Standard high frequency electrosurgical power units are used for polypectomy. These use monopolar current requiring a grounding pad which is applied to the patient's hip or upper leg. Before inserting the snare it is connected to the electrosurgical unit and can be tested by "sparking" the open snare on a metallic surface as current is applied.

A trained gastrointestinal assistant (GIA) is an important partner in the successful performance of colonoscopy and polypectomy. It is the responsibility of the GIA to ensure that the equipment is properly set up, and all precautions taken in advance to ensure patient safety. The GIA often is the person who handles the snare closure in close cooperation with the endoscopist.

One of the safety measures is to use the snare handle as an information source during polypectomy. This is accomplished during pre-procedure preparation by marking the shaft of the snare handle to indicate the position of the retracted slide-bar at which the wire snare tip is flush with the end of the plastic catheter (Fig. 4). When the slide bar is pulled back

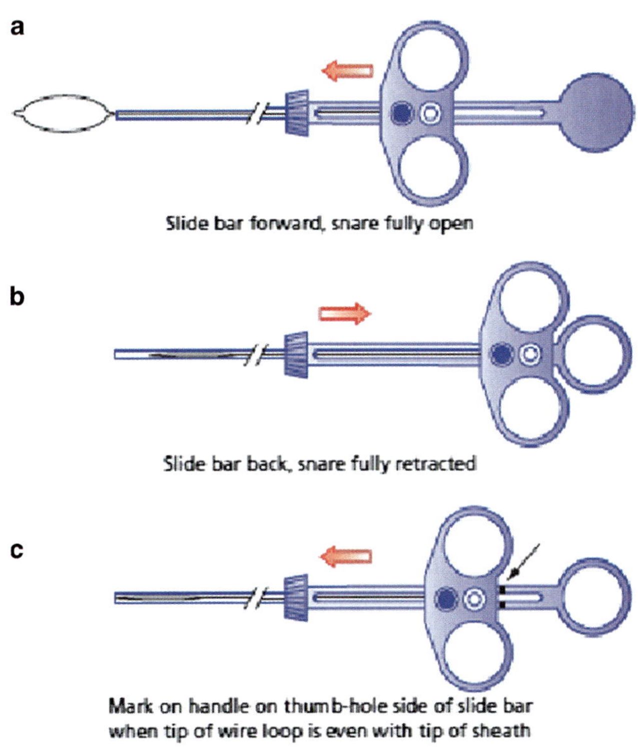

Fig. 4. Polypectomy snare. When slide bar is in the forward position, the snare is completely open. When the slide bar is pulled back, the snare is retracted completely within the sheath

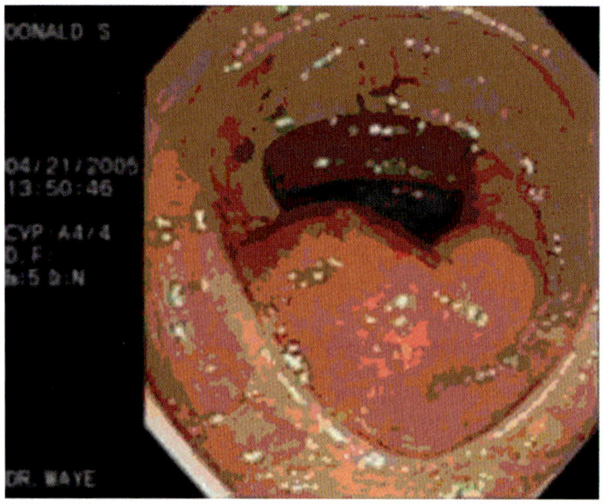

Fig. 5. Large sessile-appearing polyp. Probing with a snare will determine whether there is a stalk behind, permitting straightforward polypectomy. If it is a broad-based sessile polyp, it can be removed by piecemeal resection.

and snugly closed to a resistance sensation around a polyp, the distance from the slide bar to the previously drawn mark is an indication of the length of wire that extends beyond the tip of the plastic catheter and, thus, provides an estimate of the amount of tissue volume contained within the closed snare loop.

Polypectomy technique depends on whether the polyp is pedunculated or sessile and upon its size.

Pedunculated polyps: Polyps on a pedicle usually are removed readily with the snare and cautery technique. Some polyps may appear at first to be sessile, but are in fact large pedunculated polyps with the stalk hidden behind the polyp (Fig. 5). Other pedunculated polyps are on extremely long stalks, and pose a problem for removal because they tend to swing back and forth during the examination. They may be visible one moment and disappear suddenly from sight around a corner. Finding the pedicle and ensnaring the head of the polyp may be extremely difficult. It usually is necessary to advance the instrument beyond the polyp and proceed to the cecum to ensure that the colonoscope and the colon convolutions are straight upon withdrawal. This makes capture easier. If, however during intubation, the pedunculated polyp is lying in the right position in the visual field and seems to be relatively easy to ensnare, an attempt should be made to remove it at that time.

Sessile polyps: Polyps without stalks may be removed as well. For larger sessile polyps, injection of fluid into the submucosa beneath the polyp is useful to raise it above the deeper layers of the colon wall by creating a fluid cushion, as described in the next section.

Diminutive polyps: Tiny polyps of 2 mm or less in diameter can be removed safely and simply with conventional colonoscopy forceps, and those measuring up to 5 mm can be resected completely by a wire snare without electrocautery (cold snare technique) (Fig. 6) (Deenadayalu and Rex 2005). There is no excess bleeding from cold snare polypectomy sites.

Polyps of 1–2 cm: Intermediate sized polyps can be removed by wire snare and electrocautery, without the need for submucosal injection techniques.

Pedunculated polyps are ensnared about 2/3 of the way up the stalk and the snare tightened to snugness (Fig. 7). This position is selected so that if the stalk bleeds after

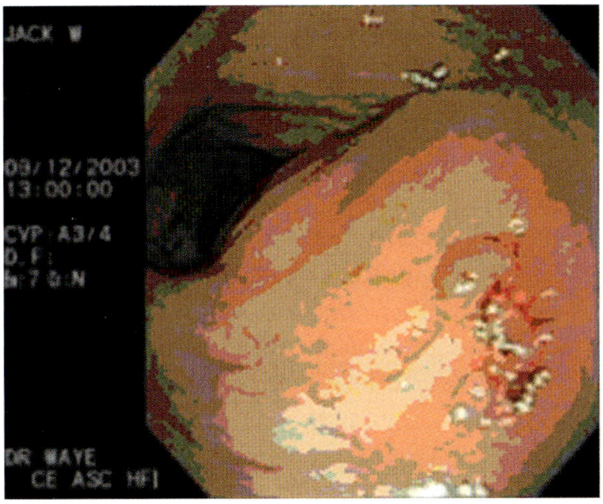

Fig. 6. Cold snare polypectomy. Polyps up to 5 mm in diameter can be safely resected with the snare, but without electrical current. Bleeding after this procedure is not common.

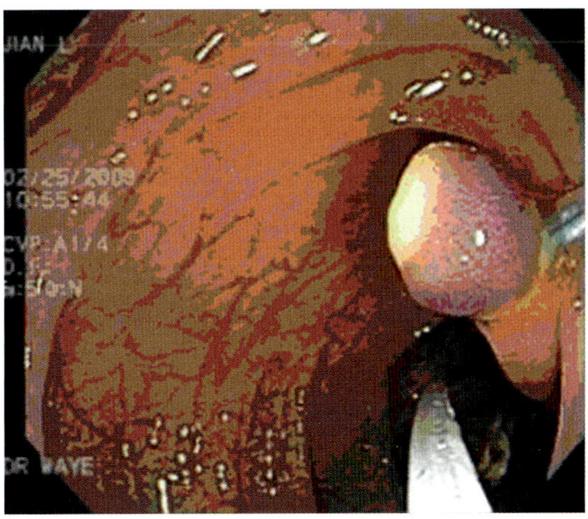

Fig. 7. Snare placement on pedunculated polyp. A wire snare had been placed about two thirds of the way up the stalk from the base, shown here with white thermocoagulation. If bleeding occurs, the stalk can be resnared and tamponaded or, as shown here, a loop can be placed adjacent to the top of the remaining stalk.

polypectomy it can again be lassoed with the snare and tamponaded. When the position of the wire snare has been judged to be satisfactory, cautery is applied and the area immediately adjacent to the wire snare observed to blanch. The snare is then closed with continued application of current. As soon as the polyp has been separated from the mucosa, the polypectomy site is inspected for bleeding.

Sessile polyps are ensnared with care taken not to entrap adjacent folds of non-polypoid mucosa. The mark previously drawn on the snare handle is checked to verify that the distance from the slide bar to the mark is an appropriate amount for the size of the polyp, and that the snare did not capture folds of normal colon. The size of the closed snare loop that extends beyond the tip of the catheter sheath can be judged by looking at the distance on the handle shaft between the mark and the slide bar. If that distance is greater than 1.5 cm, the snare should be repositioned closer to the margin of the polyp or the polyp resected in a piece-meal fashion as described in the next section. An unexpectedly large distance from the slide-bar to the previous mark on the handle should be noted by the assistant and communicated to the endoscopist.

Another method to check on whether mucosa on the far side of the polyp has been captured within the tightened wire loop is to jiggle the catheter sheath to and fro at the biopsy port, while observing the colon walls around the polyp. The polyp should be seen to move independently of the surrounding colon walls as the sheath is jiggled. If, however, both the polyp and the surrounding colon wall move simultaneously, there is a strong probability that a portion of the wall has been captured within the tip of the snare loop. Removal of the snare or partially opening the loop for repositioning should be considered before application of electrocautery current.

Once the correct snare position has been verified, the polyp is then lifted from the surrounding mucosa by deflection of the tip of the colonoscope. With application of electrocautery, a white area appears around the closed snare which is then tightened, resulting in separation of the polyp. Some physicians prefer to personally close the snare, but the usual practice is for the GIA to perform this in close cooperation with the doctor. After inspection of the polypectomy site for hemostasis, the resected polyp is retrieved.

POLYP RETRIEVAL

Polyp retrieval can be accomplished in several ways. The polyp may be aspirated through the scope into a suction trap placed between the suction nipple near the light source, and the tubing that connects it to the waste reservoir. Larger polyp pieces can be cut into smaller segments for suction retrieval. This is accomplished by using the snare to "cold-cut" the free pieces into the size that can be aspirated. Another technique is to apply continuous suction on a free piece of polyp during withdrawal, with the resected polyp held on the end of the scope. A single portion can be resnared and withdrawn with the colonoscope. A large single fragment or several pieces may be retrieved by utilizing a mesh basket device (Fig. 8) (Miller and Waye 2001) or a retrieval basket.

Polyps larger than 2 cm: Cautery injury to adjacent mucosa during resection of larger sessile polyps can be minimized by injecting fluid sub-mucosally around the perimeter of the polyp, thereby raising the polyp on a liquid "cushion" (Fig. 9) (Iishi et al. 1997). This prevents entrapment and cautery damage to the muscularis propria or serosa from the thermal energy created by the snare. The objective is to place a significant amount of fluid beneath the polyp to elevate it entirely above the normal mucosal plane. The injected solution also serves to prevent deep thermal injury as electrocautery current is applied. It is best to begin the injections on the far-side of the polyp base before injecting the base adjacent to the colonoscope tip.

This technique can be used for removal of sessile adenomas, whether small or large, but should be administered to any sessile polyp larger than 1.5 cm that is located proximal to the rectum. When current is then applied via a polypectomy snare, the lesion can be more safely removed because of a large submucosal "cushion" of fluid which prevents thermal injury to the deeper layer of the colon wall. The injected fluid may be saline (normal or

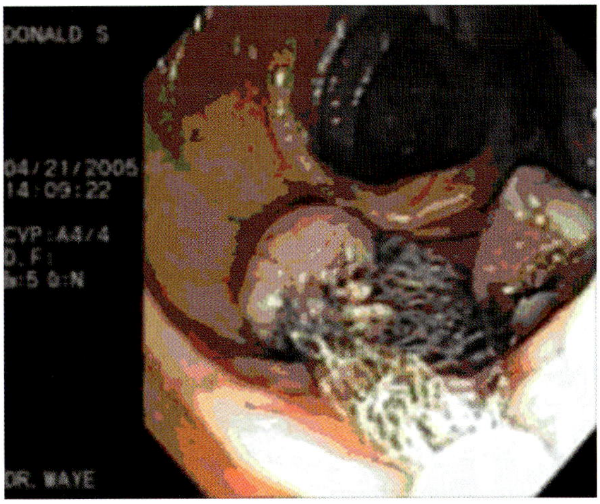

Fig. 8. Deployment of mesh basket to retrieve polyp fragments after polypectomy.

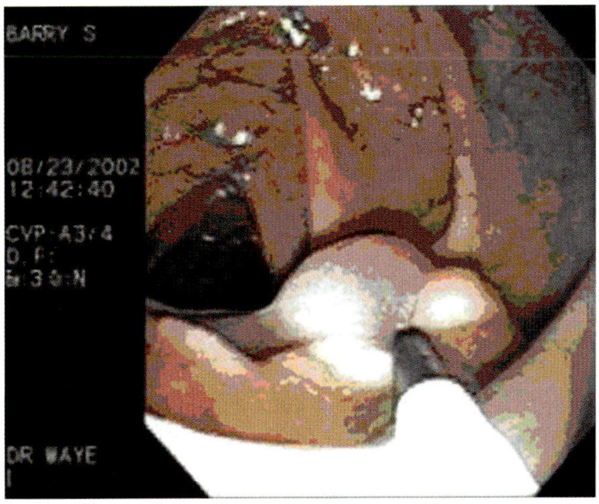

Fig. 9. Injection of saline to raise a polyp before resection. Injection begins on far side of polyp, proceeding to circumferential injections until polyp is raised on cushion of injected saline.

hypertonic), with or without methylene blue to enhance visualization with or without epinephrine (to permit the fluid to stay at the site for a longer interval than saline and to decrease immediate post-polypectomy bleeding). The addition of dye provides visual contrast between the pinkish adenomatous polyp lying on top of a bluish fluid collection.

Fluid is directly injected through a long and stiff endotherapy needle. The sheath of the endotherapy needle should be especially firm so that the needle can be pushed through the entire length of a colonoscope without crumpling, even when traversing several loops and bends in the instrument to reach a site in the right colon. The needle may be placed into the submucosa just at the edge of a polyp, or if the polyp is large and flat, multiple injections may be given around the polyp or directly into the middle of the polyp. If a bleb does not form at the injection site when 1 mL of fluid has been given, the needle should be withdrawn since the tip may have penetrated the wall, and be external to the serosal surface in the peritoneal cavity. If the needle placement is too superficial, the fluid will leak out of the beveled edge of the needle and spill into the lumen. This spilling is especially noticeable when a colored fluid, such as methylene blue is used. Multiple repeated needle placements and attempts at injection may be required to locate the correct plane for polyp elevation.

The absence of a visible bleb does not indicate that a similar bleb is forming on the serosal surface, since there is no areolar tissue in which fluid may collect except the submucosa. The injected fluid only expands the submucosal tissue layer as there is no other tissue plane in the colon wall into which the fluid will flow. If possible, the approach by the needle injection should be tangential and not perpendicular to the mucosal surface. When attempting submucosal injection for polypectomy (SIP), there is no specific volume of fluid that is used; rather, the desired end point is a large submucosal swelling beneath the polyp and adjacent portions of the mucosa. Elevation of the polyp may take 3–4 mL of saline given in several places, although some investigators use up to 30 mL of fluid.

Polyps up to 2 cm in diameter may be removed with one application of the snare, but larger polyps may require several transections in piecemeal fashion. It is permissible to remove a much larger piece with this technique than ordinarily ensnared when in the right colon without a cushion of fluid.

If a polyp fails to elevate (the "non-lifting sign") when a submucosal fluid injection is given, and fluid can be seen to elevate the adjacent mucosal space, it may be an indication of infiltration by cancer into deeper tissues, limiting the expansion of the submucosal layer. Although deep or superficial needle placement may be the cause for failure to raise a bleb under a polyp, a submucosal bulging or bleb on one side of a polyp in response to injection without any visible elevation of the tumor itself (or only minimal elevation of one portion) is a clue that there is infiltration into the submucosa. This phenomenon may also be caused by a prior attempt at polypectomy with healing and scarring of the mucosa and submucosa, preventing their separation by fluid injection.

During piecemeal polypectomy, the subsequent placement of the snare may be immediately adjacent to the first, with the edge of the wire positioned into the denuded area just created by removal of the previous piece. In this fashion, multiple portions can be sequentially resected in an orderly fashion, with removal of each succeeding piece being facilitated by its predecessor. Several deployments may be required, removing fragments until satisfactory polypectomy is achieved.

If the ensnared polyp is large, the snare may become impacted and be unable to close completely to sever the polyp. If this occurs, the electrosurgical unit can be adjusted to deliver cutting current. To avoid this complication, the polyp should be resected in a piecemeal fashion with multiple deployments of the snare to adjacent portions of the polyp. The polypectomy site should be inspected carefully for any evidence of bleeding or residual polyp.

Residual polyp fragments can be removed with either electrocautery using forceps or snare or by employing an argon plasma coagulator (Fig. 10) (Zlatanic et al. 1999; Regula et al. 2003).

Argon Plasma coagulation: The argon plasma coagulator can safely treat the base of a polypectomy site to ensure total ablation of an adenoma, once piecemeal polypectomy has been performed. The longer that the transfer of energy is directed to one area of the colon wall, the deeper will be the thermal damage. To prevent a deep burn, the tip of the probe

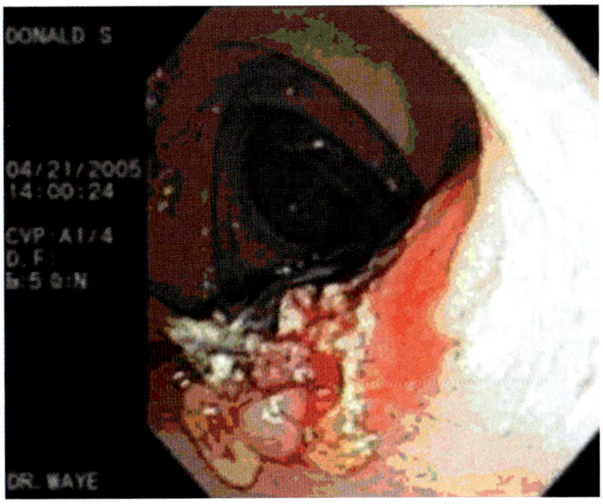

Fig. 10. Residual polyp fragments after polypectomy. These can be removed by additional snaring, or application of bicap probe or argon laser coagulation

should be kept in motion during activation. Because of the ability to maintain a superficial depth of thermal injury, the argon plasma coagulator can be successfully used to "paint" a large area of flat adenoma or residual tissue at the base of a polypectomy site, without damage to deep layers of the colon wall.

Complete resection of large sessile polyps may require several sessions and, since high rates of local recurrences are reported, it is mandatory to confirm complete removal by follow-up examinations.

COMPLICATIONS

The major complications after polypectomy are bleeding, thermal injury to the adjacent colon wall, and perforation (Nivatvongs 1986). Bleeding may be evident immediately or up to 7–10 days after polypectomy, at which time the thrombotic eschar has sloughed before adequate re-epithelialization of the polypectomy site has occurred.

If bleeding obscures vision during piecemeal polypectomy, the blood may be dispersed by flushing water through the biopsy channel or through a dedicated water channel on more advanced endoscopes. Mild bleeding may be controlled by continuation of piecemeal polypectomy where cautery of the next segment may seal the bleeding vessels at the previously cut edge.

Bleeding from an amputated pedunculated polyp stalk can be managed in a number of ways. First, the area should be lavaged to optimize identification of the bleeding site. One approach to a bleeding stalk of a pedunculated polyp is to simply repeat snaring of the remaining stalk, and closing the snare as a tourniquet or tamponade. The snare should be opened again after 5 min and closed again if oozing persists.

Alternative hemostatic techniques are application of additional coagulation to the site, injection of epinephrine, utilization of argon plasma coagulation, or deployment of endoscopic clips (Harewood 2007). A 1:10,000 solution of epinephrine can be injected directly into the site of bleeding to promote hemostasis. Another option is to employ a thermal modality such as an argon plasma coagulator, Bicap or heater probe.

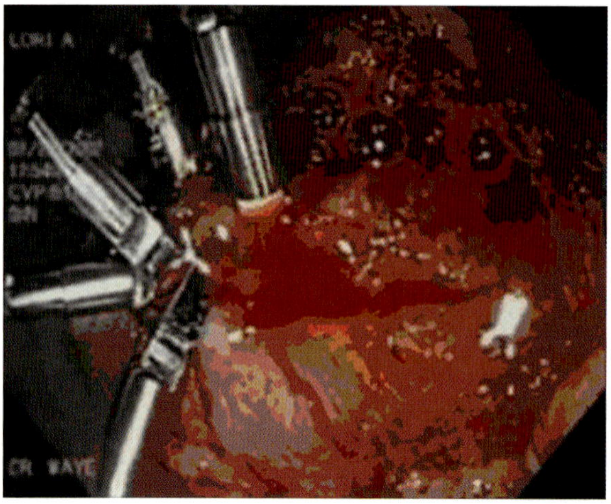

Fig. 11. Application of clips to bleeding polypectomy site. Multiple clips may be required to achieve hemostasis

Mucosal clips are small tweezer-like devices delivered through the colonoscope. They may be used also to mark mucosal lesions and identify the distance reached by the colonoscope, as well as to mark edges of tumors prior to expandable metal stent placement (Fig. 11). The clips are especially useful for bleeding from flat polypectomy sites, but have also been used successfully to stop arterial pulsatile bleeding from the severed stalk of pedunculated polyps. It is possible to apply a clip onto the base of a pedunculated polyp close to the bowel wall and snare the polyp above the clip using standard snare techniques. If electrocoagulation is used after affixing clips it is important that the wire snare does not touch the metal clip, lest an aberrant current pathway be activated, with a potential burn of the colon wall. Clips often dislodge spontaneously within several days. But, by then permanent hemostasis usually has been achieved. There is controversy concerning their use to prophylactically prevent post-polypectomy bleeding.

Transmural thermal injury to the adjacent wall presents as localized abdominal pain, tenderness, and sometimes low-grade fever. The colon wall thickness is 1.4–2.3 mm and thermal injury can extend to the serosal surface during polypectomy. Wall thermal injury usually can be managed with a liquid diet and oral broad-spectrum antibiotics and resolves within a day or so.

Perforation presents as severe abdominal pain, abdominal distension, diminished or absent bowel sounds, abdominal tenderness with rebound, elevated white blood cell count, and radiographic or CT evidence of pneumoperitoneum. This may require hospitalization, intravenous fluids, antibiotics, bowel rest, and, sometimes, surgical consultation.

POST-PROCEDURE CARE

After routine, uncomplicated polypectomy, the patient may resume a full diet, although some recommend a low-roughage diet for several days. Aspirin and nonsteroidal anti-inflammatory medication is held for at least 5 days and full therapeutic systemic anticoagulation not resumed for several days unless strongly indicated, such as for synthetic heart valves. Other medications may be resumed on the day following the procedure.

Of course, patients and their companions are routinely advised to call with any significant bleeding, pain, or temperature elevation. Arrangements are made to discuss pathology results and to answer any further questions.

RESULTS

Colonoscopic polypectomy is highly effective, but not perfect (Rex et al. 1997; Rex and Eid 2008). Large, multi-center data suggest that after successful complete polypectomy, repeat colonoscopy can be delayed for at least 3–5 years (Winawer et al. 2006). Polyps found at follow-up examinations may be recurrent at the site of former polypectomy or be new polyps. Shorter interval follow-up is indicated for incomplete colonoscopy, poor preparation of the colon for the examination, or any concern that the polyp was not completely removed.

If a large polyp resected in piecemeal fashion is found to have invasive carcinoma, the pathologist may not be able to assess the risk of residual malignancy because of inability to judge a clear margin, necessitating early surveillance or segmental resection (Robert 2007).

When the pathology of the resected polyp is hyperplastic, most gastroenterologists would agree on a 5–10 year interval for repeat examination, although there has been some evidence suggesting that there is a higher subsequent incidence of adenomatous polyps and cancer in patients who initially present with hyperplastic polyps, especially multiple and right colonic (Jass 2004).

ALTERNATIVES

Aside from colonoscopy, polyps can be detected by barium enema or CT scan with colon protocol "virtual colonoscopy." These studies are useful in patients refusing colonoscopy or in those in whom complete colonoscopy could not be accomplished due to anatomical impediments. Like colonoscopy, they require purging of colonic fecal material. Unlike colonoscopy, these alternatives may not detect small polyps and have no therapeutic (polypectomy) capability. Therefore, patients who are found to have polypoid lesions on these studies must then undergo colonoscopy for polyp removal.

Prior to colonoscopic polypectomy, laparotomy was necessary for the removal of polyps. Today, this is rarely necessary, and is reserved for invasive carcinomas, polyps that cannot technically be resected colonoscopically as described earlier, or for polyps that recur repeatedly after colonoscopic polypectomy.

Open laparotomy has been replaced in many hospitals with laparoscopic resection. Here, again, colonoscopy may be a useful or necessary adjunct by marking the polyp site by four-quadrant intra-mucosal injection of carbon particles in suspension to enable the surgeon to identify the site from the serosal surface.

COST

The cost of colonoscopic polypectomy varies significantly from region to region. Medicare and other insurance carriers readily pay for screening colonoscopies after age 50 (or after age 40 when positive family history of colon polyps or cancer). Colonoscopies with polypectomy and surveillance follow-up examinations at appropriate intervals are reimbursed as well (Robert 2007).

In conclusion, colonoscopic polypectomy remains a major tool for clearing the colon of polyps and surveying it for recurrent or additional polyps. It can be performed safely in an outpatient setting with minimal sedation.

SUMMARY OF KEY POINTS

- Most colon polyps are either hyperplastic or adenomatous.
- All polyps detected at colonoscopy can be considered for colonoscopic removal.
- Polyps on a pedicle usually are removed readily with the snare and cautery technique.
- For larger sessile polyps, injection of fluid into the submucosa beneath the polyp is useful to raise it above the deeper layers of the colon wall by creating a fluid cushion.
- Polyps up to 2 cm in diameter may be removed with one application of the snare, but larger polyps may require several transections in piecemeal fashion.
- The major complications after polypectomy are bleeding, thermal injury to the adjacent colon wall, and perforation.

REFERENCES

Boix J, Lorenzo-Zuniga V, de Moreno Vega V, Ananos FE, Domenech E, Ojanguren I, et al. Endoscopic removal of large sessile colorectal adenomas: is it safe and effective? Dig Dis Sci. 2007;52:840–4.

Butterly LF, Chase MP, Pohl H, Fiarman GS. Prevalence of clinically important histology in small adenomas. Clin Gastroenterol Hepatol. 2006;4:343–8.

Deenadayalu VP, Rex DK. Colon polyp retrieval after cold snaring. Gastrointest Endosc. 2005;62:253–6.

Doniec JM, Lohnert MS, Schneiwind B, Bokelman F, Kremer B, Grimm H. Endoscopic removal of large colorectal polyps: prevention of unnecessary surgery? Dis Colon Rectum. 2003;46:340–8.

Friedland S, Soetikno R. Colonoscopy with polypectomy in anticoagulated patients. Gastrointest Endosc. 2006;64:98–100.

Harewood GC. Prophylactic clip application after colonic polypectomy. Gastrointest Endosc. 2007;65:183.

Hui AJ, Wong RMY, Ching JYL, Hung LCT, Chung SCS, Sung JJY. Colonoscopic polypectomy bleeding with anticoagulants and antiplatelet agents: analysis of 1657 cases. Gastrointest Endosc. 2004;59:44–8.

Iishi H, Tatsuta M, Kitamura S, Narahara H, Iseki K, Ishiguro S. Endoscopic resection of large sessile colorectal polyps using a submucosal saline injection technique. Hepatogastroenterology. 1997;44:698–702.

Jass JR. Hyperplastic polyps and colorectal cancer: is there a link? Clin Gastroenterol Hepatol. 2004;2:1–8.

Lofti AM, Spencer RJ, Ilstrop DM, Meltov LJ. Colorectal polyps and the risk of subsequent carcinoma. Mayo Clin Proc. 1986;61:337–43.

Miller K, Waye JD. Polyp retrieval after colonoscopy polypectomy: use of the Roth retrieval net. Gastrointest Endosc. 2001;54:505–7.

Nivatvongs S. Complications in colonoscopic polypectomy. An experience with 1555 polypectomies. Dis Colon Rectum. 1986;29:825–30.

Regula J, Wronska E, Polkawski M, Nasierowska-Guttmeier A, Pachlewski J, Rupinski M, et al. Argon plasma coagulation after piecemeal polypectomy of sessile colorectal adenomas: long-term follow-up study. Endoscopy. 2003;35:212–8.

Rex DK, Eid E. Considerations regarding the present and future roles of colonoscopy in colorectal cancer prevention. Clin Gastroenterol Hepatol. 2008;6:506–14.

Rex DK, Cutler CS, Lemmel GI, et al. Colonoscopic miss rates of adenomas determined by back-to-back colonoscopies. Gastroenterology. 1997;112:24–8.

Robert ME. The malignant colon polyp: diagnosis and therapeutic recommendations. Clin Gastroenterol Hepatol. 2007;5:662–7.

Tolliver KA, Rex DK. Colonoscopic polypectomy. Gastroenterol Clin N Am. 2008;37:229–51.
Winawer SJ, Zaube AG, Ho MN, et al. Prevention of colorectal cancer by colonoscopic polypectomy. The National Polyp Study Workgroup. NEJM. 1993;329:1977–81.
Winawer SJ, Zauber AG, Fletcher RH, Stillman JS, ÓBrien MJ, Levin B, et al. Guidelines for colonoscopy surveillance after polypectomy: a consensus update by the US Multi-Society Task Force on Colorectal Cancer and the American Cancer Society. Gastroenterology. 2006;130:1872–5.
Zlatanic J, Waye JD, Kim PS, Baicco PJ, Glein GW. Large sessile colonic adenomas: use of argon plasma coagulator to supplement piecemeal snare polypectomy. Gastrointest Endosc. 1999;49:731–5.

19 Acute Colonic Bleeding

Gustavo A. Machicado and Dennis M. Jensen

CONTENTS

Keywords: Acute, Colonic, Bleeding, Bowel preparation, Lesions

INTRODUCTION

The term "lower gastrointestinal (LGI) bleeding" usually refers to a bleeding site starting below the ligament of Treitz (Jensen and Machicado 1988). "Hematochezia" is the clinical term applied to the passage of bright red blood or maroon colored stool, with or without clots, per rectum. We prefer to use "severe hematochezia" rather than lower gastrointestinal (LGI) or colonic bleeding, because the former is a clinically relevant term. Also, the terms "lower or colonic GI bleeding" assume that all patients with severe hematochezia have colonic bleeding sites, which is incorrect. About 15–20% of patients with severe hematochezia have upper gastrointestinal (UGI) sources of bleeding, another 4–6% have documented bleeding from the small bowel between the ligament of Treitz and the terminal ileum, and another 3–5% have no source identified (Jensen and Machicado 1988; Kovacs and Jensen 2005).

From: *Clinical Gastroenterology: Diagnostic and Therapeutic Procedures in Gastroenterology*,
Edited by: G. Y. Wu, S. Sridhar, DOI 10.1007/978-1-59745-044-7_19,

The majority of ambulatory adult patients with hematochezia present with low grade or self-limited bleeding, and do not require hospitalization or urgent intervention. Such patients can be managed in an outpatient setting. A smaller group of patients experience severe hematochezia and require hospitalization because of the volume of blood loss or symptoms due to severe anemia or comorbidity (Jensen and Machicado 1988; Kovacs and Jensen 2005). Another group of patients develop severe hematochezia while already hospitalized for other medical or surgical conditions (e.g., inpatient hematochezia). These often have very severe hematochezia, and usually require a systematic and expeditious approach to their resuscitation, preparation for colonoscopy, diagnosis, and treatment.

We recommend an aggressive and systematic approach to all patients hospitalized with severe hematochezia. This includes preparation of the patient with oral purge, while undergoing resuscitation, followed by urgent colonoscopy for diagnosis and treatment rather than angiography or elective GI procedures when the bleeding appears to stop. This endoscopic approach is similar to that used for patients with severe upper gastrointestinal hemorrhage. This approach changes outcomes of patients, particularly for those with severe or persistent hematochezia (Jensen and Machicado 1988; Kovacs and Jensen 2005).

The purposes of this chapter are to describe severe hematochezia, our approach to early resuscitative measures of the patient, our approach to the early diagnosis and treatment of the various lesions responsible for severe hematochezia (or "lower GI bleeding"), and results of this approach. We also review a traditional medical, angiographic, and surgical approach to severe hematochezia and contrast outcomes and costs of traditional and urgent endoscopic management strategies.

EPIDEMIOLOGY

Acute LGI bleeding occurs with a higher frequency in the elderly who suffer from one or more comorbid conditions. The incidence of colonic bleeding has been reported to increase from 1 in 100,000 for patients in the third decade of life to as high as 20–30 per 100,000 in patients in the eighth and ninth decades of life (Longstreth 1997). LGI bleeding is about one-fifth as common as upper gastrointestinal (UGI) bleeding (Longstreth 1997; Kollef et al. 1997; Peura et al. 1997; Velayos et al. 2004). However, this ratio may change in the future because of the decreasing incidence of peptic ulcer disease and the aging population.

Mortality rates of LGI hemorrhage are usually less than 5%, but they are higher in patients who have emergency surgery (Longstreth 1997). Similar to UGI hemorrhage, patients who start bleeding while in the hospital for an unrelated medical/surgical condition (defined as "inpatient hematochezia") have a much higher mortality rate (23%) than those who are admitted to the hospital for LGI bleeding (2.4%) (Longstreth 1997). Although the reasons for this are not completely clear, most patients with inpatient hematochezia have severe comorbid conditions and these are aggravated by severe bleeding.

RESUSCITATION AND INITIAL EVALUATION

When patients present in shock (severe volume depletion, hypotension and tachycardia), they require good intravenous access (two large bore intravenous lines) and vigorous replacement of intravenous fluids and/or blood. For patients with coagulopathies [prolonged

Table 1
Resuscitation and management of patients with severe hematochezia (Jensen and Machicado 1988, 1997; Kovacs and Jensen 2005; Jensen et al. 2000)

- Establish one or preferably two large bore intravenous lines
- Assess intravenous volume and replace vigorously
- Evaluate degree of blood loss and replace with packed RBCs
- Evaluate coagulation and correct with FFP, platelets, and/or desmopressin acetate (DDAVP)
- Place a nasogastric tube to check for a possible UGI source-blood or bile
- Treat comorbid conditions

RBC red blood cells, *FFP* fresh frozen plasma

prothrombin time (PT) or international normalized ratio (PT-INR) either from liver disease or anticoagulant therapy (warfarin)] and ongoing hematochezia, fresh frozen plasma (FFP) transfusions to normalize coagulopathies are recommended. Fresh frozen plasma replaces most liver dependent coagulation factors, thereby normalizing clotting. Patients with severe thrombocytopenia (e.g., platelet count less than 50,000) or severe chronic renal failure may require platelet transfusions for definitive hemostasis of ongoing hematochezia. Treatment of comorbidities and close monitoring in an intensive care unit or a telemetry unit by skilled nurses are also highly recommended (refer to Table 1).

The patient with severe hematochezia should have a complete medical history and careful physical examination performed. The medical history may give the physician clues as to the potential sources and location of the bleeding site. Elderly patients with heart or peripheral vascular disease who present with abdominal pain and hematochezia may have ischemic colitis. A history of cirrhosis can suggest varices, most often esophageal or gastric, but rectal varices or anastomotic varices also can present as severe hematochezia. Severe heart disease (particularly valvular), or chronic renal insufficiency can be associated with bleeding from GI angiomas. Histories of inflammatory bowel disease (IBD), peptic ulcer disease, diverticulosis, or internal hemorrhoids might indicate potential bleeding sites. A history of recent colonic polypectomy, particularly of a large sessile polyp, can suggest delayed bleeding from a post polypectomy ulcer. Abdominal pain, weight loss, fever, diarrhea or vomiting are important in the differential diagnosis of inflammatory, infectious, or malignant lesions.

As part of the medical history, it is also important to elicit and list all medicines, including over-the-counter (OTC) drugs and herbal medications, which the patient with GI bleeding has taken acutely or chronically. It is recommended that physicians or nurses speak with family members and ask them to bring in medication bottles of the patient with hematochezia, both OTC and prescription. Some of these drugs may either cause GI lesions or aggravate GI bleeding by interfering with intrinsic coagulation of the patient. Aspirin (in any dose, including 81 mg/day), non-steroidal anti-inflammatory drugs (NSAID's), antiplatelet drugs, anticoagulants, antibiotics, inflammatory bowel disease drugs, or antiarrhythmics may cause either GI lesions or cause or aggravate GI hemorrhage. Herbal medications such as gingko, echinacea, and ginseng may also cause or worsen GI hemorrhage from any pre-existing gut lesion.

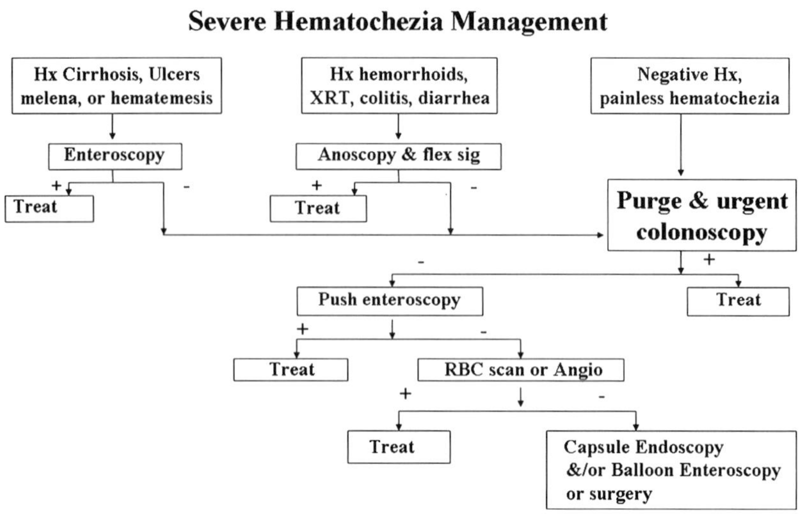

APPROACH TO THE PATIENT WITH SEVERE HEMATOCHEZIA–CLINICAL ALGORITHM

Depending on the clues obtained during the history and physical examination, one can approach the diagnostic evaluation of the patient in a more rational manner (refer to Fig. 1). Should the patient give a history of liver cirrhosis, ulcers, recent (within 30 days) aspirin or NSAID use, passage of melena or hematemesis, then an UGI source of bleeding should be excluded either by upper endoscopy or push enteroscopy. If the patient gives a history of hemorrhoids, pelvic radiation, colitis/proctitis, or diarrhea, then we first perform anoscopy and flexible sigmoidoscopy following enemas to clear the distal colon of blood and stool. If both studies prove to be negative, we purge the patient to clean the colon and perform urgent colonoscopy, whenever they are free of stool, clots, and red blood. If there is no significant history or physical findings to suggest any location for the bleeding, we use bowel preparation and urgent colonoscopy for primary diagnosis and treatment. Should urgent colonoscopy and anoscopy not yield a diagnosis, we perform push enteroscopy. Then, if the patient does not have a localization or etiologic source of severe bleeding, we recommend further workup. If the patient has continued bleeding or rebleeding, we recommend RBC scanning and/or abdominal angiography. If all these studies are negative for identification of a bleed site, then we will consider capsule endoscopy and/or either single or double balloon enteroscopy. Refer to Fig. 1 which outlines our current approach to patients with severe hematochezia.

DIAGNOSTIC EVALUATIONS

The first step to diagnosis should be to determine whether the bleeding source is likely to be upper GI, small bowel, or colonic site. We recommend placement of a nasogastric (NG) or orogastric (OG) tube for gastric lavage as 15–20% of patients with severe hematochezia bleed from an UGI tract site. Other risk factors for an UGI source include a history of UGI bleeding from ulcers, portal hypertension, inpatient hematochezia, and hypotension or shock (Jensen and Machicado 1988; Kovacs and Jensen 2005; Longstreth 1997). Although the value of a nasogastric tube aspirate has been questioned by others (Cuellar et al. 1990), we still find it useful and recommend its use to exclude an UGI bleeding source in a large proportion of patients, particularly those with a peptic ulcer history, or patients with inpatient hematochezia (Kovacs and Jensen 2001). When bile is obtained in the presence of ongoing hematochezia, there is continuity with the duodenum and an UGI lesion is unlikely as the source of the hematochezia. If no evidence can be found of UGI bleeding, then an urgent colonoscopy (within 12 h), after adequate colon preparation, is highly recommended for diagnosis and possible hemostasis. If the colonoscopy with terminal ileal entubation is negative, we recommend a careful examination of the anus and distal rectum with a slotted anoscope to evaluate for bleeding internal hemorrhoids and to exclude fissures and anal tumors. We have found this to be a safe approach and the diagnostic yield with this urgent clinical and endoscopic algorithm approaches 95% (Jensen and Machicado 1988). In contrast, colonoscopy in an unprepared colon is often non-diagnostic and can be dangerous. Urgent colonoscopy of a well-prepared patient is not only an effective diagnostic tool, but also allows for therapeutic intervention. It is a cost effective approach to the management of these patients (Jensen and Machicado 1997).

COLONOSCOPY

Colonoscopy is performed using a video-colonoscope which is a flexible tube with a miniature camera at the tip. The distal end of the instrument is maneuverable which allows the endoscopist to direct the instrument through the entire colon during insertion. In addition, colonoscopes have an irrigation port to keep the lens clear and another port for target irrigation of focal areas. An open channel is included for suctioning material during the procedure and for the passage of a variety of therapeutic tools. Through this port, the endoscopist may also obtain biopsies for pathological assessment or to perform hemostasis.

Thousands of colonoscopies are performed throughout the world every day. The procedure is performed safely and comfortably under mild sedation (e.g., conscious sedation). Complications may occur, but serious ones are rare and include bowel perforation, severe bleeding, post-coagulation syndrome, and other extremely rare and unexpected events such as splenic rupture. The incidence of colonic perforation during routine diagnostic colonoscopy is reported to be 0.01–0.2% (Rathgaber and Wick 2006; Eisen et al. 2002; Levin et al. 2006). In those undergoing polypectomy, perforation rates from 0.01% to 0.32% have been reported (Rathgaber and Wick 2006; Eisen et al. 2002; Levin et al. 2006). Bleeding following a diagnostic colonoscopy in 0.09% and a rate of 1.7% for post-polypectomy has been reported in 25,000 colonoscopies (Rathgaber and Wick 2006). Post-coagulation syndrome occurs when there has been transmural coagulation of the colonic wall, including the serosa (Rathgaber and Wick 2006; Eisen et al. 2002; Levin et al. 2006; Dominitz et al. 2003). Patients with this syndrome usually have acute localized abdominal pain, focal peritoneal signs, leukocytosis, and fever. However, there is no radiological evidence of bowel perforation or free air in the peritoneum. A CT scan may show thickening or edema of the colon wall in the area of coagulation, but no free air. Most patients fully recover with medical treatment and do not require surgery. The incidence of this complication following colonic coagulation such as during polypectomy has been reported at 0.5–1.2% (Dominitz et al. 2003).

BOWEL PREPARATION

Complete bowel cleansing is the most important aspect for successful emergency colonoscopy in patients with severe hematochezia. For a thorough examination, the colon needs to be cleared of particulate matter, including stool, clots, and blood. After excluding a UGI source of hemorrhage (refer to Fig. 1), we administer a polyethylene glycol-based balanced electrolyte purge (e.g., Golytely® or Colyte®) either orally or via an NG tube. Metoclopramide 10 mg IV may be administered 15–30 min prior to starting the purge for its prokinetic and anti-emetic effects. Because many of these patients already have an NG tube in place to check for UGI bleeding, it is easier to leave it in place for the purge. A liter of solution is administered every 30–45 min until the rectal effluent clears of solid matter and clots. In our experience, 6–8 L of this fluid are usually needed to achieve this goal, although more purge may be required in cases of severe or ongoing bleeding (refer to Table 2).

Care should be taken with those patients who have congestive heart failure, massive ascites, or chronic renal failure on hemodialysis. A careful assessment of volume status is recommended prior to starting the purge. An increase in third space fluid and intravascular volume should be treated pre-emptively. Specifically, if there is clinical evidence of congestive heart failure, diuretics are indicated. In patients with chronic renal failure on dialysis, hemodialysis concurrent with the colonic purge should be strongly considered. In patients with tense ascites, therapeutic paracentesis should be performed to diminish the risk of respiratory compromise during colonoscopy. In this subgroup of patients who are also receiving IV fluids and transfusions of blood products, as well as the colon purge, volume overload and worsening of comorbid conditions is common if diuresis, paracentesis, or dialysis are not performed before or simultaneously with the colon purge (Jensen and Machicado 1988; Kovacs and Jensen 2005).

Table 2
Colon preparation prior to urgent colonoscopy in patients with severe hematochezia (Jensen and Machicado 1988, 1997; Kovacs and Jensen 2005; Jensen et al. 2000)

- Metoclopramide (if no contraindications) 10 mg intravenously or intramuscularly 5–30 min prior to starting purge and repeat every 4–6 h for nausea.
- Polyethylene glycol based balanced electrolyte solution (Nulytely® of Colyte®) orally or via nasogastric tube at 1 L every 30–45 min until effluent is clear of clots, stool, and blood.
- Usually, 6–8 L of purge solution are required over 3–5 h to clean the colon.
- In patients with tense ascites, perform therapeutic paracentesis to prevent respiratory compromise during colonoscopy.
- If patient is in congestive heart failure, treat with intravenous diuretics or if in renal failure, use concurrent hemodialysis.

CURE HEMOSTASIS GROUP RESULTS WITH AN URGENT ENDOSCOPIC APPROACH TO SEVERE HEMATOCHEZIA

The CURE Hemostasis Research Group reported on 647 consecutive patients who were admitted to the hospital because of significant hematochezia and evaluated in a prospective cohort study (Jensen and Machicado 1997; Kovacs and Jensen 2005; Jensen et al. 2000). The patients included both those with persistent bleeding and those who stopped bleeding after hospitalization. The approach to the diagnosis in these patients was the same as with the group of persistently bleeding patients (i.e., resuscitation, placement of an NG tube to exclude an UGI bleeding site, colonic purge, and urgent colonoscopy) and this is shown in Fig. 1.

For the 647 patients with severe hematochezia in recent CURE studies (Jensen and Machicado 1988, 1997; Kovacs and Jensen 2005; Jensen et al. 2000), colonic bleeding sites were found in 75.1% (486 patients). An UGI source of the hematochezia (e.g., ulcers, varices or angiomas) was diagnosed in 17.5% (113 patients). A small bowel source was present in 4.6% (30 patients), and no source was found in 2.8% (18 patients) (refer to Fig. 2). The most common colonic sources of bleeding were diverticulosis (31.9%), internal hemorrhoids (12.8%), and ischemic colitis (11.9%) (refer to Table 3). Less common lesions included rectal ulcer, post-polypectomy ulcer, colon polyp or cancer, colon angiomas, and colitis (such as inflammatory bowel disease). Identification of major stigmata of hemorrhage (i.e., active bleeding, non-bleeding visible vessel, or adherent clot) at urgent colonoscopy after good colon preparation, and endoscopic treatment were often possible in patients with focal lesions. Low risk patients without stigmata of hemorrhage and/or severe comorbidities could be triaged to a less intensive level of care as well as to earlier discharge.

ALTERNATE PROCEDURES

Traditional Management of Severe Hematochezia in Adults

The traditional medical-surgical-angiographic management of severe hematochezia in adults is shown in Fig. 3. In this approach, patients with ongoing hematochezia have emergency angiography and, if it is positive, angiographic embolization or surgery is

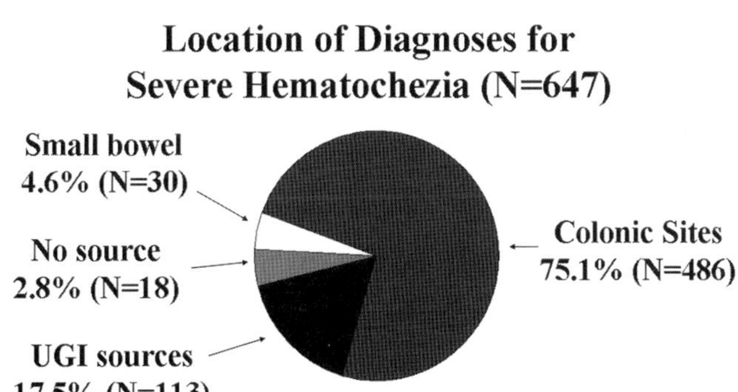

Fig. 2. For 647 patients hospitalized for severe hematochezia, the final sites (location) of hemorrhage are shown, from a large prospective CURE study, utilizing the management algorithm shown in Fig. 1 (Jensen and Machicado 1988, 1997; Jensen et al. 2000, 2008; Athanasoulis 1980; Jensen 2005).

Table 3
The eight most common colonic sources of severe hematochezia (CURE Hemostasis Research Group Study; Jensen and Machicado 1988, 1997; Kovacs and Jensen 2005; Jensen et al. 2000; Athanasoulis 1980)

Diverticulosis	31.9%
Internal hemorrhoids	12.8%
Ischemic colitis	11.9%
Rectal ulcers	7.6%
Colon angiomas or radiation telangiectasia	7.0%
UC, Crohn's disease, or other colitis	6.2%
Other LGI	5.6%
Post-polypectomy ulcer	4.7%

N=486 total severe hematochezia patients with colonic sources of bleeding
[a]Expressed as the percent of all colonic sources of severe hematochezia

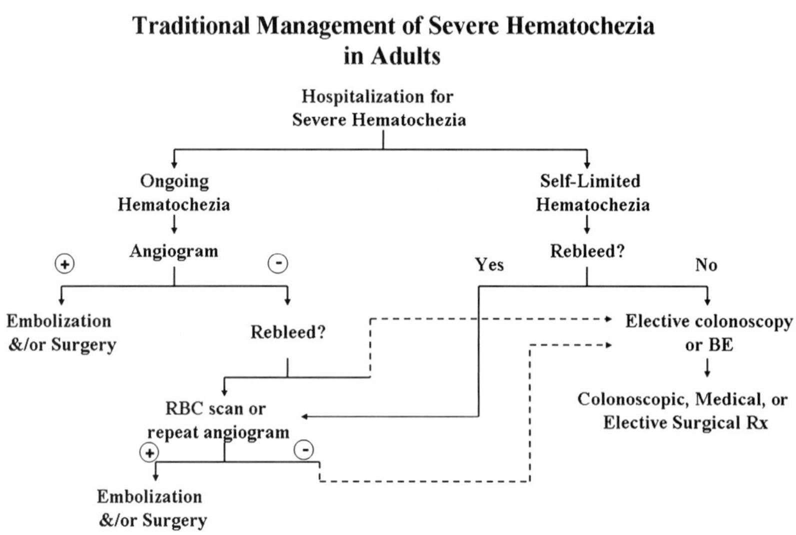

Fig. 3. Traditional medical-surgical-angiographic management of severe hematochezia in adults (Jensen and Machicado 1988, 1997; Kovacs and Jensen 2001; Savides and Jensen 1995).

performed (Jensen and Machicado 1997, 1998; Kovacs and Jensen 2001, 2005). If there is rebleeding, then the angiogram is repeated or an RBC scan is performed. For patients without rebleeding or those with self-limited hematochezia, elective colonoscopy (or in the past, barium enema) is performed. Therapy (medical, colonoscopic, angiographic, or surgical) depends upon the bleeding site localization, type, and co-morbidities of the patients (Athanasoulis 1980; Smith 2005; Green et al. 2005; Beam et al. 1992; Hunter and Pezim 1991; Jensen 2005).

Emergency Abdominal Angiography

Angiography has been reported to be useful for diagnosis and treatment of patients with severe hematochezia (Kovacs and Jensen 2001; Jensen and Machicado 1997; Athanasoulis 1980; Smith 2005; Green et al. 2005). The advantages of angiography are that skilled angiographers are able to diagnose and treat some patients with severe hematochezia. The study can be done without colonic purging, or while purging is being performed. With selective injections, visualization of hindgut, midgut, and foregut lesions (bleeding or nonbleeding) is feasible. Angiography can complement the urgent endoscopic approach (colonoscopy and enteroscopy) for diagnosis and treatment (see Fig. 1). Angiographic embolization for diverticular bleeding is reported to be 80% effective, but is not as effective for other colon lesions where rebleeding occurs in 40% of cases (Smith 2005).

The main disadvantage of angiography is that a relatively high blood flow (~ 0.5 mL/min) is required to see extravasation (e.g., active bleeding) into the gut lumen, and this is rare for colon lesions. Refer to Fig. 4 for an example of active bleeding (e.g., contrast extravasation) and presumptive diverticular hemorrhage. Indirect evidence of gut wall lesions (such as early-filling veins or neovascularity of tumors) is suggestive of potential bleeding sites. However, the examination is not definitive without extravasation into the lumen. While localization is sometimes possible, a specific etiologic diagnosis is usually not possible with angiography alone. For elderly patients, complications of angiography are also common, about 11% (Smith 2005). These include access artery occlusion, clotting, or bleeding; renal insufficiency from the contrast; bowel infarction; and volume overload from the contrast (Jensen and Machicado 1988, 1997; Smith 2005).

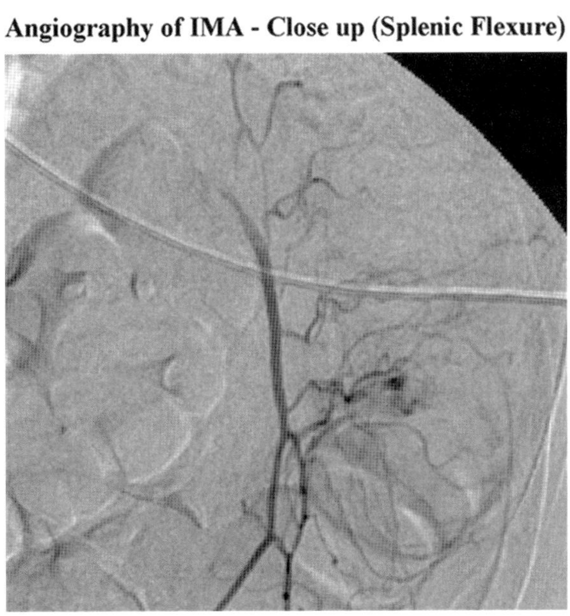

Fig. 4. Abdominal angiogram, with selective cannulation of the inferior mesenteric artery (*IMA*) and extravasation of contrast indicating active bleeding. The bleeding site was presumed to be a diverticular hemorrhage near the splenic flexure and the arteriole was embolized.

Our approach for the patient with severe hematochezia is to consider emergency angiography for patients who fail to have a diagnosis made by the urgent colonoscopy/enteroscopy approach and have ongoing or recurrent hematochezia. The endoscopic and angiographic examinations are complementary (refer to Fig. 1).

Red Cell Scanning

Technetium-labeled RBC scans have also been used for localization of potential bleeding sites in patients with severe hematochezia (Jensen and Machicado 1997; Beam et al. 1992; Hunter and Pezim 1991). Refer to Fig. 5 for a positive early RBC scan in a patient with ongoing GI bleeding.

The advantages of RBC scanning are that an early study can be done without colon preparation or while the patient with ongoing hematochezia is receiving oral purge for the colonoscopy. The threshold for detection of extravasation into the gut lumen is a 0.1 mL/min bleeding rate. Only 20% of patients who exceed this threshold show extravasation at angiography. The examination can be repeated because the RBCs and label stay in the vascular space at least 24 h. The main disadvantage is that the patients must have active bleeding when the RBC scan is done to show leakage of labeled RBC's into the bowel lumen. Also, whereas early scans (less than 4 h after baseline) may be relatively accurate for localization, delayed scans are notoriously poor for accuracy of localization. Furthermore, specific etiologic (lesion) diagnosis (as opposed to localization) cannot be made and treatment cannot be administered with RBC scanning. Definitive diagnosis and treatment of the bleeding site will depend on endoscopic/colonoscopic procedures,

RBC Scan for Ongoing Hematochezia
60 minutes

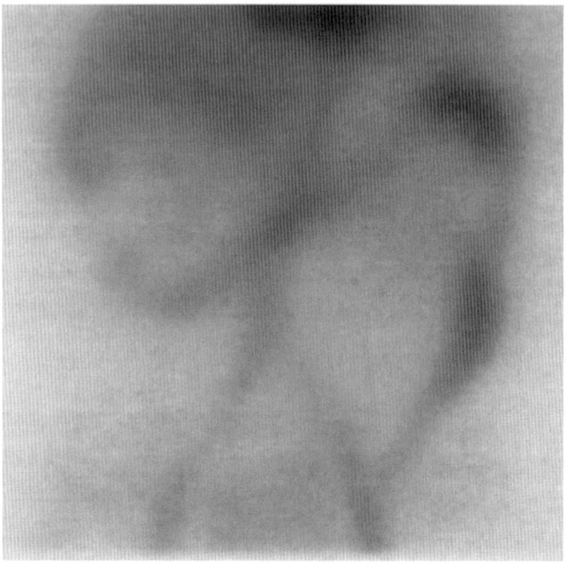

Fig. 5. Red blood cell (*RBC*) scan at 60 min, performed in a patient with ongoing hematochezia in the hospital. The subsequent angiogram was negative, but there was a clot on a diverticulum found on urgent colonoscopy.

angiography, or surgery. However, RBC scans are utilized in many hospitals as a screen before angiography. If an early RBC scan is positive, then the subsequent yield of abdominal angiography will be higher (Jensen and Machicado 1988, 1997).

We utilize RBC scans in our approach to patients with severe hematochezia (refer to Fig. 1). We recommend early RBC scans (i.e., baseline and up to 1–4 h only) in patients who are hospitalized for severe, ongoing hematochezia, before or after starting the purge. Even if the RBC scan is positive early, a confirmatory test such as angiography, urgent colonoscopy, or push enteroscopy is recommended before consideration of emergency surgery (Jensen and Machicado 1997). Emergency endoscopic hemostasis, which can be definitive or allow stabilization of the patient and elective surgery, may also be feasible (Jensen and Machicado 1988, 1997; Kovacs and Jensen 2001, 2005).

Results of Traditional Approach to Severe Hematochezia

For patients who undergo a traditional approach to severe hematochezia, we estimated that the diagnostic yield would be significantly lower and the incremental cost for patient management would be more than $10,000 per patient a decade ago (Jensen and Machicado 1997). Rockey and colleagues performed a randomized prospective study of urgent colonoscopy compared to a traditional approach (as shown in Fig. 3) for 100 patients with severe hematochezia (Green et al. 2005). They reported significantly higher rates of definitive diagnosis in the urgent colonoscopy group versus traditional management group (42% vs 22%) and lower rates of no source found (4% vs 24%). However, there were no significant differences in early rebleeding (22% vs 30%), hospital stay (5.8 vs 6.6 days), total RBC's transfused (4.2 vs 5.0 units), surgery (14% vs 12%), or death from rebleeding (2% vs 4%). Criticisms of this study are both in design of the study and in technical issues. In this study, only 4 L of colon prep were utilized and consequently many of the preps were suboptimal in the urgent colonoscopy group, new colonic hemostasis techniques (such as combination epinephrine injection and hemoclipping) of focal bleeding sites were not utilized, and test results were not utilized to triage patients to level of care or early hospital discharge (Jensen 2005).

SPECIFIC COLONIC LESIONS

Diverticular Hemorrhage

A diverticulum forms when the mucosa of the colon penetrates through an area of weakness in the muscularis and forms a balloon like structure on the outside of the colonic wall covered by serosa. Occasionally, and for unknown reasons, a small erosion will develop at the neck or the base of the diverticulum eroding into the underlying small arteriole. This can cause sudden and significant hemorrhage. Diverticular bleeding is the most frequent cause for severe hematochezia in the USA, accounting for 20–55% of all cases of lower GI bleeding in adults (Jensen and Machicado 1988, 1997; Kovacs and Jensen 2001, 2005; Longstreth 1997; Green et al. 2005).

Diverticular bleeding was the cause (including definitive diverticular or presumptive diverticular hemorrhage as defined below) of severe hematochezia in 31.9% of all patients admitted with severe hematochezia in our ongoing CURE Hemostasis study of patients with severe hematochezia (Jensen and Machicado 1988, 1997; Kovacs and Jensen 2001, 2005;

Jensen et al. 2000). However, not all patients with diverticulosis who presented with severe hematochezia were bleeding from diverticulosis. In our series, 52% of patients with known colon diverticulosis were found to have bleeding from non-diverticular sources. "Presumptive diverticular bleeding" was diagnosed when no definitive source or other potential source of hemorrhage on urgent colonoscopy, anoscopy, or push enteroscopy was found. This accounted for the bleeding site in 30.8% of patients with known colonic diverticulosis and severe hematochezia. "Definitive diverticular bleeding" was diagnosed when there was a stigma of recent hemorrhage such as active bleeding, a non-bleeding visible vessel, or an adherent clot on a diverticulum at urgent colonoscopy. This subgroup accounted for 17.2% of all patients with severe hematochezia and diverticulosis (Jensen and Machicado 1997; Jensen et al. 2000) (Fig. 6).

Treatment of patients with severe diverticular hemorrhage depends upon severity of bleeding and local expertise of gastroenterologists, interventional radiologists, and surgeons. Treatment of bleeding diverticulosis can be safe and effective by any experienced group.

Long term treatment to prevent recurrence of diverticular hemorrhage is highly recommended. Avoidance of aspirin, non-steroidal anti-inflammatory drugs (NSAIDs) and anticoagulants are the most important for prevention of rebleeding. The roles of fiber, control of constipation, and avoidance of nuts and small seeds are controversial. Contrary to common teaching about patients with diverticulosis, Strate et al. recently reported that patients who consumed nuts and seeds in their diet had no more complications of diverticular disease (hemorrhage or diverticulitis) and frequent popcorn eaters had lower rates of diverticulitis than age matched patients whose diet lacked these foods (Strate et al. 2007). Some other studies have reported an association between NSAID's use and diverticular bleeding (Aldoori et al. 1998; Laine et al. 2003).

Recently, we reported that patients with documented diverticular hemorrhage (e.g., definitive or presumptive) had low rates of recurrent diverticular hemorrhage or diverticulitis during long term follow-up after an initial severe diverticular bleed (24). The rates of severe colon rebleeding of any type were low, during a median of 3.5 years of follow-up, and were similar for patients treated initially with medical (18.9% rebled), endoscopic (18.8% rebled), or surgical therapy (25% rebled). However, the proportion of

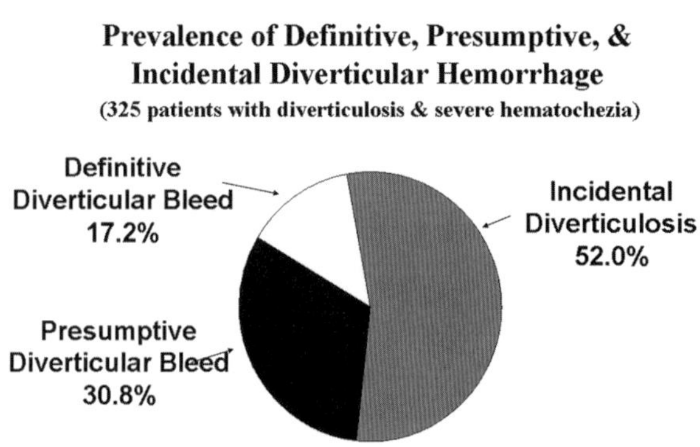

Fig. 6. Prevalence of definitive, presumptive and incidental diverticular hemorrhage in 326 patients with diverticulosis and severe hematochezia (Jensen and Machicado 1988, 1997; Jensen et al. 2000, 2008; Athanasoulis 1980; Jensen 2005).

non-diverticular sources for the rebleeding varied according to treatment, from 43% (medical) or 50% (endoscopic group) to 100% (surgical group). In other words, at least 50% of all the late rebleeding was from non-diverticular sources of LGI hemorrhage in these patients with documented colon diverticulosis (Jensen et al. 2008).

Internal Hemorrhoids

Internal hemorrhoids caused severe hematochezia in 12.8% of our patients who were hospitalized (Jensen and Machicado 1988, 1997; Kovacs and Jensen 2001, 2005; Jensen et al. 2000). Most physicians do not include internal hemorrhoids in the differential diagnosis of severe hematochezia, because the majority of internal hemorrhoidal bleeding is managed by surgeons and is perceived to be intermittent, low grade and self-limited. However, a significant proportion of patients with internal hemorrhoids have more acute severe rectal bleeding. Bleeding internal hemorrhoids constitute a significant public health problem since approximately 10.4 million people suffer from hemorrhoid symptoms annually, prompting 3.5 million physician visits per year (Johanson 1994).

We grade internal hemorrhoids with a slotted anoscope from grade I to IV (refer to Table 4), depending on the degree of prolapse through the anal sphincter. Although bleeding may occur from any grade internal hemorrhoid, severe bleeding causing anemia and hospitalization is most often from grade III or IV internal hemorrhoids. Patients having induced coagulopathies (from NSAIDs, aspirin, warfarin, or antiplatelet drugs) or intrinsic coagulopathies (from liver or hematologic disorders) may have significant rectal bleeding from lower grade internal hemorrhoids (grades I or II). Following enemas to clear the distal colon (Fleets® or tap water), bleeding hemorrhoids can be diagnosed with a flexible sigmoidoscope using a retroflexed view, but the internal hemorrhoids are always better visualized with the use of a slotted anoscope (Jutabha et al. 2001).

While outpatients with intermittent bleeding from internal hemorrhoids often have cessation of hemorrhage with medical therapy, in our experience, most of the patients with severe hematochezia require endoscopic therapy or surgery (Jensen and Machicado 1988, 1997; Kovacs and Jensen 2005; Jutabha et al. 2001). In the past, we have utilized sclerotherapy or anoscopic coagulation (such as with rigid multipolar or heater anoscopic probes) for patients with internal hemorrhoids and hematochezia (Jutabha et al. 2001; Randall et al. 1994; Jensen et al. 1997). Recently, rubber band ligation has been found to be faster and more efficient particularly for control of severe hematochezia in patients with grade II-IV internal hemorrhoids (Pfenninger 1997; Su et al. 2003). Concomitant medical therapy with fiber, stool softeners, and avoidance of aspirin, NSAID's, and anticoagulants is also highly recommended. Outpatient follow-up and further treatment to completely control bleeding and to reduce the internal hemorrhoids to grade I or less should also be considered.

Table 4
Grades of internal hemorrhoids (Jutabha et al. 2001)

Grade I: No prolapse below the dentate line
Grade II: Prolapse during defecation with spontaneous reduction
Grade III: Prolapse during defecation requiring manual reduction
Grade IV: Non-reducible prolapse below that dentate line

Surgical intervention may be indicated for those patients who prefer to have a single procedure despite discomfort and those patients with severe rectal bleeding who have failed medical and endoscopic therapy. Surgical hemorrhoidectomy is highly effective in controlling bleeding and eradicating internal hemorrhoids as well as external hemorrhoids (Senagore et al. 1993; Andrews et al. 1993; Hodgson and Morgan 1995). However, surgical hemorrhoidectomy is not free of complications (Rosen et al. 1993; Eu et al. 1995; Parickh et al. 1994; Shanmugan et al. 2005).

Ischemic Colitis

Colonic ischemia was responsible for severe hematochezia in 11.9% of our patients hospitalized with hematochezia (Jensen and Machicado 1988, 1997; Kovacs and Jensen 2001, 2005; Jensen et al. 2000). Other series report an incidence of 3–9% of severe lower gastrointestinal bleeding caused by ischemic colitis (Longstreth 1997; Peura et al. 1997; Zuckerman and Prakash 1999; Jensen et al. 2004; Gralnek and Jensen 2001; Savides and Jensen 1995). There is usually no identifiable precipitating cause for the acute onset of colonic ischemia. However, some patients with ischemic colitis have underlying atherosclerotic cardiovascular or peripheral occlusive disease. It can also be seen with acute myocardial infarction, severe heart failure, hypercoagulable states, vasculitis, sepsis, prolonged strenuous exercise, and some medications such as diuretics (Jensen et al. 2004; Savides and Jensen 1995). Some patients present with the acute onset of crampy abdominal pain, which can be localized in the right lower quadrant, epigastrium, or left lower quadrant depending on the segment of colon involved. However, the pain in severe cases tends to radiate throughout the entire abdomen. The splenic flexure and sigmoid colon, which have poor collateral blood flow (e.g., and are called "watershed areas"), are most often involved (Zuckerman and Prakash 1999; Savides and Jensen 1995). When present, abdominal pain is usually associated with bloody diarrhea. Occasionally, nausea, vomiting, and fever are present. Signs of hypovolemia, tachycardia and hypotension may be seen in very severe cases of ischemic colitis, but these are most often associated with large vessel stenosis or embolization, rather than small vessel disease or hypotension alone. Physical examination of the abdomen may be normal or have findings such as diffuse abdominal tenderness, hyperactive bowel sounds, or an abdominal bruit. No localized peritoneal signs are usually present unless there is frank colonic infarction with involvement of the serosa. Thumbprinting may be observed on plain abdominal radiographs or barium enema, but this is not a frequent finding in our experience (Jensen et al. 2004; Gralnek and Jensen 2001; Savides and Jensen 1995). In many cases of ischemic colitis that we see in elderly patients, only painless hematochezia, and no other abdominal symptom, is noted. The physical examination may reveal mild tenderness only or may be normal.

Colonoscopy is the best way to make the diagnosis of ischemic colitis of the colon (Jensen and Machicado 1988, 1997; Kovacs and Jensen 2005; Zuckerman and Prakash 1999; Gralnek and Jensen 2001; Savides and Jensen 1995). There is usually segmental involvement consisting of mucosal edema, erythema, friability, mucosal hemorrhages, mucosal necrosis and ulcerations. Colonic biopsies from the affected as well as unaffected areas are usually definitive for ischemia. Colonoscopy, stool cultures (and *Clostridium difficile* toxin assay, and ova and parasite analysis) and histopathologic findings are useful to differentiate colonic ischemia from inflammatory or infectious colitis.

Treatment consists of medical therapy and supportive care with intravenous fluids and or blood transfusions to improve tissue perfusion. Urgent treatment of comorbid conditions is also warranted, including peripheral or central vascular disease, cardiac arrhythmias, or severe anemia, which may have contributed to bowel ischemia. Antibiotics are indicated if fever or sepsis is present. If there is clinical deterioration of the patient with development or peritoneal signs, fever, leukocytosis, or evidence of bowel perforation, surgical intervention with segmental colon resection is indicated. Therapeutic colonoscopy plays no role in these patients unless a focal ulcer with stigmata of hemorrhage is found at colonoscopy, which is the case in less than 10% of our patients with severe ischemic colitis (Jensen and Machicado 1988, 1997; Kovacs and Jensen 2005; Zuckerman and Prakash 1999; Gralnek and Jensen 2001).

Solitary Rectal Ulcer Syndrome

Rectal ulcers (usually solitary, but sometimes multiple) were responsible for 7.6% of the colonic cases of severe hematochezia in our large study (Jensen and Machicado 1988, 1997; Kovacs and Jensen 2005; Jensen et al. 2000). It was the fourth most common colonic cause of severe hematochezia in the large prospective CURE Hemostasis cohort. In contrast to previous series, which reported that this syndrome occurs in younger (third and fourth decades of life) patients (Madigan and Morson 1969; Tjandra et al. 1992; Sharara et al. 2005), our patients were older, in the sixth and seventh decades of life (Gralnek and Jensen 2001; Kanwal et al. 2003; Jensen et al. 2007). This syndrome is more common in women, and is characterized by rectal bleeding and mucus discharge in 56–89% of patients (Tjandra et al. 1992; Niv and Bat 1986). The etiology of this disorder is not completely understood, but prolapse-induced rectal mucosal trauma or ischemia appear to contribute (Levine 1987). Our patients usually presented with symptoms of severe constipation and often fecal impaction. Increasingly, inpatients with prolonged hospitalization and inpatient hematochezia represent a large proportion of solitary rectal ulcer patients (Kanwal et al. 2003; Jensen et al. 2007). Pressure-induced mucosal necrosis in elderly patients with fecal impaction must also be considered. On endoscopy, one or more well-demarcated ulcerations are seen with edematous, erythematous, and nodular borders (Gralnek and Jensen 2001; Kanwal et al. 2003; Jensen et al. 2007). Active bleeding or stigmata of recent hemorrhage were found at urgent colonoscopy in most patients with severe hematochezia in our recent studies (Gralnek and Jensen 2001; Kanwal et al. 2003; Jensen et al. 2007).

Colonoscopic hemostasis of hemorrhage from rectal ulcers consists of coagulation with a large-contact thermal probe or hemoclipping, with or without pre-injection of epinephrine. After successful endoscopic hemostasis, we recommend that three to four adjacent areas be tattooed with India ink. Medical management of constipation, adequate nutritional support, and avoidance of anticoagulants, NSAIDs, and antiplatelet drugs is recommended to prevent rebleeding. Surgery is recommended for recurrent, severe bleeding.

Delayed Post-polypectomy Hemorrhage

Hemorrhage after a endoscopic polypectomy may occur immediately afterward or may be delayed hours, days, or, rarely, weeks (Levine 1987; Rex et al. 1992). Our focus in this chapter is on delayed severe post-polypectomy hemorrhage resulting in hospitalization for severe hematochezia. This is defined as occurring 1 or more days after discharge of the patient from the endoscopy unit after the polypectomy. The incidence of severe delayed post-polypectomy hemorrhage is reported as 1–6% (Gralnek and Jensen 2001; Rex et al. 1992; Jensen et al. 2001). The variation in these reported rates is most likely a function of study design, patient population (i.e., age, comorbid conditions, use of antiplatelet drugs or anticoagulants), and configuration and size of index polyps. Because of changes in colonoscopy practices (including performance of more screening colonoscopies for colorectal cancer) and with colonoscopic resection of larger sessile colonic polyps in the last two decades, including piecemeal resection or following submucosal saline injection, delayed post-polypectomy hemorrhage appears to be occurring more frequently. Severe post-polypectomy bleeding was the cause of severe hematochezia in less than 5% of colonic etiologies, in a recent study by the CURE Hemostasis Research Group (Jensen and Machicado 1988; Kovacs and Jensen 2005; Jensen et al. 2000, 2001). The mean size of the polyps was 20 mm in diameter, and most were sessile polyps without carcinoma on histopathology. Delayed hemorrhage occurred a median of 9 days (range 2–73) after polypectomy. Most patients (77%) were men with a mean age of 69 years. The majority (77%) also had taken aspirin, anti-platelet drugs, or warfarin after polypectomy for comorbid cardiac or vascular conditions. All patients required hospitalization because of severe hematochezia. After colonic purge, urgent colonoscopy revealed ulcerations with a mean diameter of 11 mm at the prior polypectomy sites. Stigmata of hemorrhage on the ulcers included active bleeding in 23%, non-bleeding visible vessel in 23%, clot in 38%, spot in 8% and clean ulcer in 8%. Ninety-two percent of patients were treated endoscopically, and only one patient rebled. One patient with cancer had surgery, and the remainder were treated medically.

Bleeding occurring immediately after polypectomy is thought to be due to inadequate cauterization of the polyp vessels during polypectomy whereas delayed post-polypectomy hemorrhage is thought to be due to sloughing of the necrotic, cauterized tissue in the induced ulcer, with exposure of an underlying blood vessel. Intrinsic (from co-morbid conditions) or extrinsic coagulopathies (from medications) can aggravate or cause the bleeding by interfering with clotting. The predominance of visible vessels with or without active bleeding or clots indicates an underlying vessel, probably similar to the anatomy of peptic ulcers as defined by Swain (Swain et al. 1986). However, to date there have been no studies reporting on the histology of stigmata of hemorrhage for delayed post-polypectomy colon ulcers, because most are now successfully treated via colonoscopy (Gralnek and Jensen 2001; Rex et al. 1992; Jensen et al. 2001). Hemostasis is performed with thermal techniques or hemoclipping with or without pre-injection with dilute epinephrine around the stigmata of hemorrhage in the post-polypectomy ulcer.

The risk of aspirin and non-steroidal anti-inflammatory drugs (NSAIDs) prior to polypectomy remains a concern. However, according to expert opinion and guidelines, no significant difference in post-polypectomy bleeding can be expected for those patients consuming these drugs and those who did not before polypectomy (Yousfi et al. 2004; Hui et al. 2004). The guidelines from the American Society for Gastrointestinal Endoscopy state that polypectomy in patients consuming standard doses of these drugs, precluding any underlying bleeding disorders, is safe (Levin et al. 2006). However, the level of scientific evidence for these guidelines is based on case reports and expert opinion rather than randomized studies. For high risk patients with coagulopathies, caution is recommended when continuing or resuming aspirin, antiplatelet drugs, and anticoagulants.

Colonic Angiomas

Colonic angiomas or radiation telangiectasia were the fifth most common colonic cause of severe hematochezia, responsible for 7% of the colonic diagnoses (Jensen and Machicado 1988; Kovacs and Jensen 2005; Jensen et al. 2000; Machicado and Jensen 2001). In contrast, the majority of patients we see (70%) with bleeding angiomas present with self-limited intermittent bleeding or occult blood-positive stools and iron deficiency anemia. These patients are usually hemodynamically stable and can undergo elective colonoscopy in the outpatient setting (Machicado and Jensen 2001). A smaller group (30%) of patients with colonic angiomas present with severe, persistent hemorrhage, may be hemodynamically unstable and/or severely anemic, and require hospitalization, blood transfusions and emergency evaluation.

The CURE Hemostasis Research Group randomized 108 prospective patients with bleeding colonic angiomas to colonoscopic treatment with bipolar coagulation (57 patients) or heater probe (51 patients). Most of these patients were elderly (>65 years) and suffered from one or more comorbid conditions (refer to Table 5). The mean follow-up of these patients was 2 years which was compared to the 2 years prior to endoscopic treatment in terms of number of bleeding episodes, number of blood transfusions, and hematocrit while on iron and not acutely bleeding (Machicado and Jensen 2001).

At colonoscopy, most angiomas (85%) were in the right colon (Machicado and Jensen 2001). The majority of angiomas (80%) were 5–10 mm in size, 18% were 11–20 mm, and 2% were greater than 20 mm. The mean number of colonoscopies to control bleeding during the follow up period was 1.4, with a range of 1–4.

Seventy percent of patients had a good outcome with colonic coagulation, experienced fewer bleeding episodes, required fewer blood transfusions, and held a higher hematocrit during follow-up (Machicado and Jensen 2001). Partial colectomies were performed in 18% of patients who had multiple colon angiomas (usually more than 25 in one segment such as the right colon). However, 38% of these operated patients continued to have recurrent bleeding, post-hemicolectomy. Complications from colonoscopic coagulation consisting of delayed hemorrhage due to ulceration (four patients) or post-coagulation syndrome due to full thickness coagulation (two patients) were observed in 5% of patients. No perforations occurred. Two of the patients with delayed hemorrhage who had coagulopathies required surgery.

Table 5
Comorbid conditions for patients with hemorrhage from colonic angiomas (*N* = 108) (see Machicado and Jensen *2001*)

Condition	*% of patients*
Severe heart disease	46
Valvular heart disease	29
Aortic stenosis	16
Aortic regurgitation	5
Mitral regurgitation	8
Chronic renal failure	
Hemodialysis	16
Cirrhosis	16
Collagen vascular disorder	5
Osler–Weber–Rendu syndrome	5

Cost Assessment

A cost analysis, comparing the urgent colonoscopy approach with a traditional medical-surgical-angiographic approach to hematochezia was previously reported by our group (Jensen and Machicado 1997). The urgent colonoscopy group had fewer hospital days, surgeries and diagnostic tests. The savings based upon 1997 estimates was a mean of $10,065 per patient. Strate and Rockey have also confirmed that early colonoscopy in patients with severe hematochezia results in shorter length of patient hospitalization (Schmulewitz et al. 2003; Strate et al. 2003).

SUMMARY OF KEY POINTS

- Severe hematochezia or lower gastrointestinal bleeding is now a more frequently encountered medical-surgical problem.
- The prevalence appears to be increasing because of recent colorectal cancer screening practices, and the aging of referral patient populations.
- Our recommended approach to these patients consists of vigorous resuscitation with intravenous fluids and blood transfusions, close monitoring in an intensive care unit or monitored bed unit, bedside evaluation with nasogastric tube lavage for signs of a possible UGI bleeding source, and urgent colonoscopy (or upper endoscopy or small bowel enteroscopy if colonoscopy is negative) following thorough colonic cleansing with a purge via oral or nasogastric tube.
- Definitive or presumptive diagnosis of the bleeding site can be made with this approach in over 95% of cases.
- In patients with severe hematochezia, a colonic bleeding site is found in 75% of cases.
- Endoscopic treatment of focal bleeding lesions in the colon or the UGI tract is highly effective and safe in these cases, thereby reducing the need for surgical or angiographic intervention.
- In patients with a definitive diagnosis and no stigmata of hemorrhage or low risk stigmata, early diagnosis may also facilitate downgrading the intensity of medical care and/or early discharge from the hospital.

REFERENCES

Aldoori WH, Giovannucci EL, Rimm EB, et al. Use of acetaminophen and nonsteroidal anti-inflammatory drugs: a prospective study and the risk of symptomatic diverticular disease in men. Arch Fam Med. 1998;7:255–60.

Andrews BJ, Layer OT, Jackson BT, et al. Randomized trial comparing diathermy hemorrhoidectomy with the scissor dissection Milligan-Morgan operation. Dis Colon Rectum. 1993;36:580–3.

Athanasoulis CA. Therapeutic applications of angiography. N Engl J Med. 1980;302:1117–25.

Beam P, Persad R, Wilson N, et al. 99 m-Technetium-labeled red blood cell scintigraphy as an alternative to angiography in the investigation of gastrointestinal bleeding: clinical experience in a district general hospital. Ann R Coll Surg Engl. 1992;74:192–9.

Cuellar RE, Gavaler JS, Alexander JA, et al. Gastrointestinal tract hemorrhage. The value of a nasogastric aspirate. Arch Intern Med. 1990;150:1381–4.

Dominitz JA, Eisen GM, Baron TH, Goldstein JL, et al. Complications of colonoscopy. Gastrointest Endosc. 2003;57:441–5.

Eisen GM, Baron TH, Dominitz JA, et al. Guideline on the management of anticoagulation and antiplatelet therapy for endoscopic procedures. Gastrointest Endosc. 2002;55:775–9.

Eu KW, Tech TA, Seow-Choen F, et al. Anal stricture following haemorrhoidectomy: early diagnosis and treatment. Aust N Z J Surg. 1995;65:101–3.

Gralnek IM, Jensen DM. An assortment of colonic lesions that present with severe hematochezia. Tech Gastrointest Endosc. 2001;3:216–20.

Green BT, Rockey DC, Portwood G. Urgent colonoscopy for evaluation and management of acute lower gastrointestinal hemorrhage: A randomized controlled trial. Am J Gastroenterol. 2005;100:2395–402.

Hodgson WJ, Morgan J. Ambulatory hemorrhoidectomy with CO_2 laser. Dis Colon Rectum. 1995; 38:1265–9.

Hui AJ, Wong RM, Ching JY, et al. Risk of colonoscopic polypectomy bleeding with anti-coagulants and antiplatelet agents: analysis of 1657 cases. Gastrointest Endosc. 2004;59:44–8.

Hunter JM, Pezim ME. Limited value of technetium 99 labeled red cell scintigraphy in localization of lower gastrointestinal bleeding. Am J Surg. 1991;159:503–6.

Jensen DM. Management of patients with severe hematochezia–with all current evidence available. Am J Gastroenterol. 2005;100:2403–6.

Jensen DM, Machicado GA. Diagnosis and treatment of severe hematochezia: the role of urgent colonoscopy after purge. Gastroenterology. 1988;95:1569–74.

Jensen DM, Machicado GA. Colonoscopy for diagnosis and treatment of severe lower gastrointestinal bleeding: routine outcomes and cost analysis. Gastrointest Endosc Clin N Am. 1997;7:477–98.

Jensen DM, Jutabha R, Machicado GA, et al. Prospective randomized comparative study of bipolar electrocoagulation versus heater probe for treatment of chronically bleeding internal hemorrhoids. Gastrointest Endosc. 1997;46:435–43.

Jensen DM, Machicado GA, Jutabha R, Kovacs TOG. Urgent colonoscopy for the diagnosis and treatment of severe diverticular hemorrhage. N Engl J Med. 2000;342:78–82.

Jensen DM, Kovacs TOG, Jutabha R, et al. Prospective study of delayed post-polypectomy bleeding compared to other causes of severe hematochezia. Gastrointest Endosc. 2001;53:182.

Jensen, DM, Zarimani AI, Kovacs TOG, Dulai G, Jutabha R, Gralnek IM, Machicado GA. Ischemic colitis is a common cause of severe hematochezia and patient outcomes are no worse than other colonic diagnoses. Gastrointest Endosc. 2004;59:AB105:536.

Jensen DM, Kovacs TOG, Jutabha R, Ohning GV, Dulai GS, Machicado GA. Rectal ulcers causing severe hematochezia: Update on diagnosis, hemostasis, healing, and outcomes. Gastrointest Endosc. 2007; 65:AB258:T1434.

Jensen DM, Singh B, Jensen ME, Sun N, Carrico M. How often do patients rebleed during long-term follow-up after an initial documented diverticular hemorrhage? Gastroenterology. 2008;134:A122(846).

Johanson JF. Hemorrhoids. In: Digestive diseases in the United States: epidemiology and impact. Washington DC: US Government Printing Office: NIH Publication 94–1447; 1994. p. 273–98.

Jutabha R, Miura-Jutabha C, Jensen DM. Current medical, anoscopic, endoscopic and surgical treatments for bleeding internal hemorrhoids. Tech Gastrointest Endosc. 2001;3:199–205.

Kanwal F, Jutabha R, Dulai D, Jensen DM. Major stigmata of hemorrhage on rectal ulcers and outcomes in patients with severe hematochezia. Gastrointest Endosc. 2003;57:462–8.

Kollef MH, ÓBrian JD, Zuckerman GR, et al. BLEED: a classification tool to predict outcomes in patients with acute upper and lower gastrointestinal hemorrhage. Crit Care Med. 1997;25:1125–32.

Kovacs TOG, Jensen DM. Upper or small bowel hemorrhage presenting as hematochezia. Tech Gastrointest Endosc. 2001;3:206–15.

Kovacs TOG, Jensen DM. Acute lower gastrointestinal bleeding. In: Weinstein WM, Hawkey CJ, Bosch J, editors. Clinical gastroenterology and hepatology. London: Elsevier Mosby; 2005. p. 127–31.

Laine L, Connors LG, Reicin A, et al. Serious lower gastrointestinal clinical events with non-selective NSAID or coxib use. Gastroenterology. 2003;124:288–92.

Levin TR, Zhao W, Conell C, et al. Complications of colonoscopy in an integrated health care delivery system. Ann Intern Med. 2006;145:880–6.

Levine DS. "Solitary" rectal ulcer syndrome. Gastroenterology. 1987;92:243–53.

Longstreth GF. Epidemiology and outcome of patients hospitalized with acute lower gastrointestinal hemorrhage: a population-based study. Am J Gastroenterol. 1997;92:419–24.

Machicado GA, Jensen DM. Bleeding colonic angiomas and radiation telangiectasias: endoscopic diagnosis and treatment. Tech Gastrointest Endosc. 2001;3:185–91.

Madigan MR, Morson BC. Solitary ulcer of the rectum. Gut. 1969;10:871–81.
Niv Y, Bat L. Solitary ulcer syndrome: clinical endoscopic and histopathological spectrum. Am J Gastroenterol. 1986;81:486–91.
Parickh SR, Molinelli B, Dailey TH. Liver abscess after hemorrhoidectomy. Report of two cases. Dis Colon Rectum. 1994;37:185–9.
Peura DA, Lanza FL, Gostout CJ, et al. The American College of Gastroenterology Bleeding Registry: preliminary findings. Am J Gastroenterol. 1997;92:924–8.
Pfenninger JL. Modern treatments for internal hemorrhoids. BMJ. 1997;314:1211–12.
Randall GM, Jensen DM, Machicado GA, et al. Prospective randomized comparative study of bipolar versus direct cost electrocoagulation for treatment of bleeding internal hemorrhoids. Gastrointest Endosc. 1994;40:403–10.
Rathgaber SW, Wick TM. Colonoscopy completion and complication rates in a community gastroenterology practice. Gastrointest Endosc. 2006;64:556–62.
Rex DK, Lewis BL, Waye JD. Colonoscopy and endoscopic therapy for delayed post-polypectomy hemorrhage. Gastrointest Endosc. 1992;38:127–9.
Rosen L, Sipe P, Stasik JJ, et al. Outcome of delayed hemorrhage following surgical hemorrhoidectomy. Dis Colon Rectum. 1993;36:743–6.
Savides TJ, Jensen DM. Endoscopic therapy for severe gastrointestinal bleeding. Adv Intern Med. 1995;40:243–71.
Schmulewitz N, Fisher DA, Rockey DC. Early colonoscopy for acute lower GI bleeding predicts shorter hospital stay: a retrospective study of experience in a single center. Gastrointest Endosc. 2003;58:841–6.
Senagore A, Mazier WT, Luchtefeld MA, et al. Treatment of advanced hemorrhoidal disease: a prospective, randomized comparison of cold scalpel vs contact Nd:YAG laser. Dis Colon Rectum. 1993;36:1042–9.
Shanmugan V, Thaha MA, Rabindranath KS, Campbell KL, Steale RJ, Loudon MA. Systematic review of randomized trials comparing rubber band ligation with excisional hemorrhoidectomy. Br J Surg. 2005;92:1481–7.
Sharara AI, Azar C, Amr SS, et al. Solitary rectal ulcer syndrome: endoscopic spectrum and review of the literature. Gastrointest Endosc. 2005;62:755–62.
Smith TP. Angiographic diagnosis and endovascular management of non-variceal gastrointestinal hemorrhage. Gastroenterol Clin. 2005;34:735–52.
Strate LL, Orav EJ, Syngal S. Early predictors of severity in acute lower intestinal tract bleeding. Arch Intern Med. 2003;163:838–43.
Strate LL, Liu YL, Syngal S, Giovannucci EL. Can patients with diverticular disease eat nuts, corn and popcorn? Gastroenterology. 2007;132:A–110.
Su MY, Chin CT, Wu CS, Ho YP, Lien SM, Tung SY, et al. Endoscopic hemorrhoidal ligation of symptomatic internal hemorrhoids. Gastrointest Endosc. 2003;58:871–74.
Swain CP, Storey DW, Bown SG, et al. Nature of the bleeding vessel in recurrently bleeding gastric ulcers. Gastroenterology. 1986;90:595–608.
Tjandra JT, Fazio VW, Church JM, et al. Clinical Conundrum of solitary rectal ulcer. Dis Colon Rectum. 1992;35:227–34.
Velayos FS, Williamson A, Sousa KH, et al. Early predictors of severe lower gastrointestinal bleeding and adverse outcomes: a prospective study. Clin Gastroenterol Hepatol. 2004;2:485–90.
Yousfi M, Gostout CJ, Baron TH, et al. Postpolypectomy lower gastrointestinal bleeding: potential role of aspirin. Am J Gastroenterol. 2004;99:1785–9.
Zuckerman GR, Prakash C. Acute lower intestinal bleeding. Gastrointest Endosc. 1999;49:228–38.

20 Complications and Their Risk Factors in Gastrointestinal Endoscopy

Koorosh MoezArdalan and Khalid Aziz

Contents

Keywords: Complications, Risk, Factors, Gastrointestinal, Endoscopy

INTRODUCTION

More than 200,000,000 gastrointestinal procedures are performed in the United States every year. As with other therapeutic modalities, complications are inherent to gastrointestinal endoscopy. Endoscopists need to be aware of the different types and the expected frequencies of these complications, in order to use strategies to minimize their occurrence and to recognize

From: *Clinical Gastroenterology: Diagnostic and Therapeutic Procedures in Gastroenterology,*
Edited by: G. Y. Wu, S. Sridhar, DOI 10.1007/978-1-59745-044-7_20,

and treat them appropriately when they occur. Furthermore, it is essential to recognize patients with a higher likelihood of developing complications. Attention must be paid to patients' preexisting medical conditions and their ability to cope with potential complications.

In this chapter, we will describe potential complications of upper and lower endoscopy, together with the adverse effects related to endoscopic retrograde cholangiopancreatography (ERCP), endoscopic ultrasound (EUS), and certain advanced therapeutic techniques such as mucosal resection.

It is important to keep in mind that one should always consider the risk benefit ratio of a procedure and make sure that the benefits outweigh the risks.

COMPLICATIONS RELATED TO PREPARATION FOR ENDOSCOPY

Upper Endoscopy

Prior to GI procedures, patients are usually asked to avoid eating and drinking about 6–8 h. This fasting period can be a potential problem for diabetics who take oral hypoglycemic medications or insulin injection. The general recommendation is that patients should stop their oral hypoglycemic drugs (Sivak 2000) and their fast acting insulin on the day of procedure. However, they will need some baseline insulin during the procedure to prevent hyperglycemia. For this purpose it has been recommended that patients receive half of their usual dose of the long acting insulin in the morning of the procedure (Ginzburg et al. 2007).

Colonoscopy

One of the essential steps before colonoscopy is bowel preparation, the lack of which can greatly hinder detection of colonic pathologies. Poor bowel preparation has a significant role in increased adenoma miss rate, prolonged procedure time, and need for repeat procedures (Ginzburg et al. 2007). Available bowel preparation regimens can be divided into two categories: isosmotic and hyperosmotic.

The isosmotics generally contain a non-absorbable solute (e.g., polyethylene glycol [PEG]) and rely on high volume to clean the bowel and, therefore, do not cause a significant shift in fluid and electrolytes. The volume used is about 2–4 L which can lead to frequent nausea, vomiting, and abdominal cramps. As a result, Mallory-Weiss tears and aspiration have been reported. Furthermore, there are isolated reports of pancreatitis and exacerbation of congestive heart failure (CHF) following large volume preparations with a polyethylene glycol (PEG)-based solution. More recent isosmotic preparations have applied a decreased volume of about 2 L together with laxatives such as bisacodyl. Bisacodyl use as a laxative has been associated with episodes of ischemic colitis in young adults (Ginzburg et al. 2007).

In contrast, hyperosmotic agents induce a net fluid shift into the bowel lumen causing significant fluid and electrolyte abnormalities, which can usually be tolerated in healthy subjects. However, in patients who have conditions more vulnerable to fluid and electrolyte shifts like renal failure, congestive heart failure (CHF), or chronic liver disease, these agents are contraindicated. A typical hyperosmotic agent is a hyperosmotic sodium phosphate solution. These solutions induce a net influx of water into the bowel lumen due to their hyperosmolar effect and the water helps with bowel cleansing. Therefore, patients are instructed to increase their fluid intake in order to prevent dehydration (Ginzburg et al. 2007).

Several case reports have described nephrotoxicity attributed to sodium phosphate based preparations in form of acute phosphate nephropathy, leading to chronic renal failure and in some cases end stage renal disease ending in hemodialysis (Markowitz et al. 2005). Furthermore, there have been reports of aphthous ulceration, similar to Crohn's disease following sodium phosphate based preparations (Ginzburg et al. 2007). Special care should be taken with older patients using diuretics, angiotensin converting enzyme (ACE) inhibitors, angiotensin receptor blockers, and possibly non-steroidal anti-inflammatory drug (NSAID). It is reasonable to avoid sodium phosphate preparations in these patients. Hyperphosphatemia following use of sodium phosphate preparations has been associated with symptomatic hypocalcemia leading to peri-oral tingling and numbness and even tetany (Ginzburg et al. 2007). As stated above an underlying renal insufficiency can predispose to these electrolyte abnormalities.

Overall, caution is reasonable when using sodium phosphate preparations especially in cases with the above mentioned risk factors. Patients should be instructed on adequate hydration during and after the procedure. Allowing a longer interval between the two doses of the preparation might further decrease the risk of complications.

COMPLICATIONS RELATED TO SEDATION AND ANESTHESIA

Sedation has been used to decrease the discomfort associated with endoscopic procedures. Sedation helps reduce patient anxiety and pain and increase the acceptability of procedures to patients, resulting in greater willingness to undergo repeat procedures. A combination of narcotics and benzodiazepines are commonly used for endoscopy. Sedation regimens include: benzodiazepines (e.g., midazolam and diazepam), opiates (e.g., morphine, meperidine, and fentanyl), and propofol.

The adverse effects range from allergic reactions to drug interactions, respiratory depression, and hypotension. A detailed history of patient's allergies together with a list of medications should be obtained prior to procedure. The spectrum of allergic reactions can include a minor local reaction, which can be controlled with IV diphenhydramine, to more severe anaphylactic reactions (Fujita et al. 1994). Anaphylaxis can present with mild dyspnea in mild cases or lead to hypotension and shock in more severe ones. Epinephrine can be used as an intramuscular injection together with IV diphenhydramine to control the anaphylactic reactions. In severe cases, patients will need to be transferred quickly to an emergency department.

Hypotension has been reported with midazolam at therapeutic doses of 0.15–0.3 mg/kg. A higher drop in blood pressure can be seen in patients with underlying cardiovascular disease. One should be cautious about combining benzodiazepines and opioids which can lead to pronounced decreases in blood pressure (Soysal et al. 2004). Furthermore, drug interactions between benzodiazepines and azole anti-fungals and protease inhibitors can lead to increase serum levels of benzodiazepines and, therefore, more exaggerated hypotension and respiratory depression.

Several studies have reported respiratory depression occurring with benzodiazepines during endoscopy which can lead to oxygen desaturation, respiratory acidosis, hyperkalemia, myocardial depression, and arrhythmias (Ginzburg et al. 2007). Consequently, routine use of supplemental oxygen during endoscopy can be beneficial. However, high levels of carbon dioxide can also occur with hypoventilation and may potentially be masked by supplemental oxygen. A study by Nelson et al. showed that adding transcutaneous CO_2 monitoring during endoscopy led to fewer episodes of severe CO_2 retention, but no clinically significant difference in the outcome (Nelson et al. 2000). Oxygen supplementation can be even more important when doing endoscopy on the elderly population due to their decreased baseline oxygen saturation, blunted cardiovascular response to hypercarbia and hypoxia and their more pronounced response to opioid induced respiratory depression.

According to American Society of Gastrointestinal Endoscopy (ASGE) guidelines, blood pressure, pulse, and oximetry monitoring are recommended in all patients undergoing a procedure with conscious sedation (Waring et al. 2003). In patients with a low baseline oxygen saturation, supplemental oxygen can be used through a nasal cannula. Transcutaneous CO_2 monitoring can be used for prolonged endoscopies. However, neither oxygen nor transcutaneous CO_2 monitoring should be used routinely. The endoscopist needs to be familiar with signs and symptoms of overdose related to sedation and be able to administer appropriate reversal agents if needed. In case of benzodiazepine overdose, flumazenil can be administered at 0.2 mg IV and can be repeated every 3–5 min up to a total dose of 3 mg. In the event of opioid overdose, naloxone can be used at 0.4 mg IV and can be repeated every 3–5 min. In patients with chronic benzodiazepine or opioid use, these reversal medications may lead to withdrawal symptoms which can manifest as seizures in chronic benzodiazepine users, and sweating, tremor, and agitation with chronic opioid users.

In cases in which local anesthetics are used in the oropharynx, attention needs to be paid during the recovery period due to impaired gag reflex. Therefore, resumption of oral intake should be delayed until the gag reflex has recovered. Furthermore, methemoglobinemia has been reported as a rare complication due to topical anesthetics (Gunaratnam et al. 2000). This should be suspected in an alert patient with a low level of oxygen after the procedure while on supplemental oxygen. Methemoglobin is a form of hemoglobin that does not bind oxygen or CO_2. When its concentration is elevated in red blood cells, tissue hypoxia can occur. It is important to be aware of this phenomenon and take prompt diagnostic action in the form of obtaining an arterial blood gas analysis. Methemoglobin concentrations as high as 15% can be managed by O_2 supplementation. However, higher concentrations (>30%) may require intravenous methylene blue (0.1–0.2 mg/kg over 5 min) every hour until the level of methemoglobin falls below 15%. In severe cases, ICU care, ventilator support, exchange transfusions may be needed.

CARDIOVASCULAR COMPLICATIONS

There are rare reports of cardiovascular complications related to upper and lower endoscopy within 24 h of procedure, including chest pain, myocardial infarction, hypotension, CHF, and arrhythmias. Gangi et al. reviewed 100,000 endoscopies and reported a rate of 0.3% complications (Gangi et al. 2004). Male gender, higher Goldman score preoperatively, and propofol use were considered independent risk factors for cardiovascular complications.

A careful history and physical before the procedure can help identify patients at higher risk for cardiovascular complications. Attention must be paid to drug interactions with sedatives. Close monitoring of cardiovascular function and blood oxygenation during the procedure is needed for early detection and prompt therapeutic action to control these complications (Arrowsmith et al. 1991). Early warning signs can include brady- or tachyarrhythmias, hypotension, and oxygen desaturation.

INFECTION

Infectious complications of endoscopy can be categorized in two main groups: one, transmission of microorganisms by contaminated endoscopy equipment "between patients," and two, "within patient" translocation of bacteria from the gastrointestinal tract to blood and then to other organs or prosthetic devices.

There are case reports of hepatitis B and C, salmonella, pseudomonas and even *Helicobacter pylori* and *Clostridium difficile* transmission through contaminated endoscopy equipments. However, HIV transmission following endoscopy has never been reported. It is worth mentioning that all of these reports were made prior to the publication of current reprocessing guidelines (ASGE 1999; Nelson et al. 2003).

In order to protect against transmission of microorganisms by an endoscopy between patients, the endoscopy team must adhere to high-level disinfection (HLD) in reprocessing of endoscopes after use, with careful adherence to the multisociety guidelines. The processing involves three major steps that begin with manual cleaning of the endoscope with detergent solution and brushes (Banerjee et al. 2008). Manual cleansing minimizes the chances of bacterial biofilm developing within the endoscope channels. It is important to keep in mind that manual cleansing is personnel-dependent and is different for each type of scope. Therefore, training and quality control is a must and manufacturers' recommendations should be adhered to for each type of endoscope. The US Food and Drug Administration (FDA) approved new labeling for an automatic endoscope reprocessor (AER) in 2006 as a "washer-disinfector" for processing endoscopes without prior manual washing and channel brushing. However, at this time, there are no independent confirmatory data regarding the efficacy of this machine. The second step is HLD which is operationally defined by the FDA as a 6-log reduction of mycobacteria (FDA. Guidance on the content and format of premarket notification [510 (k)] submissions for liquid chemical germicides. Rockville (MD): Food and Drug Administration et al. 1992). HLD is often performed using an automated washer/disinfector, and involves submerging the endoscope in a liquid chemical germicide (often 2% glutaraldehyde solution at room temperature for 20 min). Both the temperature of the solution, and the duration of the soak are critical in ensuring adequate disinfection. The third step includes proper rinsing and drying of the endoscope channels. Here, the scope will be rinsed with large volumes of water through all working channels to expel the chemical disinfectant. The importance of adequate rinsing is emphasized by a case report describing glutaraldehyde-induced colitis that was attributed to inadequate rinsing of the endoscopes. After rinsing with water, a 70% alcohol flush promotes drying and inhibits the growth of organisms in stored instruments. After the instruments are dried, they should be stored in an upright hanging position according to the manufacturers' recommendations.

In rare circumstances where sterilization of endoscopy equipment is necessary, as in the case of intraoperative endoscopy to avoid contamination of an open surgical field, ethylene oxide gas treatment has been used. Furthermore, in these cases reusable biopsy forceps, snares, sphincterotomes, and other accessories designed to breach the GI mucosal surface all require sterilization. Similarly, water bottles should also be disinfected or sterilized, and sterile water should be used in the water bottle. Overall, achieving sterilization is a difficult task due to the complex channel design of the endoscope. There is no evidence for any demonstrable benefits to the further reduction in endoscope bacterial spore counts achieved by sterilization instead of HLD (Muscarella 1996).

Another infectious complication related to endoscopy is translocation of gut bacteria to other sites in the body. Bacteremia occurring during endoscopy has been demonstrated in several reports with rates as high as 20–25% during colonoscopy and esophageal dilation (Nelson et al. 1998). According to the revised guidelines from the American Heart Association (AHA) for prevention of infective endocarditis, antimicrobial prophylaxis should be given only to patients with high-risk heart valve lesions if they undergo high risk procedures that are likely to result in a bacteremia with a microorganism that has the potential ability to cause endocarditis. *AHA no longer considers any GI procedure high risk and, therefore, does not recommend the routine use of antibiotic prophylaxis even in high-risk patients* (Wilson et al. 2007). However, some practitioners may choose to use prophylactic antibiotics for patients with high-risk cardiac lesions like synthetic vascular grafts that have been in place for less than 12 months. Furthermore, in patients undergoing ERCP for an obstructed biliary system or EUS or ERCP for a pancreatic cystic lesion, prophylactic use of an antibiotic against enterococcus is recommended. Also, for patients with ascites, procedures associated with higher rates of spontaneous and sustained bacteremia including variceal sclerotherapy, and esophageal stricture dilation, antibiotics prophylaxis is still indicated. In the setting of PEG placement, several prospective trials have shown a reduction in PEG-site infections in patients who received a single prophylactic dose of antibiotics prior to PEG insertion. Therefore, ASGE recommended that all patients undergoing PEG placement should receive antibiotic prophylaxis with cefazolin 1 g IV (or an equivalent antibiotic) 30 min prior to the procedure (Banerjee et al. 2008).

PERFORATION

Upper Endoscopy

The reported rate for perforation during upper endoscopy has been 0.02–0.2% (Ginzburg et al. 2007). In spite of the relatively rare occurrence, the mortality rate can be as high as 25%. The most common location reported is the distal third of the esophagus. However, perforations at the site of piriform sinus in patients with Zenker's diverticulum have also been reported. The risk of perforation increases in cases with underlying tissue abnormalities like cancers, and if therapeutic interventions including dilation or stent placement are performed. Blind passage of bougies carry the highest reported rate for perforation of 0.3–0.4% (Hernandez et al. 2000). In terms of the underlying pathology, caustic strictures have the highest risk of post-dilation perforation (17%), followed by malignant strictures (10%), and achalasia with pneumatic dilation (4–7%) (Ginzburg et al. 2007). It is important to inform patients about the high risk for perforation prior to dilation, and have surgical back up. A routine post-procedure esophagram has been recommended in these high-risk cases to rule out perforation. Mallory-Weiss tears have been reported as rare complications especially in the setting of large hiatal hernias. These usually present with fresh bleeding during endoscopy and resolve spontaneously.

Patients with a perforation during an upper GI endoscopy can present with severe chest pain, tachypnea, tachycardia followed by fever and leukocytosis. Crepitus may develop which can be detected by palpation of the anterior chest wall. The diagnostic test of choice is barium esophagram with a water soluble oral contrast or CT scan of chest. Treatment can range from conservative, (nothing per mouth, IV fluids, and antibiotics) to surgery in most cases. There are reports of covered metallic esophageal stents used to cover tears and facilitate healing (Gelbmann et al. 2004). Also, immediate endoscopic clipping has been reported as a possible modality in order to avoid surgery (Ginzburg et al. 2007). Clipping might be especially beneficial in cases with a retroperitoneal perforation like during endoscopic ampullectomy. In cases undergoing a non-surgical management for perforation, very close follow up with serial physical exams and CT scans is recommended and surgery needs to be considered in case of clinical deterioration.

Colonoscopy

About 0.2% of all diagnostic colonoscopies are complicated by perforation (Ginzburg et al. 2007). These can be caused by direct force from the tip of the endoscope against the mucosa, lateral pressure form a loop of colonoscope inside a loop of bowel, or excessive distention with air. Polyp removal, decompression of colonic pseudo-obstruction, or reduction of a volvulus can increase the risk of perforation. The most commonly reported sites are rectosigmoid and cecum. Polypectomy can lead to perforation especially if a large (>1 cm) sessile polyp is being removed from a portion of the colon where the wall is thin. Furthermore, using electrocautery or presence of an invasive lesion within the polyp can increase the risk of perforation during polypectomy. In these cases, injection of saline at the base of the polyp prior to polypectomy has been recommended to decrease the risk of perforation. There is also a relatively higher risk of perforation with a reported rate of 3% when colonoscopy is performed in the setting colonic pseudo-obstruction not responding to conservative measures. In the setting of sigmoid volvulus, the reported rate of perforation during colonoscopy is 5–7% (Ginzburg et al. 2007).

Patients with perforation after colonoscopy usually present with abdominal pain (acute abdomen) and distention. Fever and leukocytosis develop subsequently due to peritonitis. A plain upright X-ray of chest and abdomen will need to be obtained to look for free air under the diaphragm followed by a CT of the abdomen. Conservative management with serial abdominal exams and X-rays can only be pursued in a subset of relatively healthy patients. However, most patients will need surgical intervention for removal of the perforated segment or repair of a perforation, followed by IV antibiotics and bowel rest. As in upper endoscopy, immediate clipping of a perforation followed by frequent monitoring and IV antibiotics has been reported as an alternative to avoid surgery in patients in whom perforation was identified during the procedure (Ginzburg et al. 2007).

POST-POLYPECTOMY SYNDROME

Occasionally 1–5 days after the procedure after polypectomy, patients present with significant abdominal pain including local peritoneal signs on abdominal exam, mimicking colonic perforation. They may also develop fever and leukocytosis. However, imaging including abdominal X-ray and CT will not show any evidence of perforation. The etiology can be due to the use of electocautery during polypectomy leading to a full thickness electrical burn. The treatment is mainly supportive with IV fluids, antibiotics and bowel rest (Ginzburg et al. 2007).

BLEEDING

Upper Endoscopy

Bleeding after upper endoscopy has been reported as a relatively uncommon complication occurring in 0.15% of cases (Eisen et al. 2002). There has been no documented increase in bleeding complications in patients using aspirin or NSAIDs during a routine upper endoscopy and biopsy. Therefore, procedures can be done without any modification in these drugs. In the setting of patients with low platelets, it is believed that upper endoscopy can be performed with platelets as low as 20,000 (Silvis et al. 1976). Performing dilation during an upper endoscopy can be associated with a minor increase in the risk of bleeding.

Colonoscopy

As with upper endoscopy, colonoscopy is associated with a relatively low rate of bleeding (0.07%). However, higher rates have been reported when biopsy (0.3%) or polypectomy (1.5–2%) were performed (Waye et al. 1992). In the setting of post-polypectomy bleeding, the site can be identified by repeat colonoscopy or by tagged red blood cell nuclear scan. The bleeding can occur up to 2 weeks after polypectomy, and can usually be managed endoscopically by electrocautery or epinephrine injection and clipping. There are also reports of angiography to identify and selectively embolize the bleeding vessel (Ginzburg et al. 2007). Patients taking anti-thrombotic medications like aspirin, clopidogrel, ticlopidine, low molecular weight heparin (LMWH), and warfarin may need some modification in their drug regimen. ASGE guidelines recommend that aspirin (up to 325 mg/day) and NSIADs do not need to be stopped before any procedure. However, clopidogrel, ticlopidine, low molecular weight heparin (LMWH), and warfarin may need modification in a certain subset of patients. Table 1 shows patients with a higher risk of bleeding or thromboembolic events. Patients undergoing a procedure with low risk for bleeding need no modification in their anti-thrombotics. Patients undergoing a high risk procedure need some modification depending on their risk for thrombotic event. In those with a low risk of thrombotic events, the medication can be held for 3–5 days prior to their procedure with a high risk for bleeding; this approach might be detrimental in patients having a higher risk for thromboembolic events. In the latter group a bridge with LMWH can be provided for those on warfarin and then LMWH will be held on the day of the procedure (thus minimizing the amount of time that the patient is off anticoagulation) (Eisen et al. 2002; Zuckerman et al. 2005).

ASPIRATION

Another rare complication of upper endoscopy is aspiration of stomach contents. Older patients, and those with upper GI bleeding, altered mental status, decreased gag reflex, and hemodynamic instability are at increased risk for aspiration (Ginzburg et al. 2007). Avoiding topical anesthetics and oversedation, maintaining the head of the bed at a 30° – 45° angle, minimizing air insufflation, and thoroughly removing gastric contents prior to the procedure have been recommended to decrease the aspiration risk in these cases (Ginzburg et al. 2007). According to ASA recommendations, patients undergoing upper endoscopy will need to avoid solid food for at least 6 h and clear liquids for at least 2 h prior to their

Table 1
Bleeding and thromboembolic risks (Adapted from Eisen et al. 2002)

Procedure bleeding risk
High
Polypectomy
Biliary sphincterotomy
Pneumatic or bougie dilation
PEG placement
Endosonographic-guided fine needle aspiration
Laser ablation and coagulation
Treatment of varices
Low
Diagnostic
EGD plus or minus biopsy
Flexible sigmoidoscopy plus or minus biopsy
Colonoscopy plus or minus biopsy
Endoscopic retrograde cholangiopancreatography without sphincterotomy
Biliary/pancreatic stent without sphincterotomy
Endosonography without fine needle aspiration
Enteroscopy
Thromboembolic event risk
High
Atrial fibrillation with valvular heart disease
Mechanical valve in the mitral position
Mechanical valve in any position and prior thromboembolic event
Low
Deep vein thrombosis
Uncomplicated or paroxysmal non-valvular atrial fibrillation
Bioprosthetic valve in any position
Mechanical valve in the aortic position

procedure. Patients with massive upper GI bleeding have a higher reported risk for aspiration (1% and 4%) and, therefore, require more aggressive airway monitoring during upper endoscopy (Ginzburg et al. 2007). Prophylactic endotracheal intubation prior to endoscopy has been recommended by some, but a retrospective study by Rudolph and colleagues (Rudolph et al. 2003) on ICU patients, admitted for massive upper GI bleeding and intubated for airway protection, failed to show any significant benefit to endotracheal intubation. It is important to keep in mind that it is up to the endoscopist and the endoscopy team to ensure the adequacy of the airway during the procedure and take prompt action to secure the airway to prevent aspiration.

VASOVAGAL REACTIONS

Occasionally, patients can develop bradycardia, hypotension, or loss of consciousness during upper endoscopy or colonoscopy. This has been attributed to distention of the bowel together with pressure from looping, and possibly hypovolemia (Ginzburg et al. 2007). Therefore, partial or complete withdrawal of the scope and IV fluids will usually rectify the situation. However, severe cases might need atropine or reversal or the sedation.

SPLENIC INJURY

Injury to the spleen has been rarely reported as a complication of colonoscopy (Taylor et al. 1989). These patients can present with pain in the left upper quadrant area after the procedure. The mechanism is thought to be due to shear forces from pushing a colonoscope against splenocolic ligament leading to avulsion injury to splenic capsule. Most cases can be managed with conservative measures.

ENTRAPMENT OF THE ENDOSCOPE

There are rare case reports describing entrapment of the endoscope during upper endoscope or colonoscopy. Huang and colleagues presented a case of entrapment in a 24-year-old man which happened when the patient belched during a retroflex exam of the gastric fundus, pushing the U-turned shaft into the distal esophagus (Huang et al. 2006). Eventually, the entraped endoscope was released, using another endoscope in parallel, inserting pressure on the U-turned shaft and pushing it into the stomach.

Entrapment can also happen during a routine colonoscopy in a similar manner. Koltun and Coller have described a case with right-sided inguinal hernia (Koltun and Coller 1991). In this case, the colonoscope was entrapped in a loop of colon inside the hernia sac and the authors were not able to reduce the hernia. They eventually managed to withdraw the scope with gentle pressure support on the loop inside the hernia.

COMPLICATIONS OF PERCUTANEOUS ENDOSCOPIC GASTROSTOMY

Since its introduction in 1980 by Ponsky and Gauderer (Gauderer et al. 1980; Ponsky and Gauderer 1981) percutaneous endoscopic gastrostomy (PEG) has gained wide acceptance as a safe and efficient method of providing enteral alimentation in patients who cannot swallow due to dementia, stroke, or other causes (Ginzburg et al. 2007). The pull method, introduced by Ponsky and his colleagues, is the most widely used technique. There are several other modifications of the original procedure. The push technique differs from the pull method in that the PEG tube is pushed over a guide wire into its final position (Ginzburg et al. 2007). All of these techniques require the introduction of a flexible endoscope into the stomach and then percutaneous placement of a cannula through the abdominal wall into the stomach. Unfortunately, up to 20% of procedures can end up with complications, although most are relatively minor (Ginzburg et al. 2007).

Fistula

A rare complication of PEG placement involves development of a fistula between the stomach, colon, and skin or the so called gastrocolocutaneous fistula. This can be prevented by careful identification of the site by transillumination, and positioning of the PEG tube to provide good apposition of the stomach with the anterior abdominal wall. The presentation can range from an acute manifestation with peritonitis or colonic obstruction to a more chronic picture with leakage of stool from the stoma or diarrhea resembling tube feeds. This can be diagnosed radiographically. The fistula usually resolves with removal of the tube. However, surgery needs to be considered if the patient develops signs of peritonitis.

Buried Bumper Syndrome

Occasionally, the gastric mucosa can grow over the internal bolster (bumper) after PEG placement and result in migration of the internal bumper along the length of the sinus tract in 1–2% of cases (Venu et al. 2002). These patients can present with multiple episodes of abdominal pain, tube blockage, or leakage around the tube during feedings. This can be managed by removing the old PEG tube and placing a new one. A new location should be tried if the bumper is completely covered by the mucosa.

Stoma Leak or Enlargement

Another common problem with PEG tubes is leakage around the stoma which has been reported in 1–3% of patients (Ginzburg et al. 2007). Several factors have been associated with this condition including infection at the PEG site, high gastric acid output, loose or absent external bolster, torsion of the tube, buried bumper, or excessive cleaning with hydrogen peroxide. The treatment mainly involves correcting the underlying factors and proper site care. Depending on the cause, these patients can benefit from acid suppression with a proton pump inhibitor, antibiotics to control infection, and increasing tension on the tube by adjusting the external bolster (Ginzburg et al. 2007). In cases where stoma enlargement has lead to leakage, some authors have recommended replacing the PEG with a large size tube. However, based on our experience, when the above mentioned measure to control the leakage fail, the original PEG will has to be removed and a new site for a new PEG will need to be chosen. Another proposed method involves leaving a smaller sized catheter at the old PEG site, allowing partial closure of the site and then placing a new replacement tube when the stoma enlargement has resolved (Ginzburg et al. 2007).

Wound/Tube Infection

Infection around the PEG site has been reported in about one third of cases (Ginzburg et al. 2007). In most of these patients, infection is minor and can be managed by 1 week of oral antibiotics. However, IV antibiotics or tube removal may be necessary in certain situations. Gossner and colleagues have demonstrated that prophylactic antibiotics prior to the procedure (a single dose of a first-generation cephalosporin, e.g., cefazolin or an equivalent antibiotic) can reduce the rate of infection following PEG placement (Gossner et al. 1999). This has been further emphasized by a meta-analysis demonstrating a significant decrease in the rate of peri-stomal wound infection when antibiotics were given at the time of the procedure (24% infection without prophylaxis versus 6.4% with prophylaxis) (Sharma and Howden 2000). Additional attention will need to be paid to patients with a higher risk of infection such as those with diabetes mellitus, renal insufficiency, and alcohol abuse, where necrotizing fasciitis has been reported as a result of severe infection at the PEG site (Ginzburg et al. 2007).

Tube Dislodgement

Occasionally, PEG tubes may be removed accidentally (up to 5%). Generally, in cases where the tube was placed more than 4 weeks prior to an accidental removal, the sinus tract has matured. Therefore, a new replacement PEG tube can be placed at the bedside through the original tract without need for endoscopy. However, this reinsertion should be done within 24 h of the original tube removal. Otherwise, the tract may close which may necessitate dilatation or an endoscopic replacement. The tube insertion should be verified by aspiration of gastric contents and if there is any doubt about the tube placement, a gastrografin study via the new gastrostomy tube should be performed.

Pneumoperitoneum

More than one-third of PEG insertions have been reported to show some evidence of pneumoperitoneum on radiology. In the setting of a clinically stable patient, the finding of pneumoperitoneum does not appear to have any clinical significance. In fact, it has been shown that these patients can be fed and discharged uneventfully within 24 h (Ginzburg et al. 2007). However, the presence of peritoneal signs points to the possibility of clinically significant perforation and will require more aggressive evaluation.

Hemorrhage

Bleeding from the wound has also been reported following PEG placement. As expected, bleeding is more common in patients on anticoagulation or those with an underlying coagulopathy. The treatment is usually conservative including local pressure and adequate external bolster placement. A hematoma may form in some cases due to injury to abdominal wall vessels. Spontaneous resolution happens in most cases. However, there has been a case report of massive ulcerated hematoma following PEG placement that eventually led to a partial gastrectomy in order to stop the bleeding (Chikamori et al. 2003).

ENDOSCOPIC RETROGRADE CHOLANGIOPANCREATOGRAPHY

ERCP has been widely used as both a diagnostic and therapeutic modality in pancreaticobiliry disorders. There are many reports of ERCP complications providing a rate of 5–10%, which is higher compared to other endoscopic procedures (Wang et al. 2009). The majority of these complications are of mild to moderate severity. However, a significant number can be severe leading to a reported mortality rate of about 1% (Wang et al. 2009). Andriulli and colleagues performed a systematic review of 21 prospective studies covering 16,800 patients undergoing ERCP (Andriulli et al. 2007). Overall, complications attributed to ERCP occurred in 1,154 patients (6.8%), including in a decreasing order of frequency: pancreatitis 585 cases (3.5%), infection in 242 cases (1.4%), bleeding in 226 (1.3%), and perforations in 101 (0.6%). 173 cases (1.3%) developed cardiovascular and/or analgesia related complications. The overall mortality rate was 0.07% (9 cases).

Pancreatitis

Pancreatitis has been reported as the most common ERCP related complication in 1–7% of cases (Andriulli et al. 2007). It is important to keep in mind that transient elevation of amylase and lipase, which is extremely common after ERCP, does not necessarily constitute pancreatitis. According to the standards of practice committee statement of ASGE, the consensus definition for ERCP pancreatitis is a new or worsened abdominal pain with a serum amylase that is three or more times the upper limits of normal 24 h after the procedure that requires at least 2 days of hospitalization (Mallery et al. 2003). Pancreatitis is usually of mild to moderate severity in more than 80% of cases. However, severe pancreatitis has been reported in up to 11% of all post-ERCP pancreatitis cases (Andriulli et al. 2007).

Several factors have been attributed to increased risk of post-ERCP pancreatitis. Based on a recent prospective study by Wang and colleagues involving 14 centers in China over the course of 1 year, the younger age of the patient (< 60 years), female gender, presence of periampullary diverticulum, cannulation time of more than 10 min, more than one pancreatic deep wire pass, and performing needle-knife precut were found to play a significant role in the development of post-ERCP pancreatitis (Wang et al. 2009).

Infection

The main infectious complications reported after ERCP include cholangitis (up to 1%) and cholecystitis (up to 0.5%) (Mallery et al. 2003). Several factors have been considered to increase the rate of post-ERCP cholangitis including use of combined percutaneous-endoscopic procedures (rendezvous technique), stent placement in malignant strictures, presence of jaundice, low case volume, and incomplete or failed biliary drainage. Accordingly, placement of plastic stents has been proposed as a means of reducing cholangitis in cases with incomplete or unsuccessful stone extraction. In cases involving a malignant hilar obstruction, some endoscopists have recommended to avoid filling all intrahepatic segments and to try to drain all intrahepatic segments that are filled with contrast.

Several studies have evaluated the role of antibiotic prophylaxis in decreasing post-ERCP cholangitis. Most studies including a meta-analysis failed to show any benefit for routine prophylaxis with antibiotics (Harris et al. 1999). However, in cases with known cholangitis, incomplete drainage, or inadvertent filling of a pancreatic pseudocyst, prophylactic use of antibiotics is recommended (Mallery et al. 2003).

Cholecystitis has also been reported as a post-ERCP complication. The presence of stones in the gallbladder and filling of the gallbladder with contrast during ERCP have been proposed as possible factors that increase the risk of cholecystitis (Freeman et al. 1996).

Hemorrhage

Post-ERCP hemorrhage has been reported in 0.7–2% of patients (Mallery et al. 2003). It usually happens in the setting of sphincterotomy and can present as melena, hematochezia, or hematemesis. Half of these cases present with delayed bleeding that can happen up to 1–2 weeks after the procedure. The majority are of mild to moderate severity with severe hemorrhage (i.e., requiring two or more units of blood, surgery, or angiography) occurring in 0.1–0.5% (Andriulli et al. 2007; Mallery et al. 2003). Similar to other procedures, the presence of an underlying coagulopathy and anticoagulants used within 72 h can increase the risk of bleeding. Furthermore, the presence of acute cholangitis or papillary stenosis, use of precut sphincterotomy, and low case volume of the endoscopist (one sphincterotomy per week or fewer) have been considered as risk factors. Use of aspirin or NSAIDs does not appear to significantly increase the risk of bleeding.

Perforation

Reported rates for perforation range from 0.3% to 0.6% (Freeman et al. 1996; Mallery et al. 2003). Three different types of perforation have been reported post-ERCP: guidewire-induced perforation, periampullary perforation during sphincterotomy, and perforation at a site remote from the papilla (Howard et al. 1999). Early diagnosis of periampullary perforations is important, since prompt initiation of biliary and duodenal drainage (nasobiliary and nasogastric tubes) together with broad spectrum antibiotics can prevent more aggressive operative interventions in up to 86% of cases (Enns et al. 2002).

Other types of perforations, that are remote from the papilla, are frequently diagnosed later and will need surgery. Several factors have been recognized to increase the risk of post-ERCP perforation including history of a Billroth II partial gastrectomy, performance of a sphincterotomy, intramural injection of contrast, duration of procedure, biliary stricture dilation, and SOD (Enns et al. 2002).

Cardiopulmonary Complications

Although rarely reported, cardiopulmonary complications can lead to a significant number of mortalities from ERCP (Mallery et al. 2003). These may arise from arrhythmias, hypoventilation, aspiration, or other underlying conditions. Furthermore, medications used for sedation and analgesia might play a role in precipitating these complications. Such complications might be reduced by careful preoperative evaluation and collaboration with anesthesiologists for high-risk or difficult-to-sedate patients.

Mortality

Death associated with ERCP has been reported in about 0.2% of cases (1 in 500) (Andriulli et al. 2007). Mortality rate is twice more frequent after therapeutic compared with diagnostic ERCP (Andriulli et al. 2007; Freeman et al. 1996). Any of the above mentioned complications can be associated with mortality.

Miscellaneous Complications

There are several other complications reported to be associated with ERCP including: ileus, antibiotic-related diarrhea, hepatic abscess, pneumothorax/pneumomediastinum, perforation of colonic diverticula, duodenal hematoma, portal venous air, and impaction of therapeutic devices such as stone retrieval baskets (Masci et al. 2001). Infection of pseudocysts has been reported especially after filling of pseudocysts during ERCP. Therefore, it is recommended to avoid filling of pseudocysts in the absence of subsequent drainage.

ENDOSCOPIC ULTRASOUND

EUS shares the risks and complications of other endoscopic procedures including risks of conscious sedation, cardio-respiratory events and allergic reaction to medication. There are other complications specifically associated with performance of EUS due to unique properties of echoendoscopes along with risks of fine needle aspiration (FNA), true cut biopsy (TCB) and other therapeutic interventions.

Perforation

The reported frequency of GI perforation during EUS range between 0.03% and 0.4% with a mortality rate of 0.002% (O'Toole et al. 2001). The increased risk is partly due to long non-flexible rigid transducers, and oblique viewing optics of both radial and linear echoendoscopes. The risk of perforation is particularly higher in patients with esophageal cancer and esophageal strictures, if dilation is performed to traverse the obstructing esophageal tumor. Initial studies reported perforation rates as high as 24%. But, recently sequential dilation to no more than 16 mm without use of undue force has been reported to be safe without any perforation in 120 patients (Pfau et al. 2000). The risk can be reduced if a mini-probe or a small caliber echoendoscope is used. But, the depth of penetration of the tumor cannot be assessed accurately with these instruments.

Bleeding

Clinically significant bleeding is rare with EUS and EUS guided FNA as most endosonographers use Doppler to avoid path of visible vessel when FNA is performed. The incidence of EUS related bleeding was 0.4% in two prospective studies and 1.3% in a retrospective analysis. FNA of pancreatic cystic lesions is associated with 6% rate of self limited bleeding (Wiersema et al. 1997).

Infection

The frequency of bacteremia as a complication of EUS and EUS-FNA was reported in three prospective studies which collectively included over 250 patients (Wiersema et al. 1997). These studies did not find a statistically significant increase in the rate of bacteremia when compared with that seen after upper endoscopy, and none of the patients who developed bacteremia manifested clinical signs or symptoms of illness. Similarly, a study of 52 patients who underwent EUS–FNA of solid lesions of upper GI tract showed bacteremia in 6% of patients. None of these patients developed signs or symptoms of infection. However, an infection rate of 9% was reported after EUS-guided FNA of cystic lesions of pancreas, mediastinum and other areas, and pre-procedure antibiotics administration has been recommended in these cases (Ryan et al. 2002). At present, there are no guidelines regarding antibiotics prophylaxis by ASGE or American Heart Association in patients undergoing EUS or EUS guided FNA of solid lower GI lesions and non-pancreatic cystic lesions, although antibiotic prophylaxis is recommended by ASGE for FNA of pancreatic cystic lesions, but not for solid upper GI lesions.

Pancreatitis

Pancreatitis may occur after EUS- FNA of both cystic and solid lesions with the incidence rate of 0.3–0.6% in two prospective studies. EUS-FNA-induced pancreatitis is usually mild, but severe pancreatitis with fatal complications has been reported. The risk is higher if multiple passes are made, or large amount of pancreatic parenchyma or the pancreatic duct is traversed (Eloubeidi et al. 2004).

Miscellaneous

Other rare complications reported with EUS include bile peritonitis and tumor seeding of the needle track. EUS-guided celiac block and neurolysis is associated with transient diarrhea (4–15%), orthostasis (1%), transient increase in pain (9%), abscess formation as well as lower extremity weakness with or without paresthesias, paraplegia, perforation and chronic gastroparesis (Shah et al. 2004; Chen et al. 2002).

ADVANCED THERAPEUTIC TECHNIQUES

Endoscopic Mucosal Resection

Endoscopic mucosal resection (EMR) first introduced in Japan, has been shown to be a promising therapeutic option for removal of superficial benign, potentially malignant and malignant gastrointestinal tract lesions. EMR allows histologic assessment of the entire specimen, in contrast to other ablative methods such as photodynamic therapy (PDT) and argon plasma coagulation (APC). In cases of malignant lesions, patients need to be carefully selected to include only those with superficial lesions and no lymph node involvement. In comparison to other endoscopic procedures, EMR carries higher complication rate. Bleeding and perforation are the most common complications. Overall, bleeding has been reported in 4–20% of esophageal squamous cell carcinomas, 10% of patients with Barrett's esophagus, and 12% of early gastric cancers (EGC) (Conio et al. 2006). In the colon, bleeding has been reported in 1–9% of cases, although rates as high as 12–45% have been recorded (Conio et al. 2006). Most of the bleeding occurs during the procedure, but sometimes it is delayed. Bleeding after polypectomy using EMR has been reported to occur after a median of 5 days with a range of 0–17 days (Sorbi et al. 2000). Gastroenterologists will need to have more training and experience in the procedure and be able to cope with its procedural complications including bleeding and perforation.

Radiofrequency Ablation

Radiofrequency ablation (RFA) entails using high frequency alternating current to ablate dysfunctional tissue. It has been used in a variety of clinical situations including management of tumors, abnormal electrical pathways in heart tissue in cases of arrhythmias, and more recently in eradication of Barrett's esophagus. In a recent study comparing RFA with sham procedure in ablative therapy for dysplastic Barrett's esophagus, 77% patients in the RFA group had complete eradication of intestinal metaplasia, as compared with 2.3% in the control group ($P<0.001$) and patients in the RFA group had less disease progression (3.6% vs. 16.3%, $P=0.03$) and fewer cancers (1.2% vs. 9.3%, $P = 0.045$). The side effects of RFA reported in this study of 127 patients included chest pain (two patients), upper gastrointestinal hemorrhage (in one patient on anti-platelet therapy for heart disease), and esophageal stricture (6%). No perforations or procedure-related deaths were reported. Overall, RFA appears to be a relatively safe method for ablation of Barrett's esophagus and treatment of various gastrointestinal tumors (Pouw et al. 2008). Further studies regarding the long term efficacy and safety of RFA will need to be performed.

ENDOSCOPY IN PREGNANT OR LACTATING WOMEN

Most of the studies on pregnant women are limited to case series. The general consensus is that endoscopy in pregnancy is safe when the indication for endoscopy is appropriate, and care is taken with sedation. However, a number of potential risks have been reported for endoscopy during pregnancy. Oversedation may cause maternal hypotension and hypoxia which can lead to fetal hypoxia and potentially fatal consequences. The fetus can be exposed to potentially teratogenic drugs and radiation (ERCP). Fetal hypoxia can occur due to inappropriate maternal positioning leading to compression of inferior vena cava by the pregnant uterus, therefore compromising uterine blood flow.

According to ASGE guidelines for endoscopy during pregnancy or lactation, (Qureshi et al. 2005) the clinician should always have a strong indication for the procedure especially in high risk pregnancies. Whenever possible the procedure should be deferred to the second trimester. The lowest possible dose of sedative medications (category A or B drugs) should be used during the procedure. The procedure time should be minimized; the patient should be positioned in the left pelvic tilt or left lateral position to avoid vena caval or aortic compression, and fetal heart sounds should be monitored before the initiation of sedation and at the completion of the procedure. Obstetric support should be available in the event of a pregnancy-related complication. Finally, endoscopy is contraindicated in the setting of obstetric complications such as placental abruption, imminent delivery, ruptured membranes or pre-eclampsia.

Cappell et al. (1996a) reported on safety and diagnostic yield of upper endoscopy in 83 pregnant women. The diagnostic yield was 95%, and there were no cases of premature labor or other complications related to the fetus. The same group reported the outcomes of 48 sigmoidoscopies (46 patients) and eight colonoscopies (eight patients) during pregnancy (Cappell et al. 1996b). They reported no adverse effect or complications related to the procedures. However, it seems a reasonable recommendation to try to avoid excessive abdominal pressure during colonoscopy (especially during late pregnancy) and prone or decubitus positioning of the pregnant patient. There are no reports on the safety of different bowel preparation agents during pregnancy. Therefore, polyethylene glycol solutions are considered category C.

Jamidar et al. (1995) reported 29 ERCPs in 23 pregnant patients (only three diagnostic ERCPs). There was only one post-procedure complication (acute pancreatitis), and no adverse effects on the fetus. It is important to protect the fetus from radiation by lead sheets placed under the pelvis and the lower abdomen. The fluoroscopy time should be minimized with the X-ray beam strictly focused on the area of interest. To confirm successful bile duct cannulation, one can demonstrate bile aspirate instead of fluoroscopy. Overall, fetal exposure should be kept below 5–10 rad level which is the level associated with radiation induced teratogenesis.

Sedation for endoscopy has also been addressed in the 2005 ASGE guidelines. Generally, sedation should be attempted with the lowest effective dose of the safest medication available. To avoid the critical time of organogenesis, all endoscopic procedures should be deferred to the second trimester if possible. Meperidine (category B) is preferred over fentanyl (category C) for initial sedation. Benzodiazepines are uniformly classified as category D; however, in cases where meperidine alone is insufficient, benzodiazepines may be added. There are no reports of midazolam causing congenital abnormalities or fetal demise, making midazolam a preferred adjunct to meperidine.

In the case of lactating women, the main concern is drug excretion in breast milk. In this case fentanyl appears to be the preferred opiate since it is only excreted in pharmacologically insignificant quantities in breast milk. Midazolam may be used as an adjunct, but breastfeeding should be avoided for 4 h afterwards. In cases where meperidine is used, the drug can be detected in breast milk up to 24 h after administration.

SUMMARY OF KEY POINTS

- Endoscopy is an important diagnostic and therapeutic modality.
- The spectrum of complications can range from adverse effects related to preparation and anesthesia to procedure related complications including: cardiovascular, infection, bleeding, perforation, postpolypectomy syndrome, aspiration, vasovagal reactions, and splenic injury.
- Percutaneous endoscopic gastrostomy (PEG) can be associated with fistula, buried bumper syndrome, stoma leak and/or enlargement, tube dislodgement, wound/tube infection, pneumoperitoneum, and bleeding.
- Endoscopic retrograde cholangiopancreatography (ERCP) can lead to similar pattern of complications as upper endoscopy together with an added risk of pancreatitis.
- EUS also shares the complications of other upper endoscopic procedures together with an added risk associated with fine needle aspiration (FNA) and true cut biopsies and mildly increased risk of perforation due to long nonflexible rigid transducers, and oblique viewing optics.
- The major complications attributed to endoscopic mucosal resection are infection and bleeding.
- The main reported complications of radiofrequency ablation are chest pain, upper GI bleeding and esophageal stricture.
- Overall endoscopy during pregnancy is a safe procedure when done with appropriate indication and careful sedation.
- The risks from endoscopy can be minimized by careful patient selection, extensive training, and adherence to proper techniques.
- Prompt recognition and appropriate management of complications are essential to ensure the best patient outcomes.

REFERENCES

Andriulli A, Loperfido S, Napolitano G, et al. Incidence rates of post-ERCP complications: a systematic survey of prospective studies. Am J Gastroenterol. 2007;102:1781–8.

Arrowsmith JB, Gerstman BB, Fleischer DE, Benjamin SB. Results from the American Society for Gastrointestinal Endoscopy/U.S. Food and Drug Administration collaborative study on complication rates and drug use during gastrointestinal endoscopy. Gastrointest Endosc. 1991;37:421–7.

ASGE. Infection control during gastrointestinal endoscopy: guidelines for clinical application. From the ASGE. American Society for Gastrointestinal Endoscopy. Gastrointest Endosc. 1999;49:836–41.

Banerjee S, Shen B, Nelson DB, et al. Infection control during GI endoscopy. Gastrointest Endosc. 2008;67:781–90.

Cappell MS, Colon VJ, Sidhom OA. A study of eight medical centers of the safety and clinical efficacy of esophagogastroduodenoscopy in 83 pregnant females with follow-up of fetal outcome with comparison control groups. Am J Gastroenterol. 1996a;91:348–54.

Cappell MS, Colon VJ, Sidhom OA. A study at 10 medical centers of the safety and efficacy of 48 flexible sigmoidoscopies and 8 colonoscopies during pregnancy with follow-up of fetal outcome and with comparison to control groups. Dig Dis Sci. 1996b;41:2353–61.

Chen HY, Lee CH, Hsieh CH. Bile peritonitis after EUS-guided fine-needle aspiration. Gastrointest Endosc. 2002;56:594–6.

Chikamori F, Kuniyoshi N, Kawashima T, Takase Y. Huge submucosal hematoma of the stomach after accidental removal of the percutaneous endoscopic gastrostomy tube. Dig Endosc. 2003;15:341–3.

Conio M, Ponchon T, Blanchi S, Filiberti R. Endoscopic mucosal resection. Am J Gastroenterol. 2006;101:653–63.

Eisen GM, Baron TH, Dominitz JA, et al. Guideline on the management of anticoagulation and antiplatelet therapy for endoscopic procedures. Gastrointest Endosc. 2002;55:775–9.

Eloubeidi MA, Gress FG, Savides TJ, et al. Acute pancreatitis after EUS-guided FNA of solid pancreatic masses: a pooled analysis from EUS centers in the United States. Gastrointest Endosc. 2004;60:385–9.

Enns R, Eloubeidi MA, Mergener K, et al. ERCP-related perforations: risk factors and management. Endoscopy. 2002;34:293–8.

FDA. Guidance on the content and format of premarket notification [510 (k)] submissions for liquid chemical germicides. Rockville: Food and Drug Administration, Infection Control Devices Branch, Division of General and Restorative Devices, Office of Device Evaluation; 1992.

Freeman ML, Nelson DB, Sherman S, et al. Complications of endoscopic biliary sphincterotomy. N Engl J Med. 1996;335:909–18.

Fujita Y, Ishikawa H, Yokota K. Anaphylactoid reaction to midazolam. Anesth Analg. 1994;79:811–2.

Gangi S, Saidi F, Patel K, Johnstone B, Jaeger J, Shine D. Cardiovascular complications after GI endoscopy: occurrence and risks in a large hospital system. Gastrointest Endosc. 2004;60:679–85.

Gauderer MW, Ponsky JL, Izant Jr RJ. Gastrostomy without laparotomy: a percutaneous endoscopic technique. J Pediatr Surg. 1980;15:872–5.

Gelbmann CM, Ratiu NL, Rath HC, et al. Use of self-expandable plastic stents for the treatment of esophageal perforations and symptomatic anastomotic leaks. Endoscopy. 2004;36:695–9.

Ginzburg L, Greenwald D, Cohen J. Complications of endoscopy. Gastrointest Endosc Clin N Am. 2007;17:405–32.

Gossner L, Keymling J, Hahn EG, Ell C. Antibiotic prophylaxis in percutaneous endoscopic gastrostomy (PEG): a prospective randomized clinical trial. Endoscopy. 1999;31:119–24.

Gunaratnam NT, Vazquez-Sequeiros E, Gostout CJ, Alexander GL. Methemoglobinemia related to topical benzocaine use: is it time to reconsider the empiric use of topical anesthesia before sedated EGD? Gastrointest Endosc. 2000;52:692–3.

Harris A, Chan AC, Torres-Viera C, Hammett R, Carr-Locke D. Meta-analysis of antibiotic prophylaxis in endoscopic retrograde cholangiopancreatography (ERCP). Endoscopy. 1999;31:718–24.

Hernandez LV, Jacobson JW, Harris MS. Comparison among the perforation rates of maloney, balloon, and savary dilation of esophageal strictures. Gastrointest Endosc. 2000;51:460–2.

Howard TJ, Tan T, Lehman GA, et al. Classification and management of perforations complicating endoscopic sphincterotomy. Surgery. 1999;126:658–63. discussion 64–5.

Huang PM, Wang HP, Chen CN, Chen LH, Lee YC. Impaction of an upper gastrointestinal endoscope in the distal esophagus: alternative method of removal by double endoscopy without fluoroscopic assistance. Endoscopy. 2006;38:293.

Jamidar PA, Beck GJ, Hoffman BJ, et al. Endoscopic retrograde cholangiopancreatography in pregnancy. Am J Gastroenterol. 1995;90:1263–7.

Koltun WA, Coller JA. Incarceration of colonoscope in an inguinal hernia. "Pulley" technique of removal. Dis Colon Rectum. 1991;34:191–3.

Mallery JS, Baron TH, Dominitz JA, et al. Complications of ERCP. Gastrointest Endosc. 2003;57:633–8.

Markowitz GS, Stokes MB, Radhakrishnan J, D'Agati VD. Acute phosphate nephropathy following oral sodium phosphate bowel purgative: an underrecognized cause of chronic renal failure. J Am Soc Nephrol. 2005;16:3389–96.

Masci E, Toti G, Mariani A, et al. Complications of diagnostic and therapeutic ERCP: a prospective multicenter study. Am J Gastroenterol. 2001;96:417–23.

Muscarella LF. High-level disinfection or "sterilization" of endoscopes? Infect Control Hosp Epidemiol. 1996;17:183–7.

Nelson DB, Sanderson SJ, Azar MM. Bacteremia with esophageal dilation. Gastrointest Endosc. 1998;48:563–7.

Nelson DB, Freeman ML, Silvis SE, et al. A randomized, controlled trial of transcutaneous carbon dioxide monitoring during ERCP. Gastrointest Endosc. 2000;51:288–95.

Nelson DB, Jarvis WR, Rutala WA, et al. Multi-society guideline for reprocessing flexible gastrointestinal endoscopes. Society for Healthcare Epidemiology of America. Infect Control Hosp Epidemiol. 2003;24:532–7.

O'Toole D, Palazzo L, Arotcarena R, et al. Assessment of complications of EUS-guided fine-needle aspiration. Gastrointest Endosc. 2001;53:470–4.

Pfau PR, Ginsberg GG, Lew RJ, Faigel DO, Smith DB, Kochman ML. Esophageal dilation for endosonographic evaluation of malignant esophageal strictures is safe and effective. Am J Gastroenterol. 2000;95:2813–5.

Ponsky JL, Gauderer MW. Percutaneous endoscopic gastrostomy: a nonoperative technique for feeding gastrostomy. Gastrointest Endosc. 1981;27:9–11.

Pouw RE, Sharma VK, Bergman JJ, Fleischer DE. Radiofrequency ablation for total Barrett's eradication: a description of the endoscopic technique, its clinical results and future prospects. Endoscopy. 2008;40:1033–40.

Qureshi WA, Rajan E, Adler DG, et al. ASGE guideline: guidelines for endoscopy in pregnant and lactating women. Gastrointest Endosc. 2005;61:357–62.

Rudolph SJ, Landsverk BK, Freeman ML. Endotracheal intubation for airway protection during endoscopy for severe upper GI hemorrhage. Gastrointest Endosc. 2003;57:58–61.

Ryan AG, Zamvar V, Roberts SA. Iatrogenic candidal infection of a mediastinal foregut cyst following endoscopic ultrasound-guided fine-needle aspiration. Endoscopy. 2002;34:838–9.

Shah JN, Fraker D, Guerry D, Feldman M, Kochman ML. Melanoma seeding of an EUS-guided fine needle track. Gastrointest Endosc. 2004;59:923–4.

Sharma VK, Howden CW. Meta-analysis of randomized, controlled trials of antibiotic prophylaxis before percutaneous endoscopic gastrostomy. Am J Gastroenterol. 2000;95:3133–6.

Silvis SE, Nebel O, Rogers G, Sugawa C, Mandelstam P. Endoscopic complications. Results of the 1974 American Society for Gastrointestinal Endoscopy Survey. JAMA. 1976;235:928–30.

Sivak M, editor. Gastroenterologic endoscopy. Philadelphia: WB Saunders; 2000.

Sorbi D, Norton I, Conio M, Balm R, Zinsmeister A, Gostout CJ. Postpolypectomy lower GI bleeding: descriptive analysis. Gastrointest Endosc. 2000;51:690–6.

Soysal S, Karcioglu O, Demircan A, et al. Comparison of meperidine plus midazolam and fentanyl plus midazolam in procedural sedation: a double-blind, randomized controlled trial. Adv Ther. 2004;21:312–21.

Taylor FC, Frankl HD, Riemer KD. Late presentation of splenic trauma after routine colonoscopy. Am J Gastroenterol. 1989;84:442–3.

Venu RP, Brown RD, Pastika BJ, Erikson Jr LW. The buried bumper syndrome: a simple management approach in two patients. Gastrointest Endosc. 2002;56:582–4.

Wang P, Li ZS, Liu F, et al. Risk factors for ERCP-related complications: a prospective multicenter study. Am J Gastroenterol. 2009;104:31–40.

Waring JP, Baron TH, Hirota WK, et al. Guidelines for conscious sedation and monitoring during gastrointestinal endoscopy. Gastrointest Endosc. 2003;58:317–22.

Waye JD, Lewis BS, Yessayan S. Colonoscopy: a prospective report of complications. J Clin Gastroenterol. 1992;15:347–51.

Wiersema MJ, Vilmann P, Giovannini M, Chang KJ, Wiersema LM. Endosonography-guided fine-needle aspiration biopsy: diagnostic accuracy and complication assessment. Gastroenterology. 1997;112:1087–95.

Wilson W, Taubert KA, Gewitz M, et al. Prevention of infective endocarditis: guidelines from the American Heart Association: a guideline from the American Heart Association Rheumatic Fever, Endocarditis, and Kawasaki Disease Committee, Council on Cardiovascular Disease in the Young, and the Council on Clinical Cardiology, Council on Cardiovascular Surgery and Anesthesia, and the Quality of Care and Outcomes Research Interdisciplinary Working Group. Circulation. 2007;116:1736–54.

Zuckerman MJ, Hirota WK, Adler DG, et al. ASGE guideline: the management of low-molecular-weight heparin and nonaspirin antiplatelet agents for endoscopic procedures. Gastrointest Endosc. 2005;61:189–94.

21 Documentation and Description of Endoscopic Procedures

Shannon Marek, Sreeram V.J. Parupudi, and Subbaramiah Sridhar

CONTENTS

Keywords: Documentation, Description, Endoscopic, Procedures, Lesions

INTRODUCTION

Quality assurance in endoscopic practice has become a standard requirement in most countries. In an era of liability and malpractice, ensuring quality in endoscopic practice is the only dependable strategy to reduce risk of litigation. One of the measures of quality of endoscopic procedures is appropriate documentation of lesions and completeness of the procedure. To maintain higher standards of practice and to train junior gastroenterologists, a physician should make every attempt to complete a thorough endoscopic examination, document the procedure with accurate vocabulary, take appropriate photographs of every step of the procedure, and specifically describe the presence or lack of abnormalities. This stepwise approach is helpful for comparison with follow-up examinations and serves to guide referring physicians for subsequent patient care. An endoscopist should note whether the given procedure was complete, and if not, the reason for its incompleteness; i.e., non-cooperative patient, inadequate sedation, retained food in the stomach, sub-optimal or poor preparation, stricture, loop formation etc.

From: *Clinical Gastroenterology: Diagnostic and Therapeutic Procedures in Gastroenterology*,
Edited by: G. Y. Wu, S. Sridhar, DOI 10.1007/978-1-59745-044-7_21,

Photographic documentation of endoscopic procedures may be evolving from still photographs to video recording. All examination findings at endoscopy and subsequent recommendations are based on images, which are created during the procedure. This allows a physician to maintain an accurate record for future use, comparison purposes, and research.

PHOTODOCUMENTATION OF ENDOSCOPIC PROCEDURES

In order to obtain the most helpful photographs, physicians must make every attempt to:

1. Clean the lens of endoscopes and the region of interest before taking a photo.
2. Adequately inflate the lumen of the organ.
3. Avoid close lateral proximity with the mucosa to avoid over illumination of the area of interest.
4. Freeze the frame to focus before storing the picture of interest.
5. Select images to archive.

It is important to include a sufficient number of images to document complete endoscopic examination. On the other hand, video recording (if available) of the entire procedure or specific important segments of the procedure can also be done. Newer technologies may also provide more accurate images. The addition of narrow band imaging technology built into modern endoscopes enhances the visibility of some mucosal lesions. All negative examinations should also contain standard photographic documentation of specific structures.

UPPER GASTROINTESTINAL ENDOSCOPY

Routinely, upper gastrointestinal endoscopies are done using forward viewing endoscopes. The newer equipments have a wider-angle lens and greater degree of tip movement (or deflection), allowing for more efficient examination and survey of the

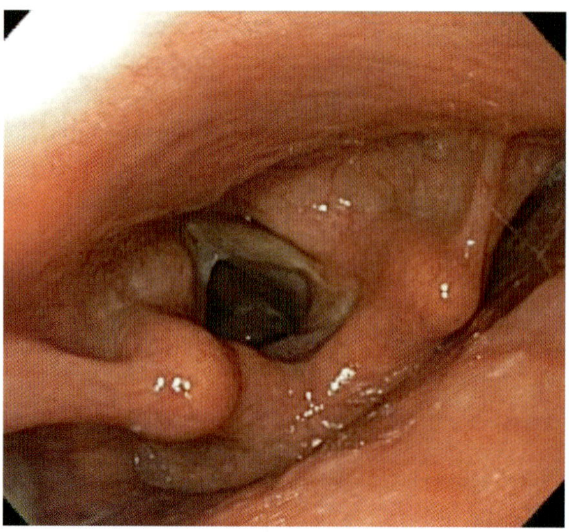

Fig. 1. Upper endoscopic view of the hypopharynx.

stomach and the duodenum. Some areas are routinely difficult to examine, treat, or even obtain tissue samples. These areas, called "review areas," are: (1) just distal to the upper esophageal sphincter, (2) the proximal lesser curve, (3) proximal duodenal bulb, (4) medial aspect of the second part of the duodenum, and (5) areas immediately distal to surgical anastamoses. The European Society of Gastrointestinal Endoscopy (ESGE) has proposed and recommended that at least eight images of the upper gastrointestinal tract be performed to constitute a complete examination, and additional images should be taken as necessary. These are the minimal recommendations for a normal examination, and any abnormalities should also be well documented with photos and/or video. For upper endoscopy, the areas of documentation include the hypopharynx to evaluate the vocal cords and the epiglottis (we propose this is *in addition* to ESGE recommendation) (Fig. 1); the upper esophagus just below the upper sphincter, which also usually demonstrates a forward view of the proximal half of the esophagus (Fig. 2); just above the lower esophageal sphincter, allowing proper examination for intestinal metaplasia or esophagitis (Fig. 3a); the Z-line should be visualized

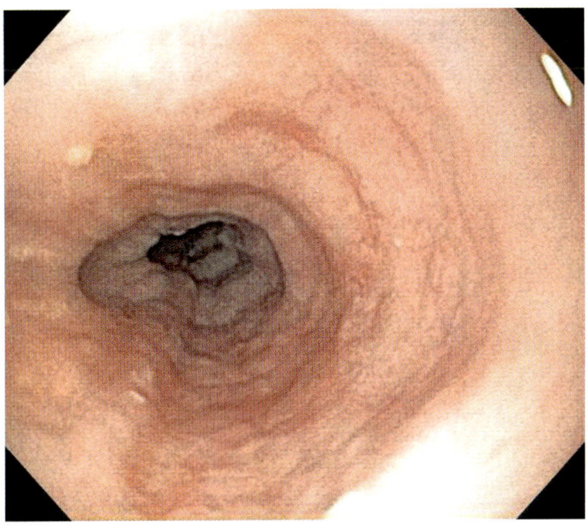

Fig. 2. The upper esophagus.

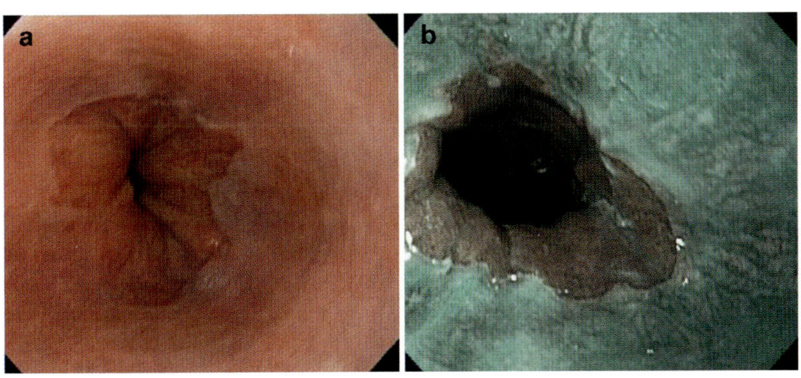

Fig. 3. (**a**) The gastroesophageal junction. (**b**) The gastroesophageal junction visualized by narrow band imaging (*NBI*).

noting the approximate distance from incisors, preferably with a narrow-band image (we propose this *in addition* to ESGE recommendation to better define the demarcation of the squamo-columnar junction and facilitate identification of Barrett's esophagus) (Fig. 3b); a retroflexed view of the cardia and a part of the fundus (we propose two photographs of this area by torquing the endoscope by 180° in the retroflexed

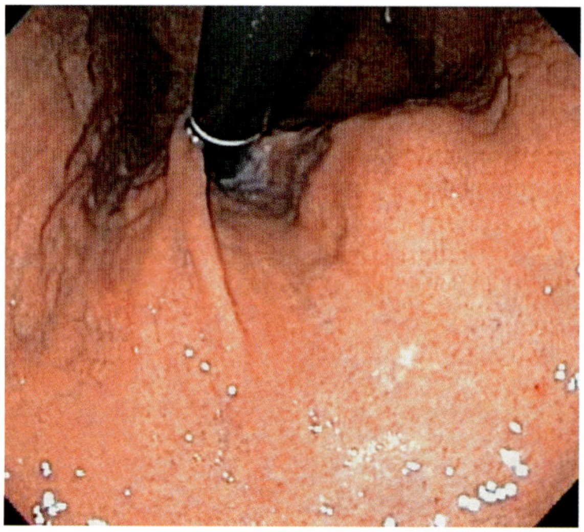

Fig. 4. The cardia viewed by retroflexion of the upper endoscope.

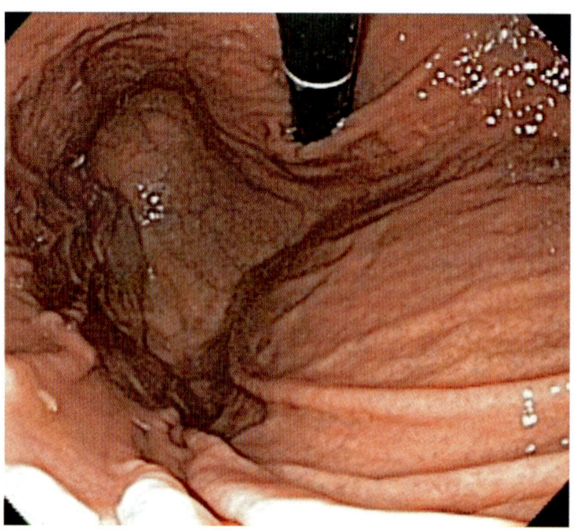

Fig. 5. The fundus viewed by retroflexion of the upper endoscope.

view, an area also amenable to video recording. This would help define lesions close to GE junction and high on the lesser curve with a closer view of cardia by retroflexion) (Figs. 4 and 5); the upper part of the lesser curve (Fig. 6); the angulus of the stomach from a partially retroflexed view (Fig. 7); the antrum (Fig. 8); the duodenal bulb photographed from the pylorus (an additional photo of the retroflexed view of the

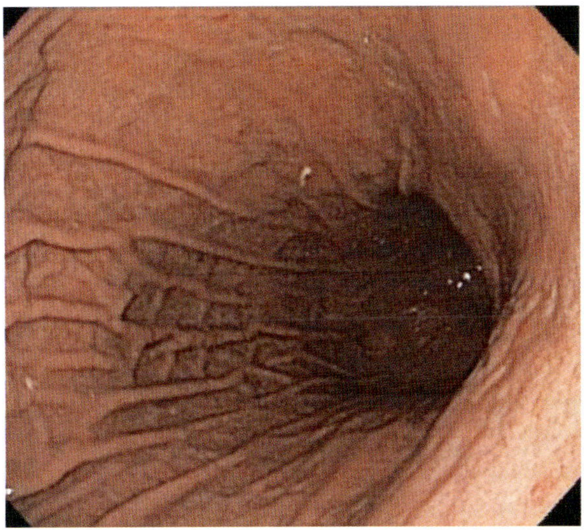

Fig. 6. The lesser curvature of the stomach.

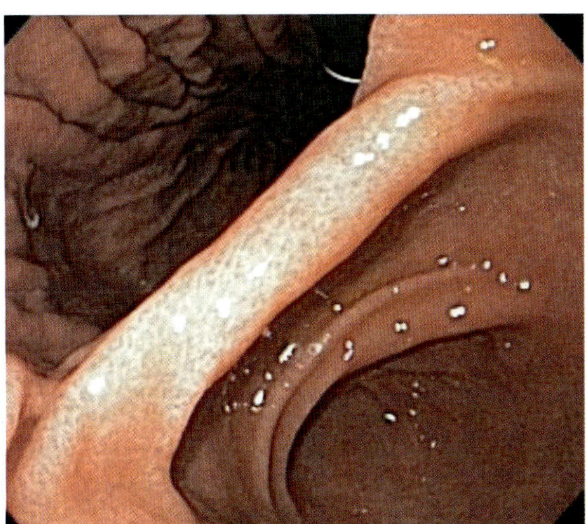

Fig. 7. The angulus of the stomach viewed by retroflexion of the upper endoscope.

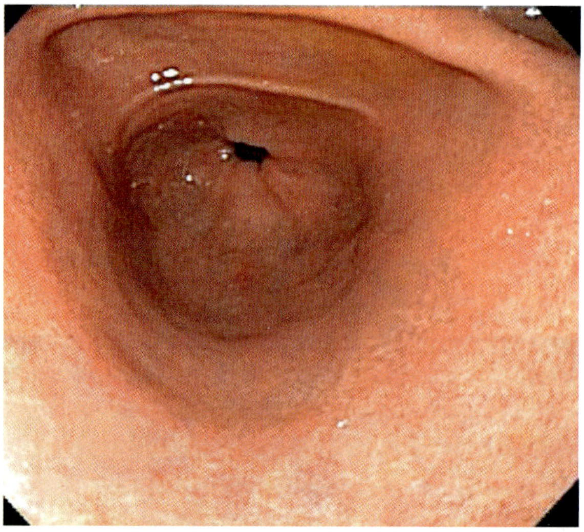

Fig. 8. The antrum of the stomach.

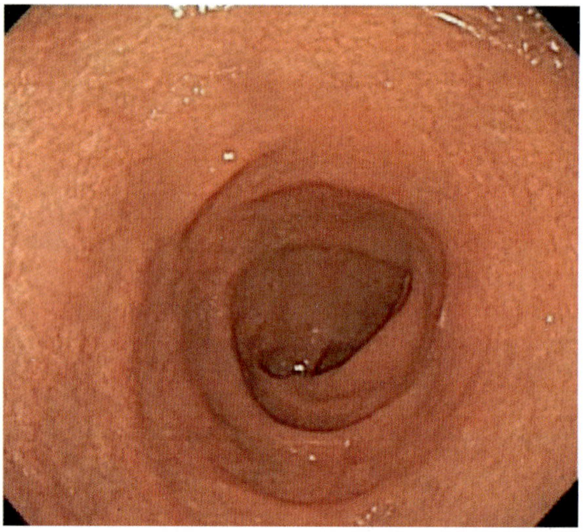

Fig. 9. The duodenal bulb.

duodenal bulb may also be taken with extreme degree of caution to avoid trauma) (Fig. 9); the second part of the duodenum with specific attention to the medial wall of this area to confirm a complete examination. The Ampulla of Vater is often visualized in this photo (Fig. 10).

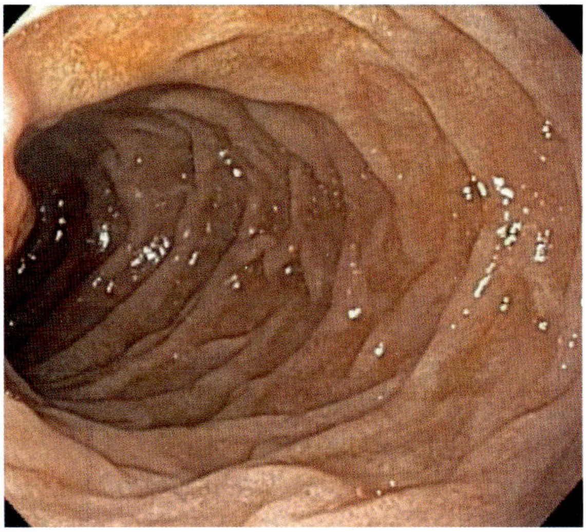

Fig. 10. Second part of duodenum (Ampulla of Vater is partially visualized along the medial wall).

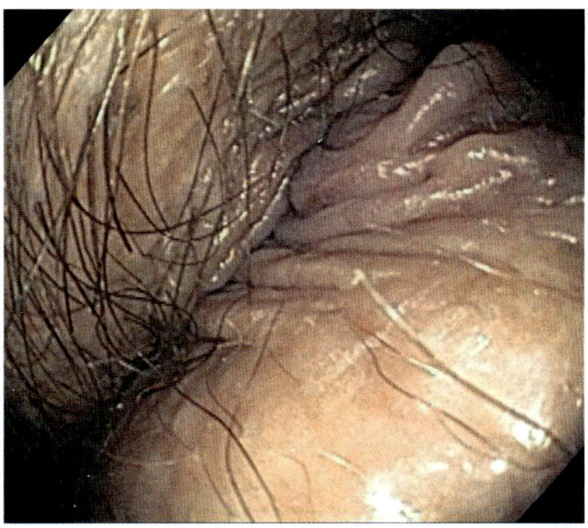

Fig. 11. External view of the anus viewed with a colonoscope.

COLONOSCOPY

Similar to upper gastrointestinal endoscopies, colonoscopies are performed using forward viewing equipment. Similar to upper gastrointestinal endoscopies, some areas are relatively difficult to examine and treat or even for tissue sampling. These "review areas" are (1) sigmoid colon, (2) inferior aspect of the splenic flexure, (3) medial aspect of the colon just proximal to the hepatic flexure, and (4) areas immediately distal to surgical anastamoses. Physicians should make every attempt to take appropriate numbers of photographs for a complete examination. The ESGE has recommended at least eight images of the lower

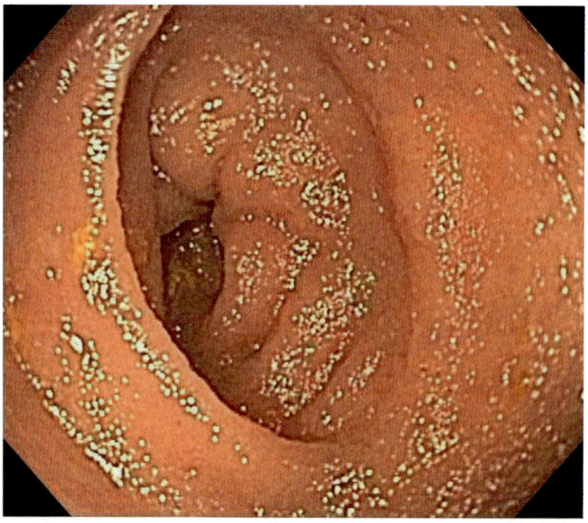

Fig. 12. The terminal ileum viewed with a colonoscope.

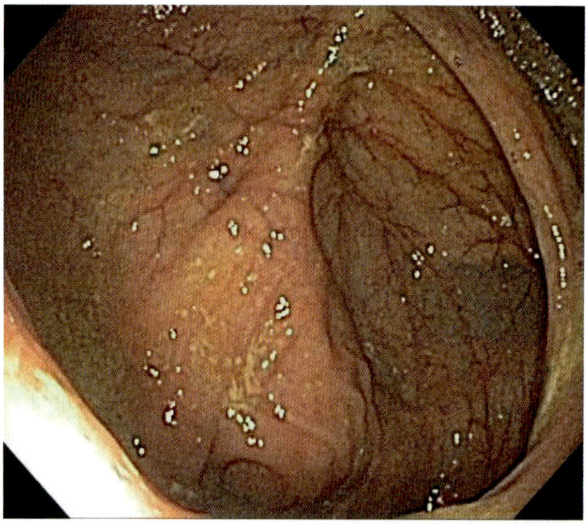

Fig. 13. The cecum.

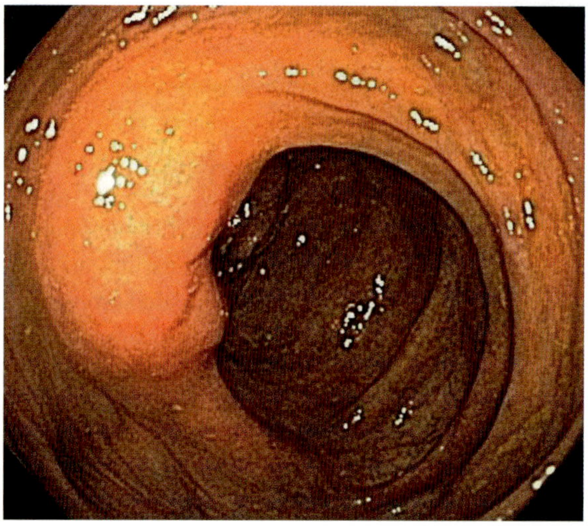

Fig. 14. The ileocecal valve.

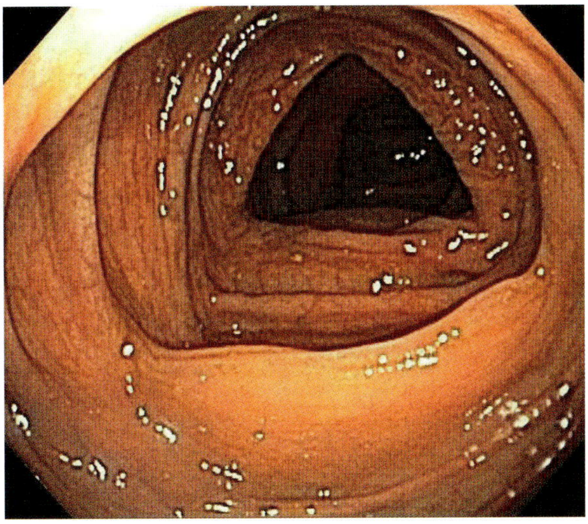

Fig. 15. The ascending colon.

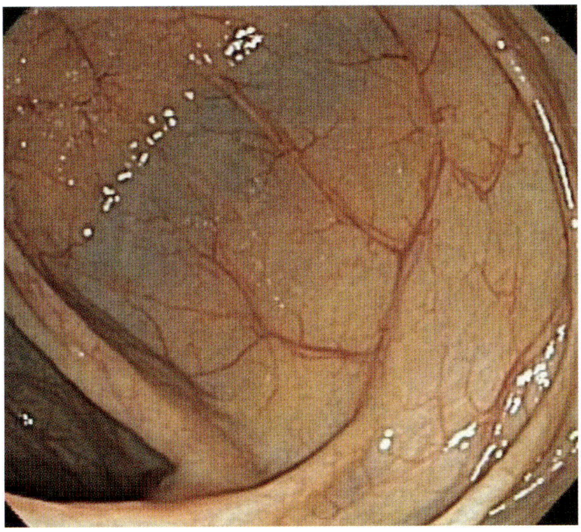

Fig. 16. The hepatic flexure.

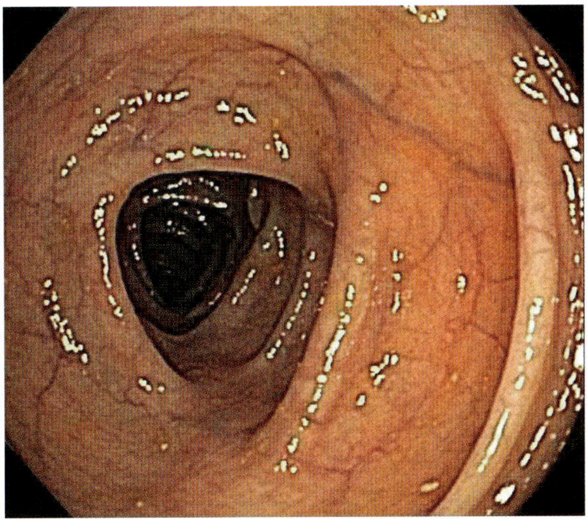

Fig. 17. Proximal to the splenic flexure.

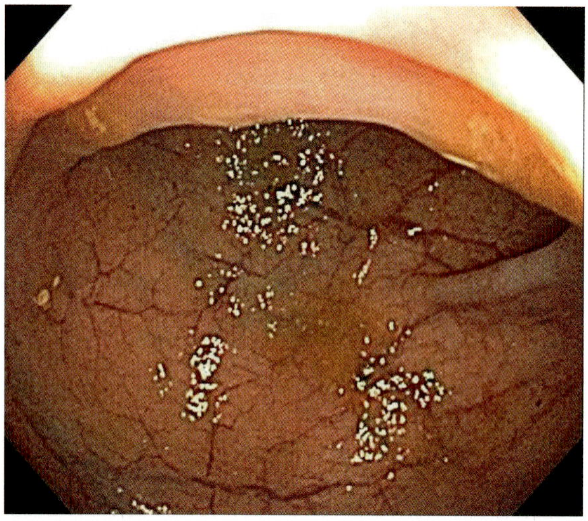

Fig. 18. The splenic flexure.

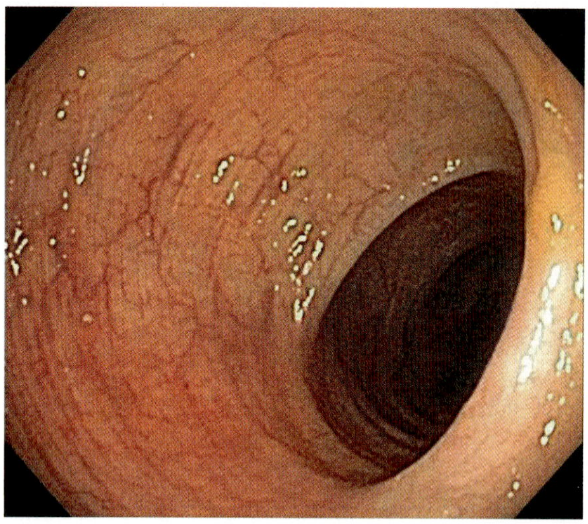

Fig. 19. The descending colon.

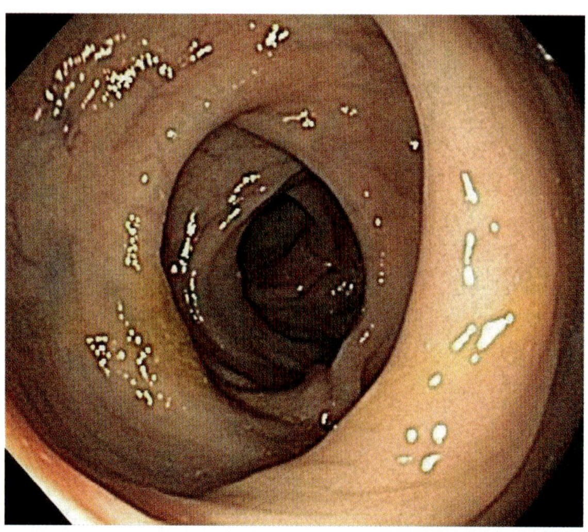

Fig. 20. The sigmoid colon.

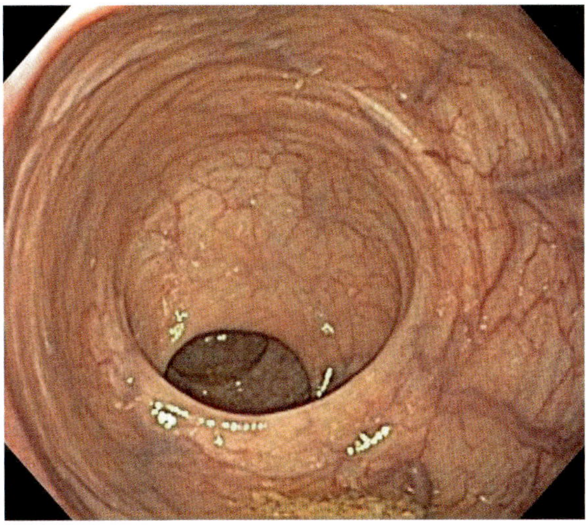

Fig. 21. The rectal vault.

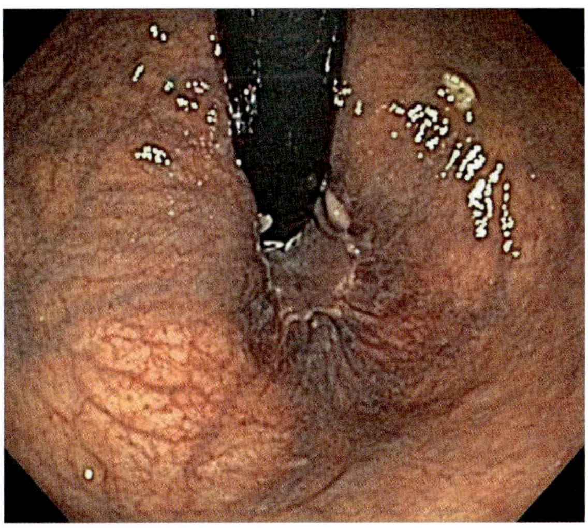

Fig. 22. The rectum viewed by retroflexion of a colonoscope.

gastrointestinal tract to constitute a complete examination and additional images may be taken as necessary to document pathology. When colonoscopy is being performed for screening purposes, careful examination of the mucosal details for difficult-to-diagnose flat polyps becomes extremely important in high risk groups. Documentation of the effort involved in such careful examination is possible only when a report is accompanied by appropriate pictorial records. For colonoscopy, the areas of documentation include the anal opening prior to insertion (we propose this *in addition* to ESGE recommendation. This would help documenting perianal pathology.) (Fig. 11); the terminal ileum when appropriate (we propose this *in addition* to ESGE recommendation, and suggest attempting terminal ileal intubation routinely as an added measure of quality to confirm the completeness of colonoscopy) (Fig. 12); the cecum with appendiceal opening to confirm a complete examination (Fig. 13); the ileocecal valve (Fig. 14); the ascending colon just proximal to the hepatic flexure (Fig. 15); the hepatic flexure (Fig. 16); the mid-transverse colon (we propose this additional image to document the diligence in examining mucosal detail) (Fig. 17); just

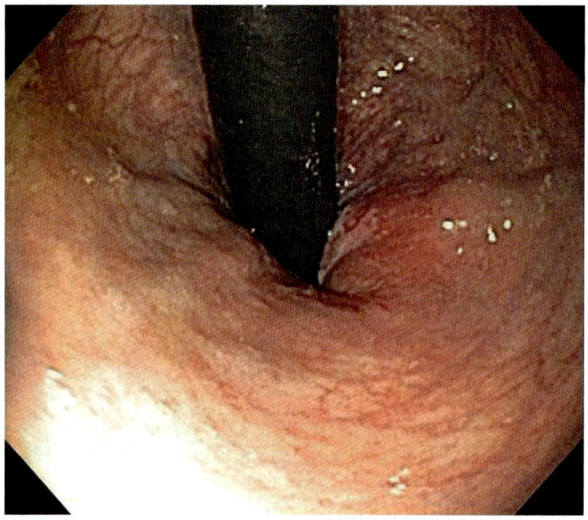

Fig. 23. The rectum viewed in retroflexion after torquing the colonoscope.

proximal to the splenic flexure (Fig. 17); the splenic flexure (Fig. 18); the descending colon (we propose this additional image) (Fig. 19); the mid-sigmoid colon (Fig. 20); the rectal vault, forward view (Fig. 21); the rectum, retroflexed view (we propose these additional images to document the completeness of examining the mucosal detail in distal rectum). The second image in the retroflexed view should be taken after torquing the shaft of the colonoscope to 180°) (Figs. 22 and 23).

ACCURATE DESCRIPTION OF ENDOSCOPIC FINDINGS

It is extremely important to describe what exactly one sees rather than making interpretations while reporting a procedure. The endoscopic procedure findings should be concise, using words and phrases to describe the abnormality as accurately as possible. Descriptions of endoscopic findings in a structured manner using terminology based on the World Congress Working Party Report (Crespi et al. 1996) is reasonable. The format of endoscopic reporting is outlined in Table 1.

Table 1
Documentation and description of endoscopic procedures (Modified from Crespi et al. *1996*)

Format	*Comment*
Patient demographic data	
Date of the procedure	
Endoscopist (s)	
Type of the procedure	
Instruments used	There is much variation among endoscopic instrument capabilities
Reasons for the procedure	This has replaced indications. One may use symptoms, diseases, for assessment of a condition or diagnostic sampling of a particular organ, etc.

Format	*Comment*
Medications used	Should include dose and route of administration. May also state "per anesthesia" if an anesthesiologist was involved and kept separate records of sedation
Anatomical extent of the examination	Including for the identifying anatomical landmark feature e.g., cecum, verified by cecal strap, ileocecal valve, and appendiceal orifice
Ease of examination	Degree of difficulty in passing the scope. External pressure used or patient position changed
Patient toleration	
Limitation (s) of the examination	Document the quality of the patient's colon prep
Findings	Use specific terminology as referenced elsewhere in this chapter
Specimens obtained and anatomical location	Document whether lesions were completely or only partially removed
Therapeutic intervention	
Images taken	Include images with the report
Complications	
Suspected diagnosis (conclusion)	This is not a final diagnosis. This may mean conclusion, negative or positive
Discharge plan and follow up	Guide referring physicians with specific recommendations
Copy(s) to the referring doctor	Communication of the findings to the referring doctor

TERMINOLOGY

The description of the examinations should be detailed enough using acceptable jargon to make a report easy to read and understand. The terminology used in the report should closely follow recommendations laid by the World Organization for Digestive Endoscopy (OMED) (Table 2).

LOCATION OF THE LESION

Description of the location of the lesion of interest is extremely important for the referring physicians, the surgeons and also for the pathologists. Describing a lesion with reference to incisor teeth or the anal verge is rather imprecise, but can be helpful if documented in conjunction with anatomical location (Table 3).

DESCRIPTION OF LESIONS

At times, the endoscopist may find it difficult to describe the lesion of interest because of ambiguity in terms of description. Certain terms are acceptable in common usage (Table 4). Pathologists may prefer certain terminologies to describe a lesion. It is better to describe the

Table 2
Terminology (Modified from Crespi et al. *1996*)

Impression	*Meaning*
Normal	Examination is complete and everything is normal
Lumen	Contains all terms regarding an abnormality of the size of the organs, any deformity, compression and any evidence of previous surgery
Contents	Presence of various materials within the organ
Mucosa	Patterns of the mucosa that are mainly diffuse, and may involve all the mucosa of one limited area
Flat lesions	Lesions that remain in the plane of the mucosa
Protruding lesions	Lesions growing above the plane of the mucosa
Excavated lesions	Lesions whose surface is beneath the plane of the mucosa

Table 3
Description of lesion location (Modified from Crespi et al. *1996*)

Impression	*Meaning*
Cardia of the stomach	Used to replace hiatus. It is important to indicate the location of Z-line (distance from the incisors) vis-à-vis the proximal extent or the origin of the gastric folds
Gastric fundus	Anatomical part of the stomach that lies under the diaphragm
Gastric body	The area of the stomach above the angulus lined by linear gastric folds

Table 4
Description of lesions (Modified from Crespi et al. *1996*)

Impression	*Meaning*
Red mucosa, erythema, congested mucosa or hyperemia	Hyperemia is equivalent to erythema. Edema is equivalent to congested mucosa
Mucosal sclerosis	Post-sclerotherapy or post-band ligation related mucosal changes
Aptha	Small superficial defect in the mucosa, white or yellow in color, surrounded by red halo. They are single of multiple, frequently seen within erythematous mucosa
Erosion	Small superficial defect in the mucosa, white or yellow in color, with a flat edge. Frequently seen in Crohn's disease
Stenosis	Narrowed segment of the gut by stricture or stenosis or compression
Mass	Preferred to tumor
Angioectasia	Telangiectasia or angiodysplasia
Scar	Preferred to fibrosis. This may be related healed ulcer or effect of radiotherapy, mucosal ablation or mucosal resection
Obstruction	Blockage by intraluminal obstacle (foreign body)
Occlusion	Complete closure of the lumen by an intrinsic lesion

Table 5
Description of lesion characteristics (Weinstein and Hill *1985*)

Terminology	*Should be replaced by*
-Itis	Absent vascular pattern, erythema, friability, subepithelial hemorrhages, exudates, erosions
Edema	Swelling, cobblestone appearance, prominent folds
Scar	Depressed or non depressed, white, stellate or linear streak
Atrophy	Thin folds, pallor, prominent vessels
Ectasia or angiodysplasia	Better to describe the actual lesion (smooth, non raised or raised red lesion)

Table 6
Localization of lesions (Weinstein and Hill *1985*)

Organ/site	*Location*
Esophagus	State the number of centimeters from the incisor teeth
Stomach	Mention whether the biopsies were obtained from the fundus or the body (proximal or mid or distal, and whether anterior or posterior) or the antrum
Duodenum	Bulb (anterior or posterior), second part or third or the fourth part
Colon	Cecum, ascending colon, hepatic flexure, transverse colon (proximal, mid or distal), descending colon (proximal and then as number of centimeters from the anal verge. Sigmoid colon (in centimeters from the anal verge). Rectum (centimeters from the anal verge)

lesion with reference to its size, and the extent. Certain benign appearing lesions are better described by stating characteristics (Table 5). When biopsies from a particular organ are taken, the endoscopist should document location from which the biopsies were obtained. This enables the pathologist to interpret the abnormality, and the referring physician to understand the implications. Table 6 refers to how to report the sites of the biopsies

SUMMARY OF KEY POINTS

- Image documentation and appropriate reporting is an extremely important permanent part of the patient's record, which can be referenced at a later date.
- Consistency, specificity, and accuracy in descriptions are essential.
- The European Society of Gastrointestinal Endoscopy (ESGE) has proposed and recommended that at least eight images of the upper gastrointestinal tract, and at least eight images of the lower gastrointestinal tract to constitute complete examinations and additional images may be taken as necessary to document pathology.
- Endoscopic reports can help to provide better care for our patients, which is the most important priority.

REFERENCES

Crespi M et al. Working Party Report by the Committee for Minimal Standards of Terminology and Documentation in Digestive Endoscopy of the European Society of Gastrointestinal Endoscopy. Minimal standard terminology for a computerized endoscopic database. Ad hoc Task Force of the Committee. Am J Gastroenterol. 1996;91(2):191–216.

Weinstein WM, Hill TA. Gastrointestinal mucosa biopsy. In: Berk J, editor. Bockus Textbook of Gastroentreology. Philadelphia: W. B. Saunders; 1985. p. 626–44.

22 Ultrasound-Guided/Assisted Percutaneous Liver Biopsy

Kristin Loening MacArthur and George Y. Wu

Contents

Keywords: Ultrasound-Guided/Assisted Percutaneous, Liver, Biopsy

INTRODUCTION

Liver disease can now be evaluated by a variety of advanced serological and imaging methods. However, histological assessment continues to provide valuable diagnostic and prognostic information that cannot be obtained in any other way. Many physicians have tended to be hesitant to perform liver biopsies due to the inherent risks of the procedure. However, when performed correctly, liver biopsy is a safe and invaluable tool for clinical decision-making, especially in complex conditions that involve the liver. This chapter will discuss the indications and contraindications for liver biopsy, provide a step-by-step approach to the decision-making process with detailed instructions and technical tips, and offer practical information for safe and effective performance of ultrasound-guided percutaneous liver biopsy.

From: *Clinical Gastroenterology: Diagnostic and Therapeutic Procedures in Gastroenterology*,
Edited by: G. Y. Wu, S. Sridhar, DOI 10.1007/978-1-59745-044-7_22,

INDICATIONS

The primary indication for liver biopsy is to provide diagnostic information when serological tests and imaging have not led to a diagnosis, and when histological data in a specific disease will alter management. It is also indicated in established liver disease when severity or rate of progression will influence prognosis or treatment (Campbell and Reddy 2004). The various approaches to liver biopsy and their relative indications are displayed in Table 1 (Bravo et al. 2001).

Table 1
Various options for liver biopsy

Approach	*Description*	*Indications*	*Performed by*
Transthoracic, palpation/percussion guided	The biopsy site is determined by manual palpation of the liver edge and percussion during exhalation	Uncommon. Use of ultrasound provides reliable, non-invasive beneficial guidance	Gastroenterologist/ hepatologist
Transthoracic, ultrasound assisted	The biopsy site is confirmed by ultrasound before the biopsy	No contraindications to blind biopsy. Simple and cost-effective approach	Gastroenterologist/ hepatologist
Transthoracic, ultrasound guided	The needle and biopsy placement is guided in real-time by ultrasound	Presence of focal lesions identified by prior imaging studies. Prior abdominal surgery with adhesions	Radiologist
Subcostal ultrasound assisted/ guided	The same procedures as above except from a subcostal approach rather than transthoracic	Hepatomegaly that extends below the costal margin	Radiologist
Transjugular or transvenous	The biopsy is approached either through the jugular or femoral vein using fluoroscopy	Coagulopathy, ascites, morbid obesity, vascular hepatic lesions, fulminant hepatic failure, indication for concomitant procedure (e.g., TIPS)	Interventional radiologist
Laparoscopic/surgical	The biopsy is approached via laparoscopy and surgical excision	Suspected metastases, unexplained ascites, staging of hepatocellular carcinoma, large biopsy required	Surgeon

One of the most common indications is abnormal liver enzymes, where histological information may aid in obtaining a diagnosis. Other examples include cholestatic liver disease, steatosis, steatohepatitis, drug-induced liver disease, viral hepatitis, autoimmune hepatitis, cholangitis, and neoplastic lesions. In addition, liver biopsy provides diagnostic value in less common diseases such as Wilson's disease, alpha antitrypsin-1 deficiency, congenital metabolic storage diseases, mucopolysaccharidosis, hemochromatosis, granulomatous disease, amyloidosis and other infiltrative diseases (Rockey et al. 2009).

Liver biopsy offers direct information on the grade and stage of liver disease. It provides information regarding the extent of inflammation and fibrosis in diseases such as hepatitis B and C viral infections. This information is essential to prognosis and will help influence treatment selection (Bravo et al. 2001). It is particularly useful when diseases overlap, such as concomitant hemochromatosis and steatohepatitis, where staging may govern the aggressiveness of management (Siegel et al. 2005). Sequential biopsies may offer information on the progression of disease as in cases of methotrexate treatment (Campbell and Reddy 2004; Siegel et al. 2005) or liver transplants where the etiology of transplant dysfunction is unclear (Rockey et al. 2009).

It should be noted that liver biopsy is not usually indicated for the diagnosis of suspected hepatocellular carcinoma, although controversy exists (Campbell and Reddy 2004; Siegel et al. 2005). In these cases, liver biopsy may increase the risk of needle track seeding and sampling error may lead to an incorrect diagnosis. Therefore, imaging followed by surgical biopsy may be a safer option. Many non-malignant focal liver lesions such as hemangioma, focal nodular hyperplasia, and cysts have characteristic findings on imaging studies or serological markers for diagnosis, making these modalities preferred over liver biopsy (Rockey et al. 2009). However, when there is doubt, and especially if growth rates are uncharacteristically rapid, liver biopsy may be helpful.

CONTRAINDICATIONS

Contraindications for percutaneous liver biopsy include those that may increase the risk for post-procedure bleeding as well as characteristics that hinder proper and safe mechanics of the procedure. Absolute contraindications include coagulopathy, an uncooperative patient, impaired mental status, infection of the hepatic bed, or extrahepatic biliary obstruction with cholangitis (Rockey et al. 2009). It is recommended that the prothrombin time (PT) be less than 3–5 s prolonged and the International Normalized Ratio (INR) be less than 1.6 (Siegel et al. 2005; Thampanitchawong and Piratvisuth 1999). Additionally, the platelet count should be greater than 60,000–80,000 and there should be no recent NSAID or anticoagulant use, renal failure or severe illness (Rockey et al. 2009; Siegel et al. 2005). Relative contraindications include a difficult body habitus (i.e., morbid obesity) or ascites, in which cases a transjugular biopsy approach is preferred. Previous surgery in the area with the possible presence of adhesions is also a relative contraindication. Possible vascular lesions, hemangiomas, amyloidosis and hydatid disease are also relative contraindications to a percutaneous approach (Rockey et al. 2009).

The American College of Physicians and Patient Care Committee of American Gastroenterology Association recommend that patients live within a 30 mile radius of the procedure site, be accompanied by a chaperone that can supervise them for the 24 h following the procedure and should be directly observed for 6 h post-biopsy at the procedure center where there is access to appropriate treatment for major complications (Jacobs and Goldberg 1989). It is notable that most centers offer a 2–4 h direct observation period after the procedure in accordance with evidence of safety with this protocol (Howard et al. 2008).

PROCEDURE TECHNIQUE: PERCUTANEOUS ULTRASOUND-ASSISTED LIVER BIOPSY

Patient preparation begins with obtaining informed consent and ensuring that the patient will be compliant with instructions during the procedure. A thorough explanation of the procedure in a step-by-step manner including what the patient may expect to feel at each step is valuable in allaying fear and anxiety. Particular attention should be devoted to peri- and post- procedural pain concerns. The patient must stop all anti-platelet medications at least 10 days prior and all anti-coagulant medications at least 5 days prior (warfarin) or 12–24 h prior (heparin). PT, INR and platelet count results should be routinely obtained within a week of the procedure (Rockey et al. 2009).

Percutaneous liver biopsy can be completed with several different needle types, all of which have individual advantages and disadvantages as shown in Table 2. The needle type should be selected according to the suspected disease process as well as relevant patient risk factors (Sporea et al. 2008). While some institutions use re-usable needles, commercial kits and guns are so convenient and reliable that at most institutions, the latter have largely supplanted the former. Regardless of the type of needle used, certain supplies are required as shown in Fig. 1a. These include sterile gloves, a straight edge, an extra bottle of 10 mL of 1% lidocaine, a specimen container and a typical liver biopsy kit with either a Jamshidi-Menghini needle (Fig. 1b) or a Menghini needle (Fig. 2a). A liver biopsy gun is shown in Fig. 2b. The additional 1% lidocaine is useful in ensuring adequate local anesthesia.

BIOPSY WITH A JAMSHIDI-MENGHINI NEEDLE KIT

The patient is placed supine with the right side of the body placed at the edge of the procedure table. The right arm is placed with the hand behind the head or the neck with torsion of the thorax about 5° to the left. The legs and hips are then pivoted approximately 15° toward the left. These positional maneuvers widen the right intercostal spaces. The liver and right thoracic area are palpated and percussed at the 8–10th intercostal spaces along the midaxillary line (Fig. 3a). The patient is instructed to give full inspiration

Table 2
Percutaneous biopsy needles

	Suction	*Cutting*
Types	Jamshidi, Klatskin, Menghini	Tru Cut, Vim-Silverman
Advantages	Good sample size	Smaller sample size, no fragmentation
Disadvantages	Fragmentation	Risk of bleeding

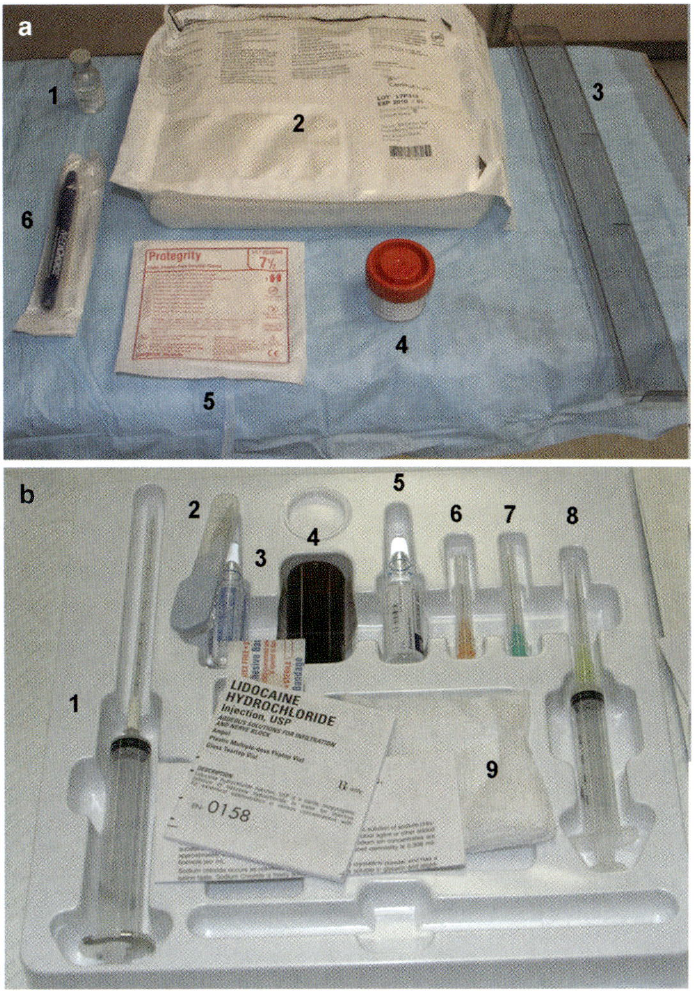

Fig. 1. (**a**) Preparatory materials for percutaneous liver biopsy: *1* lidocaine 1% 10 mL *2* Jamshidi (Menghini) liver biopsy kit, *3* plastic ruler, *4* specimen container with 10% neutral buffered-formalin, *5* sterile gloves, *6* surgical marker. (**b**) Jamshidi (Menghini) liver biopsy kit: *1* Jamshidi (Menghini) needle, 9.8 cm, 17 G (1.47 mm) beveled tip, *2* #11 surgical scalpel, *3* normal saline 5 mL, *4* alternate specimen container, *5* lidocaine 1% 5 mL, *6* 25 G needle, *7* 22 G needle, *8* 18 G needle, *9* sterile gauze.

followed by full expiration, with a 2–3 s hold at full expiration (Fig. 3b). The point of maximum dullness during full expiration is determined and confirmed by diaphragmatic excursion. This preliminary site is marked as a potential biopsy location (Fig. 3c). Next, ultrasound is used to visualize the liver location, borders, characteristics and presence of hepatic lesions. A 19 khz handheld probe is most convenient. The probe is held in the appropriate orientation, usually with a marker on the probe pointing upward. The probe is glided over areas of interest including the site of preliminary mark (Fig. 3d). The gallbladder and its location should be identified and made certain that this structure is distant and caudad from the potential biopsy site. The gain should be adjusted to show optimal contrast between solid and fluid regions. The site of the maximum diameter of the liver is

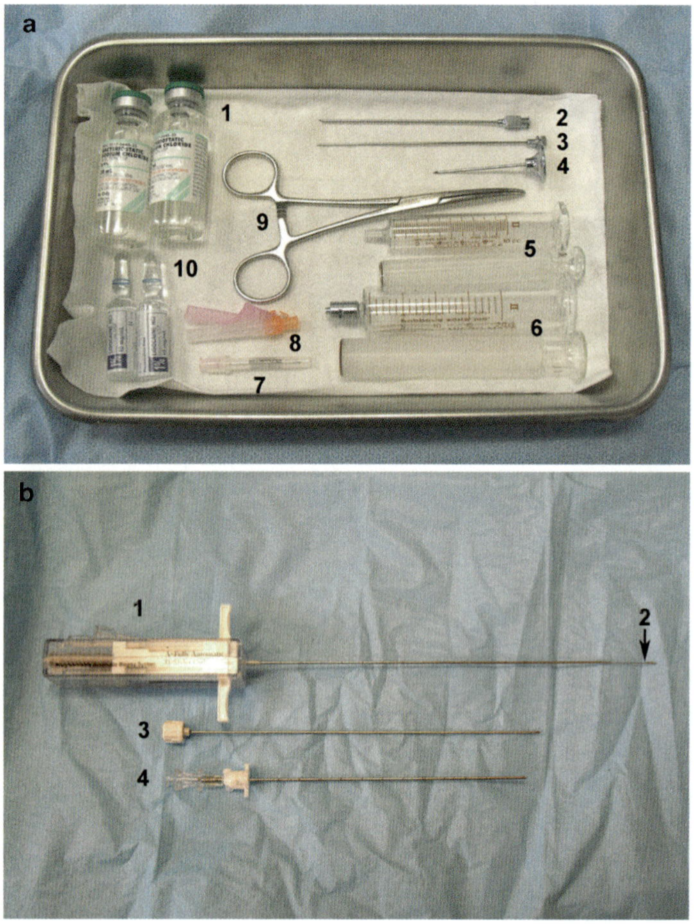

Fig. 2. (**a**) Menghini liver biopsy kit**:** *1* bacteriostatic sodium chloride 60 mL, *2* Menghini needle, 7.0 cm, 16 G (1.65 mm) beveled tip, *3* stylette, *4* trocar, *5* syringe for anesthesia, *6* syringe for biopsy, *7* 20 G needle, *8* 25 G needle, *9* forceps, *10* lidocaine 1% 10 mL. (**b**) Liver biopsy gun, *1* liver biopsy gun, 18 G, *2* biopsy site, *3* trocar, *4* sheath.

determined and marked if different from the preliminary mark (Fig. 4a). Doppler imaging at the site ensures avoidance of large peripheral hepatic vessels and bile ducts (Fig. 4b). Both the B-mode and Doppler images can be captured for the medical record. The puncture site is selected in the inferior portion of the intercostal space to avoid the intercostal nerves and vessels. With the ultrasound probe in place, a straight edge is placed over the chest and a line is drawn from the mark along the direction of the ultrasound beam (Fig. 3e).

The ultrasound jelly is removed and an antiseptic solution is applied to the marked site spiraling from the center outward. A piece of tape is folded over to make a double stick surface and is used to anchor a drape that is placed over the surgical field, aligning a prominent crease in the paper with site and line drawn on the chest. Local anesthesia, 1% lidocaine, is injected tangential to the skin with a 25 G needle infiltrating intradermally to raise a bleb, then aiming perpendicular to the skin penetrating 2–3 mm at a time progressively deeper into the subcutaneous tissue and intercostal muscles to anesthetize the path of entry

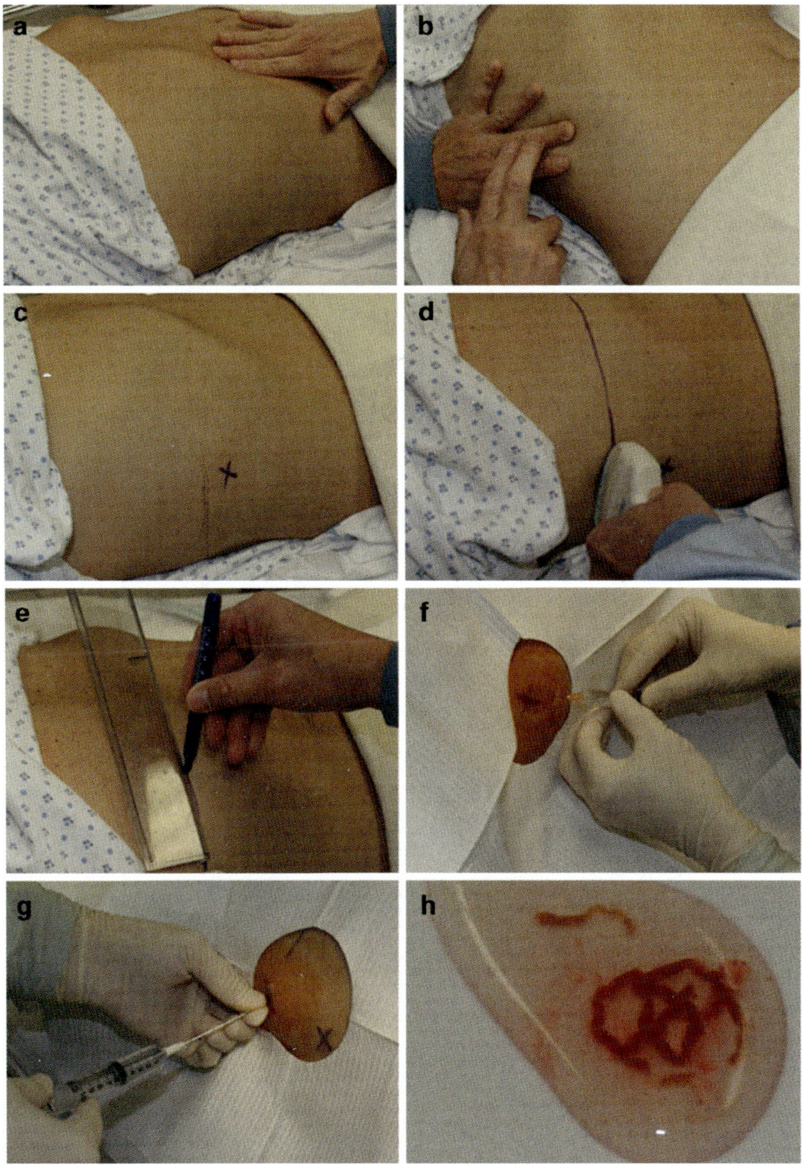

Fig. 3. (**a**–**h**) Stepwise process of percutaneous liver biopsy with ultrasound assistance: (**a**) palpation, (**b**) percussion, (**c**) marking potential site, (**d**) ultrasound examination of biopsy path (see Fig. 4 for examples of ultrasound images), (**e**) marking direction of biopsy, (**f**) administration of anesthesia, (**g**) insertion of biopsy needle, (**h**) sample of liver biopsy in saline.

(Fig. 3f). The plunger is withdrawn each time prior to injection to determine if a blood vessel has been punctured. The needle is changed to a 21 G needle and the process is repeated injecting 2.5 mL in the process. If blood is obtained during the infiltration, it usually indicates that the surface of the liver has been reached. The needle should be withdrawn and the angle changed to 15° from perpendicular aiming caudad, and another 2.5 mL should be injected in an attempt to spray the Glisson's capsule. Satisfactory infiltration is the key to minimize discomfort of the liver biopsy. There should be little hesitation to use more

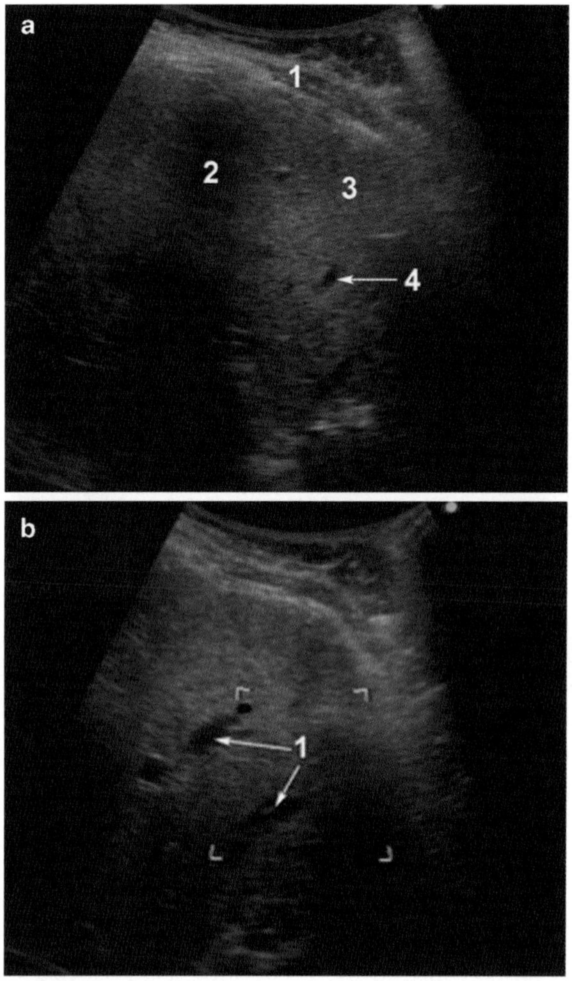

Fig. 4. (**a**) B-mode ultrasound image of target area for liver biopsy: *1* Glisson's capsule, *2* rib shadow, *3* liver, *4* blood vessel or bile duct. (**b**) Doppler mode ultrasound image of target area for liver biopsy: *1* hepatic blood vessels. Doppler mode can be used to differentiate between blood vessels (red and blue structures) and bile ducts (no color). Colors have intentionally not been reproduced in this figure.

than the 5 mL of lidocaine provided in the kit, in order to ensure proper anesthesia especially in individuals who are obese or more sensitive to pain. A number 11 surgical blade is used to make a 1–2 mm nick in the skin at the site for introduction of the biopsy needle.

The biopsy device is prepared by removing the biopsy needle from the syringe and aspirating 3–4 mL of sterile saline into the barrel. Then, the biopsy needle is replaced securely with a firm, twisting motion.

To perform the biopsy, the needle shaft is held with one hand, and the needle is slowly advanced 1–2 mm at a time through the chest wall (Fig. 3g), until the penetration of the peritoneum is felt. There is usually a "popping" sensation transmitted through the needle at this time. A small amount of saline is expressed through the needle to confirm the position of the needle in the peritoneum and to flush out any tissue present in the needle. If the needle is in the peritoneum, no resistance will be felt and the saline will be expelled easily. If resistance is felt, it may indicate that the needle is at or in the liver edge or still in the chest wall. In this case, the needle should be withdrawn slightly and saline again injected. If resistance to injection is still felt, the needle should be advanced slowly until the peritoneum is pierced, and the injection procedure repeated. Once it is certain that the needle has entered the peritoneum, suction is applied to the syringe, and locked or held in a way to maintain vacuum. One hand holds the needle with the thumb and fingers at the desired depth, and the other hand adjusts the direction, making sure that the needle is aimed along the crease of the drape and that the needle is level to the table. The patient is instructed to inspire fully, then expire fully and hold exhalation until directed otherwise. At full exhalation held for 1–2 s, the needle is rapidly advanced into the liver along the marked direction in an even and fluid motion, followed by rapid withdrawal all occurring in about 1 s. The sample is expelled into a clean flat surface of the kit, and carefully placed into a screw-capped container containing 10% neutral buffered-formalin (Fig. 3h). A typical sample will be 2.5–4 cm in length.

For ultrasound-guided biopsies, sterile jelly and a probe covered with sterile plastic is used and held by an assistant while the biopsy is performed. The optimal location is determined and the site is anesthetized with lidocaine as described above.

As soon as possible after the biopsy, the patient should be bandaged and instructed to lie on his/her right side and remain in that position for 2–4 h to prevent bleeding. Blood pressure, pulse, heart rate, and symptoms are monitored every 15 min for the first hour, every 30 min for the second hour and then hourly until discharge (Arora 2009). If all is well after 3 h of observation, the patient can be discharged. At home, patients are instructed to remain at bed rest for the remainder of the day and should stay in the right lateral decubitus position as much as possible. Patients should avoid intense activity, exercise and heavy lifting the day after the procedure. Over-the-counter pain medicines are commonly used for pain. Prescription narcotics can be used, but if the procedure is performed properly and local anesthesia adequate, this is rarely necessary. NSAIDS or anticoagulants should be avoided for at least 48 h.

The ideal size of a liver biopsy specimen has been shown to be approximately 1.5 cm in length, although studies show adequacy anywhere between 1 and 3 cm (Bravo et al. 2001; Rockey et al. 2009). The diameter should be between 1.2 and 2 mm and the sample should include at least 6–8 portal triads. This represents 1/50,000 of the adult liver size (Bravo et al. 2001; Sporea et al. 2008) Sampling error has been shown to approach 20–30% (Campbell and Reddy 2004). This can be decreased by multiple samples of different lobes, although this is rarely done in clinical practice. Note that staging and grading of chronic viral hepatitis has been shown to require a minimum of 2 cm in biopsy length with at least 11 portal triads (Guido and Rugge 2004)

ALTERNATE DEVICES

A Menghini needle kit (Fig. 3c) is used following the same procedure as with the Jamshidi-Menghini needle kit, with two exceptions. The first is that the Jamshidi-Menghini has a lock to maintain suction in the syringe. This allows for a more controlled grip on the needle shaft and syringe when taking the biopsy. The second is that the Jamshidi-Menghini needle is designed to prevent aspiration of the sample into the barrel of the syringe and thus, ensures easy removal of the sample from the needle. With the Menghini needle, the biopsy sample is retained either within the needle or within the barrel of the syringe. Depending on its location, the sample can be poured out from the syringe after removing the plunger or can be pushed out of the needle using the stylette. Sometimes it is difficult to retrieve the sample from the syringe barrel. For this reason, some Menghini needle kits supply a blunt stopper to be inserted into the proximal end of the needle before taking the biopsy to prevent the sample from entering the barrel of the syringe.

LIVER BIOPSY GUN

Radiologists often use a liver biopsy gun (Fig. 3d) for ultrasound-guided biopsies. The biopsy gun is best used for sampling focal rather than generalized liver lesions. Additionally, the gun is unique in that it allows for multiple passes to be completed at low risk until an adequate sample is obtained, and guide-devices are available to maintain the gun in a particular position for sampling specific lesions. The biopsy gun technique is similar to the procedure described above, with the exception of the use of real-time ultrasound, and a slightly different method of entry and biopsy. After preparation and local anesthesia, a 17 G needle is inserted into the sheath and twisted to lock into place. The sheath and needle are inserted percutaneously into the liver and guided to the appropriate depth by ultrasound. The 17 G needle is removed, while the sheath is held carefully in position. The biopsy gun is loaded to engage the 18 G needle and then is inserted into the sheath with the bevel of the needle facing toward the ultrasound probe. The tip of the bevel is visualized on ultrasound to confirm appropriate placement within the liver. The biopsy gun trigger is pressed and the biopsy is taken. The gun is removed keeping the sheath held in place. The sample is removed and visualized and if inadequate, the gun can be reinserted to obtain another sample. Once an adequate sample is obtained, the sheath can be removed and the patient prepared for recovery.

COMPLICATIONS

Most complications from percutaneous liver biopsy occur shortly after the procedure. The overall rate of major or life-threatening complications has been shown to be between 0.09% and 2.3% (Adams and Lewis 2002). This rate has been shown to be dependent on the experience and training of the operator (Froehlich et al. 1993). Sixty-one percent of complications occur in the first 2 h, and 96% occur in the first 24 h (Piccinino et al. 1986). One to three percent of patients are hospitalized for an adverse event, most commonly for vasovagal hypotension or post-procedure pain (Bravo et al. 2001). The most common complication of the procedure is pain. Pain is usually described as a dull ache in the right upper quadrant of the abdomen or in the right shoulder. It typically lasts less than 2 h and responds to analgesics (Montalto et al. 2001). Moderate or severe pain should raise suspicion for bleeding or biliary leak and indicates the need for further investigation through ultrasound or abdominal CT with contrast.

Bleeding is the most significant complication of liver biopsy and may be subcapsular, intrahepatic, free intraperitoneal hemorrhage or hemobilia. Most severe bleeding occurs within 4 h, but may occur up until 1 week after the procedure (Terjung and Lemnitzer 2003). Risk factors for severe hemorrhage include older age, greater than three passes, or presence of cirrhosis or liver cancer (Piccinino et al. 1986). Signs of severe bleeding include abdominal pain and hemodynamic instability. It should be managed with aggressive fluid support and blood transfusions as needed. Vascular embolization or surgical repair are options if the bleeding continues (Bravo et al. 2001) Percutaneous liver biopsy poses a risk of death, mainly due to bleeding, with a mortality rate of approximately less than or equal to 1/10,000 (Rockey et al. 2009).

Additional complications include gall bladder puncture or bile leak, pneumothorax, hemothorax, bowel or kidney perforation and infection (Bravo et al. 2001). Biliary leak is usually minor, but may require surgery if severe. Pneumothorax or hemothorax may require chest tube drainage. Bowel perforation carries the risk of infection and may require the use of antibiotics. These complications can usually be monitored expectantly and supportively, although close observation is required to monitor the need for rapid intervention if severity worsens (Rockey et al. 2009).

COSTS

An example of costs for various methods of liver biopsy are presented in Table 3. Percutaneous liver biopsy is the least expensive method comparatively. Additionally, ultrasound guidance has been shown to be both beneficial (Lindor et al. 1996) and cost effective (Younossi et al. 1998) when performing percutaneous liver biopsies. These figures should be considered examples of relative costs of the different methods rather than typical charges as these will vary considerably between institutions.

Table 3
An example of costs[a] of various methods of liver biopsy

Approach	*Physician's fees*	*Hospital fees*	*Total*
Percutaneous US-guided/ assisted	$1,030[b]	$823[c]	$1,853
Transjugular/transvenous	$1,355	$596	$1,951
Laparoscopic	$1,635	$1,113[d]	$2,748
Open surgical wedge	$1,885	$596	$2,481

[a]These figures should be considered examples of relative costs of the different methods rather than typical charges because these will vary considerably among institutions
[b]Includes ultrasound reading fee of $145
[c]Fees are per 30 min of GI suite time
[d]Fees are per 30 min of OR time

SUMMARY OF KEY POINTS

- Liver biopsy continues to be indicated in cases where non-invasive testing is inconclusive or when histologic information will influence management or prognosis.
- Absolute contraindications to percutaneous liver biopsy include coagulopathy, altered mental status or serious illness. Relative contraindications include a difficult body habitus, presence of abdominal adhesions or known vascular hepatic lesions.
- The primary methods of liver biopsy are ultrasound assisted/guided percutaneous, transvenous, laparoscopic or open surgical wedge.
- Complications of percutaneous liver biopsy usually occur in the immediate hours following the procedure and include pain, bleeding and nearby visceral organ damage.
- When performed correctly, percutaneous liver biopsy is a safe and cost effective tool for definitive diagnosis of liver disease.

REFERENCES

Campbell MS, Reddy KR. The evolving role of liver biopsy. Aliment Pharmacol Ther. 2004;20:249–59.

Bravo AA, Sheth SG, Chopra SC. Liver Biopsy. N Engl J Med. 2001;344(7):495–500.

Rockey DC, Caldwell SH, Goodman ZD, Nelson RC, Smith AD. Liver biopsy. AASL position paper. Hepatology. 2009;49(3):1017–44.

Siegel CA, Suriawinata AA, Silas AM, Van Leeuwen DJ. Liver biopsy 2005: when and how? Cleve Clin J Med. 2005;72(3):199–201. 206, 208 passim.

Thampanitchawong P, Piratvisuth T. Liver biopsy: complications and risk factors. World J Gastroenterol. 1999;5:301–4.

Jacobs WH, Goldberg SB. Statement on outpatient percutaneous liver biopsy. Dig Dis Sci. 1989;34:322–3.

Howard R, Karageorge G, van Harselaar K, Bell M, Basford P, Schultz M, et al. Post-procedure surveillance in liver biopsy: how long is long enough? N Z Med J. 2008;121(1280):8–14.

Sporea I, Popescu A, Sirli R, et al. World J Gastroenterol. 2008;14(21):3396–402.

Arora G. Percutaneous liver biopsy, April 5, 2009, Emedicine.

Guido M, Rugge M. Liver biopsy sampling in chronic viral hepatitis. Semin Liver Dis. 2004;24:89–97.

Adams T, Lewis JH. Percutaneous liver biopsy. Clin Perspect Gastroenterol. 2002;2:117–21.

Froehlich F, Lamy O, Fried M, Gonvers JJ. Practice and complications of liver biopsy. Results of a nationwide survey in Switzerland. Dig Dis Sci. 1993;38(8):1480–4.

Piccinino F, Sagnelli E, Pasquale G, Giusti G. Complications following percutaneous liver biopsy: a multicentre retrospective study on 68, 276 biopsies. J Hepatol. 1986;2:165–73.

Montalto G, Soresi M, Carroccio A, et al. Percutaneous liver biopsy: a safe outpatient procedure? Digestion. 2001;63:55–60.

Terjung B, Lemnitzer I. Bleeding complications after percutaneous liver biopsy, an analysis of risk factors. Digestion. 2003;67:138–45.

Lindor KD, Bru C, Jorgensen RA, et al. The role of ultrasonography and automatic-needle biopsy in outpatient percutaneous liver biopsy. Hepatology. 1996;23:1079–83.

Younossi ZM et al. Ultrasound-guided liver biopsy for parenchymal liver disease an economic analysis. Dig Dis Sci. 1998;43(1):46–50.

Index

From: *Clinical Gastroenterology: Diagnostic and Therapeutic Procedures in Gastroenterology*,
Edited by: G. Y. Wu, S. Sridhar, DOI 10.1007/978-1-59745-044-7,

Printed in the United States of America